Practical Evidence-Based Physiotherapy

Rob Herbert BAppSc MAppSc PhD

Associate Professor, School of Physiotherapy, University of Sydney, Sydney, Australia

Gro Jamtvedt PT MPH

Researcher, Norwegian Health Services Research Centre, Oslo, Norway

Judy Mead MCSP

Head of Research and Clinical Effectiveness,
The Chartered Society of Physiotherapy, London, UK

Kåre Birger Hagen PT PhD

Senior Researcher, National Resource Centre for Rehabilitation in Rheumatology,
Diakonhjemmet Hospital, Oslo, Norway

Foreword by
Sir Iain Chalmers

Editor, James Lind Library, Oxford, UK

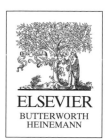

ELSEVIER
BUTTERWORTH
HEINEMANN

EDINBURGH   LONDON   NEW YORK   OXFORD   PHILADELPHIA   ST LOUIS   SYDNEY   TORONTO   2005

ELSEVIER
BUTTERWORTH
HEINEMANN

© 2005, Elsevier Limited

First published 2005
 Reprinted 2007

ISBN 978 0 7506 8820 8

British Library Cataloguing in Publication Data
A catalogue record for this book is available from the British Library.

Library of Congress Cataloging in Publication Data
A catalog record for this book is available from the Library of Congress.

Notice
Knowledge and best practice in this field are constantly changing. As new research and experience broaden our knowledge, changes in practice, treatment and drug therapy may become necessary or appropriate. Readers are advised to check the most current information provided (i) on procedures featured or (ii) by the manufacturer of each product to be administered, to verify the recommended dose or formula, the method and duration of administration, and contraindications. It is the responsibility of the practitioner, relying on his or her own experience and knowledge of the patient, to make diagnoses, to determine dosages and the best treatment for each individual patient, and to take all appropriate safety precautions. To the fullest extent of the law, neither the publisher nor the authors assume any liability for any injury and/or damage.

The Publisher

The
Publisher's
policy is to use
**paper manufactured
from sustainable forests**

Printed in China

Contents

Foreword

A few years ago, I wrote an article about what I want from health research when I am a patient (Chalmers 1995). I tried to make clear that I want decisions about my care to be based on reliable evidence about the effects of treatments. I can't imagine that many patients or health professionals would suggest that this is an unreasonable wish, but they might well vary quite a lot in what they regard as 'reliable evidence'.

I illustrated the issue by noting that, after about five treatments from a chiropractor to whom she had been referred by her general practitioner, my wife believed that she had reliable evidence that chiropractic could help relieve her chronic shoulder and back pain. By contrast, although I was delighted that her longstanding symptoms had subsided, I noted that I would begin to believe in the benefits of chiropractic when a systematic review of the relevant controlled trials suggested that it could be helpful.

Sometimes the effects of treatments are dramatic, as they had been for my wife. For example, after my general practitioner referred me for physiotherapy for a very painful right shoulder injury, the experienced physiotherapist tried a number of technological approaches using some impressive-looking kit; nothing seemed to be helping. Then she decided to treat my right supraspinatus tendon with what I understand are called Cyriax's frictions. The relief was instantaneous and dramatic, and I needed no persuasion that it was as the result of the treatment.

If treatments never did any harm and were universally available in unlimited variety and supply, basing decisions in health care on the individual experiences of patients and professionals would not present any problems. But treatments do have the capacity for doing harm. Chest physiotherapy in very low birthweight infants, for example, came under suspicion of causing brain damage (Harding et al 1998). Even though doubt remains as to whether the associations observed at the time reflected an adverse effect of neonatal physiotherapy (Knight et al 2001), it would have been reassuring if it had been possible to point to a strong evidence base justifying the use of physiotherapy in these fragile infants. Even if treatments don't harm the people for whom they are prescribed, if they don't do any good they use limited resources that could be deployed more profitably elsewhere.

I don't know how frequently physiotherapy has dramatic effects. But if it is anything like medical care, dramatic effects of treatment are very rare. In these circumstances, it is important to assess whether particular forms of care are likely to do more good than harm, and this entails doing carefully designed research.

A decade ago, I sustained a fractured fibula while on holiday in the USA. The orthopaedic surgeon there advised me that, when the swelling had subsided after my impending return to the UK, I would have a plaster cast applied for 6 weeks. Two days later a British orthopaedic surgeon said that the advice that I had received was rubbish, and that I was to have a supportive bandage and to walk on the ankle until it hurt, and then some more! When I asked whether I might be entered into a randomized trial to find out whether he or his 'colleague' across the Atlantic was correct, he told me dismissively that randomized trials were for people who were uncertain whether or not they were right, and he was certain that he was right!

Several questions were posed in the account of this experience published in the *Journal of Bone and Joint Surgery* (Chalmers et al 1992). Which of these orthopaedic surgeons was right? Were they both right, but interested in different outcomes of treatment? What were the consequences, in terms of short term and long term pain and function (and the costs of treatment), of acquiescing in the advice of the second rather than the first? And what was known about the effects of the various forms of physiotherapy which were subsequently prescribed (Chalmers et al 1992)? In the decade since that experience, there has been a welcome increase in the likelihood of patients and professionals obtaining answers to questions like these, and this impressive new book constitutes an important milestone in these developments.

Reliable identification of modest but worthwhile effects of physiotherapy poses a substantially greater challenge than reliable evaluation of the effects of most drugs and some other forms of health care. Not only is it often difficult to characterize physiotherapy interventions in words that allow readers to understand what was done, but taking account of the social and psychologically mediated effects of physiotherapists themselves may also pose interpretive conundrums. I remember being impressed by the results of a randomized comparison of routine instruction for post-natal pelvic floor exercises with personal encouragement from a physiotherapist, done by colleagues in a unit where I worked at the time (Sleep & Grant 1987). No differences were detected in the frequency of urinary or faecal incontinence between the two groups of women 3 months after delivery, but those who had received personal advice and encouragement from the physiotherapist were less likely to report perineal pain and feelings of depression.

Physiotherapists who recognize that they have a professional responsibility to do their best to ensure that their treatments are likely to do more good than harm, and that they are a sensible use of limited resources for health care, will find that *Practical Evidence-Based Physiotherapy* is a veritable goldmine of useful information. I am confident that next time I am referred for physiotherapy this book will have helped to ensure that I will be offered treatment that is likely to be good value for both my time and my taxes.

Sir Iain Chalmers

References

Chalmers I 1995 What do I want from health research and researchers when I am a patient? BMJ 310:1315–1318

Chalmers I, Collins R, Dickersin K 1992 Controlled trials and meta-analyses can help to resolve disagreements among orthopaedic surgeons. Journal of Bone and Joint Surgery 74-B:641–643

Harding JE, Miles FK, Becroft DM et al 1998 Chest physiotherapy may be associated with brain damage in extremely premature infants. Journal of Pediatrics 132:440–444

Knight DB, Bevan CJ, Harding JE et al 2001 Chest physiotherapy and porencephalic brain lesions in very preterm infants. Journal of Paediatrics and Child Health 37:554–558

Sleep J, Grant A 1987 Pelvic floor exercises in postnatal care. Midwifery 3:158–164

Preface

How does it come to happen that four physiotherapists from three countries write a book together? We first met at the World Confederation of Physical Therapy's (WCPT) Expert Meeting on Evidence-Based Practice in London in 2001. By then we knew of each others' work, but at that meeting we discovered kindred spirits who had been thinking about similar issues, albeit from quite different perspectives.

We had all been thinking and writing about evidence-based practice. Judy Mead had co-edited and co-authored the first textbook on evidence-based health care in 1998 (Bury & Mead, 1998). Kåre Birger Hagen and Gro Jamtvedt were working on a Norwegian textbook on evidence-based physiotherapy (subsequently published as Jamtvedt et al, 2003). And Rob Herbert and his colleagues at the Centre for Evidence-Based Physiotherapy had launched the PEDro database on the internet late in 1999. Together we had been teaching skills of evidence-based practice, carrying out clinical research and advising health policy makers. The ground had been laid for collaboration on a text with a broader perspective than any of us could write on our own.

The catalyst for the book was Heidi Harrison, commissioning editor at Elsevier. During the WCPT Congress at Barcelona in 2003, Heidi twisted eight arms and extracted four commitments to the writing of this book. We are grateful to Heidi for getting us started, and for providing ongoing support over the year that it took to write the book.

Is there a need for another textbook on evidence-based practice? We think so. Few textbooks on evidence-based practice have been written with physiotherapists in mind. This book considers how physiotherapists can use clinical research to answer questions about physiotherapy practice. In that respect at least we think this book is unique.

We hope this book can meet the needs of a diverse readership. We want it to provide an introduction to the skills of evidence-based practice for undergraduate students and practising physiotherapists who have not previously been exposed to the ideas of evidence-based practice. Throughout the book we have highlighted critical points in the hope that those who are new to these ideas will not 'lose the forest for the trees'. We also hope to provide a useful resource for those who already practise physiotherapy in an evidence-based way. We do that by providing a more detailed presentation of strategies for searching for evidence, critical appraisal of evidence, and using clinical practice guidelines than is available in other texts. We have gone beyond the boundaries that usually encompass texts on evidence-based practice by considering how evidence about feelings and experiences can be used in clinical decision-making. There is an extensive use of footnotes that we hope will stimulate the interest of advanced readers.

Some books are great labours. This one was exciting, challenging and fun. It has been a shared process in which all contributed their different perspectives. We have discussed, struggled with difficult ideas, resolved disagreements, and learned a lot. We also learned about each other and became good friends. For two wonderful weeks we met and worked together intensively: first in the snowy mountains of Norway in mid-winter, and later in a quiet village near Oxford in spring.

We would like to thank the people who reviewed part or all of the manuscript and gave useful feedback. They are, in alphabetical order, Trudy Bekkering, Mark Elkins, Claire Glenton, Mark Hancock, Hans Lund, Sue Madden, Chris Maher, Anne Moore, Anne Moseley and Cathie Sherrington. All remaining shortcomings are our own.

Rob Herbert, Gro Jamtvedt,
Judy Mead and Kåre Birger Hagen, 2005

References

Bury TJ, Mead JM (eds) 1998 Evidence based healthcare: a practical guide for therapists. Butterworth-Heinemann, Oxford

Jamtvedt G, Hagen KB, Bjørndal A 2003 Kunnskapsbasert Fysioterapi. Metoder og Arbeidsmåter. Gyldendal Akademisk

Chapter **1**

Evidence-based physiotherapy: what, why and how?

OVERVIEW

This chapter introduces the authors' interpretation and rationale for the term 'evidence-based physiotherapy'. Evidence-based physiotherapy is physiotherapy informed by relevant, high quality clinical research. The *practice* of evidence-based physiotherapy should involve the integration of evidence (high quality clinical research), patient preferences and perspectives, practice-generated knowledge and other factors. The chapter provides a brief outline of the history of evidence-based health care and why it is important. Steps for practising evidence-based physiotherapy are described, setting out a preview of the rest of the book.

WHAT IS 'EVIDENCE-BASED PHYSIOTHERAPY'?

The aim of this book is to give physiotherapists a practical guide to evidence-based physiotherapy.

What do we mean by 'evidence-based physiotherapy'?

Evidence-based physiotherapy is physiotherapy informed by relevant, high quality clinical research.

This implies that when we refer to 'evidence' we mean high quality clinical research.

High quality clinical research ⟶ Evidence-based physiotherapy

Although evidence-based physiotherapy must be informed by high quality clinical research, we do not believe that high quality clinical research is the only information required for practice. There are several reasons for this. The most obvious is that research alone does not make good or bad decisions – people do. When patients, health professionals and policy makers make health care decisions, they bring to their decisions a range of values, preferences, experiences and knowledge. Thus decision-making in physiotherapy, as with any other aspect of health care, is a complex process involving more than just research. Decisions should be informed by patient preferences and physiotherapists' practice knowledge. High quality clinical research is therefore essential for evidence-based practice, but practice should be based on more than just evidence.

The practice of evidence-based physiotherapy should be informed by relevant, high quality clinical research, patients' preferences and physiotherapists' practice knowledge.

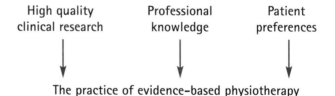

High quality   Professional   Patient
clinical research   knowledge   preferences

The practice of evidence-based physiotherapy

Our definition of evidence-based physiotherapy differs from earlier definitions, because in earlier definitions evidence was considered to be more than just high quality clinical research. Previous authors considered evidence-based physiotherapy involved the use of 'the best available evidence' (Bury & Mead 1998, Sackett et al 2000), which includes high quality clinical research or, where high quality clinical research is not available, lower quality clinical research, consensus views and clinical experience. In our view, practice can only be evidence-based when it uses high quality clinical research. However, we do not deny the legitimate basis of areas of physiotherapy where there is a lack of high quality clinical research. Where high quality clinical research does not exist, good practice *must* be informed by knowledge derived from other sources of information, such as experts or trusted colleagues, personal or shared practice experience (practice-generated knowledge), patient preferences and lower quality research.

We recognize that physiotherapists live with uncertainty because there is often a lack of reliable, relevant evidence. But decisions still have to be made, and physiotherapists need to use the best information that is available to them when making clinical decisions. Our position is simply that we should reserve the term 'evidence-based physiotherapy' for physiotherapy practice that is based on high quality clinical research. The need to include patient preferences and practice knowledge in decision-making is relevant to all practice, whether evidence-based or not.

WHAT DO WE MEAN BY 'HIGH QUALITY CLINICAL RESEARCH'?

The term clinical research is usually used to mean research on patients, conducted in clinical settings.[1] It is empirical in nature, which means that it generates knowledge with experiment or observation rather than theory. There is an enormous volume of clinical research, but not all of it is of high quality. From the point of view of consumers of research, high quality clinical research is that which is carried out in a way that allows us to trust the results (it has a low risk of bias[2]) and is relevant to our questions. This book is designed to help you appraise the validity or trustworthiness of qualitative and quantitative clinical research, and to assess its relevance to you and your patients, and apply the evidence to your practice.

The book will focus on studies that provide answers to questions that arise in physiotherapy practice. We are most interested in those studies whose results impact directly on decisions that need to be made by physiotherapists and patients. We will not focus on practice epistemology[3] or on questions that researchers might ask to develop practice knowledge, or on research into the processes of generating the knowledge or theories that underpin practice. Nor will this book focus in detail on how physiotherapists learn and develop practice-generated knowledge, skills and experience, or how to develop theories.

WHAT DO WE MEAN BY 'PATIENT PREFERENCES'?

The traditional clinical model has been one in which physiotherapists make decisions about therapy for their patients. In recent years there has been a movement towards consumer involvement in decision-making and patients have developed expectations that they will be given an opportunity to contribute to, and share, decisions involving their health (Edwards & Elwyn 2001). In contemporary models of clinical decision-making, patients are encouraged to contribute information about their

---

[1] Clinical research may not always be carried out on patients. It could include in-depth interviews with carers, for example. Similarly, the setting may not always be a clinical one – it could include patients' homes or other community environments, or public health activities such as community-based health promotion programmes.

[2] One way of defining bias is that it is a systematic deviation from the truth.

[3] Epistemology is the branch of philosophy that investigates the origins, nature, methods and limits of human knowledge. Practice epistemology refers to study of the nature of knowledge and the processes of generating knowledge that underlie practice (Richardson et al 2004).

experience, their preferences and what is most important to them. There is a move away from the situation where the physiotherapist or the doctor alone makes decisions for the patient, towards the situation in which the patient makes informed choices or decisions that are shared between the health professional and the patient. Patients are invited to contribute their experiences, preferences and values to the decision-making process. This is an important cultural change. It requires that physiotherapists are able to communicate to patients the risks and benefits of alternative actions, and it requires communication skills, empathy and flexibility from physiotherapists.

WHAT DO WE MEAN BY 'PRACTICE KNOWLEDGE'?

Practice knowledge is knowledge arising from professional practice and experience (Higgs & Titchen 2001). Consciously or subconsciously, physiotherapists add to their personal knowledge base during each patient encounter. This knowledge is used on a day-to-day basis, along with many other sources of information, including high quality clinical research, to inform future practice. Practice knowledge is created through reflective processes that enable practitioners to evaluate their practice and learn from their experience. Practice knowledge is used in clinical reasoning and the highly skilled judgements that have to be made in patient encounters. Titchen & Ersser (2001) comment that practice knowledge 'underpins the practitioner's rapid and fluent response to a situation'. It is what differentiates competent well-educated new graduates and experienced physiotherapists.

Practice knowledge is not 'evidence' as we have defined it. Nonetheless, practice knowledge should always be brought to the decision-making process. Practice knowledge contributes to the professional judgements that have to be made with patients. For example, practice knowledge might suggest alternative interventions even if the evidence indicates a particular intervention is effective. There is some evidence that upper extremity casting for children with cerebral palsy may increase the quality and range of upper extremity movement (Law et al 1991). However, an experienced physiotherapist might suggest alternative interventions if his or her practice knowledge indicates that casting will cause the child distress, or if the child or the child's parents are unlikely to tolerate the intervention well.

ADDITIONAL FACTORS

According to our definition, the practice of evidence-based physiotherapy involves integration of three elements: high quality clinical research, patient preferences and practice knowledge. But other factors influence practice as well. Any decision or action will always take place within a particular context, and this context interacts with the availability of research, patient preferences and practice knowledge. The context includes culture, setting, resources and politics. We all work within different settings and work environments and these influence both our way of posing practice-related questions and the way we communicate with patients and populations. Good practice is responsive to a range of contextual factors.

The availability of resources often influences clinical decisions. For example, the most effective intervention for a particular problem could require an expensive piece of equipment that is not available, in which case a less effective intervention would have to be used. Another resource to be considered may be the skills of the physiotherapist. In making shared decisions about an appropriate intervention, physiotherapists need to judge whether they have the skills and competence needed to provide treatment safely and effectively. If not, the patient should be referred to another physiotherapist who does have the necessary skills and expertise. When considering how services should be provided for your patients you may also need to consider whether services are available in other settings (for example, in the community instead of a hospital) and, if there is a choice, which setting would provide the greater benefit for the patient.

If we look at physiotherapy from a global perspective we can see huge variations in the spectrum of conditions that are treated and in the resources provided for health care. Comparisons of morbidity and mortality worldwide clearly show how important these factors are. This also has implications for what kinds of patients and problems physiotherapists are concerned with, and how they make clinical decisions.

In addition, there are important cultural influences that shape how physiotherapy should be practised. Culture affects patient and physiotherapist expectations, attitudes to illness and the provision of health care, communication and patient–physiotherapist interaction, and the ways in which interventions are administered. This means that it might be quite appropriate for physiotherapy to be practised very differently in different countries. We acknowledge that some cultures, particularly those with strong social hierarchies, provide contexts that are less conducive to evidence-based practice or shared decision-making. In multicultural societies physiotherapists may need to be able to accommodate to the range of cultural backgrounds of their patients.

THE PROCESS OF CLINICAL DECISION-MAKING

At the heart of the practice of evidence-based physiotherapy is the process of clinical decision-making. Clinical decision-making brings together information from high quality clinical research, information from patients about their preferences, and information from physiotherapists within a particular cultural, economic and political context.

Clinical decision-making is complex. It requires clinical reasoning to analyse, synthesize, interpret and communicate relevant information from and to the patient in a dynamic and interactive way. Practice knowledge, evidence and information from patients are integrated using professional judgement. 'Clinical reasoning needs to be seen as a pivotal point of knowledge management in practice, utilizing the principles of evidence-based practice and the findings of research, but also using professional judgement to interpret and make research relevant to the specific patient and the current clinical situation' (Higgs et al 2004). Only when physiotherapy is practised in this way can we 'claim to be adopting credible practice that is not only evidence-based, but also client-centred and context-relevant' (Higgs et al 2004).

While acknowledging the importance of clinical reasoning and the development of practice knowledge, the focus of this book is narrower – we aim to help physiotherapists inform their practice with relevant, high quality clinical research. Readers who are specifically interested in clinical reasoning and development of practice knowledge could consult Higgs & Jones (2000) and Higgs et al (2004).

WHY IS EVIDENCE–BASED PHYSIOTHERAPY IMPORTANT?

FOR PATIENTS

Evidence-based physiotherapy is important for patients because it implies that, within the limitations of current knowledge they will be offered the safest and most effective interventions. The expectation is that this will produce the best possible clinical outcomes.

Patients are increasingly demanding information about their disease or clinical problem and the options available for treatment. Many patients have access to a wide range of information sources, but not all of these sources provide reliable information. The most widely used source of information is probably the internet, but the internet provides the full spectrum of information quality, from reliable to spurious data. If patients are to make informed contributions to decisions about the management of their conditions they will need assistance to identify high quality clinical research.

In some countries, such as the United Kingdom, patients' demands for information have been nurtured and encouraged. A number of high priority government programmes have promoted shared decision-making and choice by giving people reliable evidence-based information (National Institute for Clinical Excellence; Coulter et al 1999), and by supporting patients to help each other understand about disease processes (NHS Executive 2001).

FOR PHYSIOTHERAPISTS AND THE PROFESSION

Physiotherapists assert that they are 'professionals'. Koehn (1994) argues that a particularly unique characteristic of being a professional is trustworthiness – the expectation is that professionals strive to do good, have the patient's best interests at heart and have high ethical standards. A tangible demonstration of a profession's interests in the welfare of its patients is its preparedness to act on the basis of objective evidence about good practice, regardless of how unpalatable the evidence might be. A prerequisite is that the profession must be aware of what the evidence says. If we don't know whether the evidence indicates that the interventions we offer are effective, or might cause harm, or just make no difference, our claim to be 'professionals' is questionable. Physiotherapy qualifies as a profession in so far as practice is informed by evidence. And in so far as it is not, there is a risk of losing the respect and trust of patients and the public at large.

The profession of physiotherapy has changed enormously in the last 60 years. There has been a transition from doing what doctors told physiotherapists to do, which was usually accepted quite uncritically, to using experience and intuition on which to base decisions, to the current position where evidence-based practice has been promoted as a model for physiotherapy practice (Gibson & Martin 2003). Our new-found professional autonomy should be exercised responsibly. With autonomy comes responsibility for ensuring that patients are given accurate diagnoses and prognoses, and are well-informed about benefits, harms and risks of intervention.

FOR FUNDERS OF PHYSIOTHERAPY SERVICES

Whether physiotherapy services are funded by the public, through the taxes they pay, or by individuals in a fee-for-service or insurance payment, we want to be confident that health care does good, and not harm. Policy-makers, managers and purchasers of health services have an interest in ensuring value for money and health benefits in situations where health resources are always scarce. Decisions have to be made about where and how to invest to benefit the health of the population as a whole. Decisions on investment of health services need to be based on evidence (Gray 1997).

HISTORY OF EVIDENCE–BASED HEALTH CARE

The term 'evidence-based medicine' was first introduced in 1992 by a team at McMaster University, Canada, led by Gordon Guyatt (Evidence-Based Medicine Working Group 1992). They produced a series of guides to help those teaching medicine to introduce the notion of finding, appraising and using high quality evidence to improve the effectiveness of the care given to patients (Oxman et al 1993, Guyatt et al 1994, Jaeschke et al 1994).

Why did the term evolve? What were the drivers? There had been growing concern in some countries that the gap between research and practice was too great. For example, in 1991, the Director of Research and Development for the Department of Health in England noted that 'strongly held views based on belief rather than sound information still exert too much influence in health care' (Department of Health 1991). High quality medical research was not being used in practice even though evidence showed the potential to save many lives and prevent disability. For example, by 1980 there were sufficient studies to demonstrate that prescription of clot-busting drugs (thrombolytic therapy) for people who had suffered heart attacks would produce a significant reduction in mortality. But in the 1990s, thromobolytic therapy was still not recommended as a routine treatment except in a minority of medical textbooks (Antman 1992). Similarly, despite high quality evidence that showed bed rest was ineffective in the treatment of acute back pain, physicians were still advising patients to take to their beds (Cherkin et al 1995).

Another driver was the rapidly increasing volume of literature. New research was being produced too quickly for doctors to cope with it. At the same time, there was a recognition that much of the published research was of poor quality. Doctors had a daily need for reliable information about diagnosis, prognosis, therapy and prevention (Sackett et al 2000).

One way of dealing with the growing volume of literature has been the development of systematic reviews, or systematically developed summaries of high quality evidence, which will be discussed in many chapters in this book. In 1992 the Cochrane Collaboration[4] was established. The Cochrane Collaboration's purpose is the development of high quality systematic reviews, which are now carried out through 50 Cochrane Review Groups, supported by 12 Cochrane Centres around the world. The Collaboration has had a huge impact on making high quality evidence more accessible to large numbers of people.

One of the early drivers of evidence-based physiotherapy was the Department of Epidemiology at the University of Maastricht in the Netherlands. Since the early 1990s this department has trained several 'generations' of excellent researchers who have produced an enormous volume of high quality clinical research relevant to physiotherapy. In 1998, the precursor to this book, *Evidence-based Healthcare: a practical guide for therapists* (Bury & Mead 1998), was published, providing a basic text to help therapists understand what evidence-based practice was and what it meant in relation to their clinical practice. And from 1999 PEDro, a database of randomized trials, has given physiotherapists easy access to high quality evidence about effects of intervention.

Now every physiotherapist has heard of evidence-based practice, and evidence-based practice has initiated much discussion and also some scepticism. Some feel the concept threatens the importance of skills, experience and practice knowledge and the pre-eminence of interaction with individual patients. We will discuss these issues further in this book.

HOW WILL THIS BOOK HELP YOU TO PRACTISE EVIDENCE–BASED PHYSIOTHERAPY?

This book provides a step-by-step explanation of how to practise evidence-based physiotherapy. The focus is on using evidence to support decision-making that pertains to individual patients or small group of patients, but much of what is presented applies equally to decision-making about physiotherapy policy and public health issues.

STEPS FOR PRACTISING EVIDENCE–BASED PHYSIOTHERAPY

Evidence-based practice involves the following steps (Sackett et al 2000):

Step 1   Convert information needs into answerable questions.
Step 2   Track down the best evidence with which to answer those questions.
Step 3   Critically appraise the evidence for its validity, impact and applicability.

---

[4] The Cochrane Collaboration was named after Archie Cochrane, a British epidemiologist who was driven by the need to assess the effectiveness and efficiency of medical treatments and procedures. More information about Archie Cochrane and the Cochrane Collaboration can be found at www.cochrane.org/index0.htm.

Step 4 Integrate the evidence with clinical expertise and with patients' unique biologies, values and circumstances.

Step 5 Evaluate the effectiveness and efficiency in executing steps 1–4 and seek ways to improve them both for next time.

These steps form the basis for the outline of this book.

Chapter 2: What do I need to know?

Evidence-based physiotherapy will only occur when two conditions are met: there has to be a sense of uncertainty about the best course of action, and there has to be recognition that high quality clinical research could resolve some of the uncertainty. Once these conditions are met, the first step in delivering evidence-based physiotherapy is to identify, often with the patient, what the clinical problem is. Framing the problem or question in a structured way makes it easier to identify the information you need. Chapter 2 is designed to help you to frame answerable questions. We focus on four types of clinical questions: those about the effects of intervention; attitudes and experiences; prognosis; and the accuracy of diagnostic tests.

Chapter 3: What constitutes evidence?

Each type of clinical question is best answered with a particular type of research. Chapter 3 considers the types of research that best answer each of the four types of clinical question.

Chapter 4: How can I find relevant evidence?

You will need to do a search of relevant databases to find evidence to answer your clinical questions. Chapter 4 tells you about which databases to search, and how to search in a way that will be most likely to give you the information you need in an efficient way.

Chapter 5: Can I trust this evidence?

Not all research is of sufficient quality to be used for clinical decision-making. Once you have accessed the research evidence, you need to be able to assess whether or not it can be believed. Chapter 5 describes a process for appraising the trustworthiness or validity of clinical research.

Chapter 6: What does this evidence mean for my practice?

If the research is of high quality, you will need to decide if it is relevant to the particular clinical circumstances of your patient or patients, and, if so, what the evidence means for clinical practice. Chapter 6 considers how to assess the relevance of clinical research and how to interpret research findings.

Chapter 7: Clinical practice guidelines

Properly developed clinical guidelines provide recommendations for practice based on a synthesis of the research evidence that is integrated with contributions from clinical experts and patients. Chapter 7 describes how to decide whether clinical practice guidelines are sufficiently trustworthy to apply in practice.

Chapter 8: Making it happen

It can be hard to get high quality clinical research into practice. Chapter 8 discusses barriers to changing practice and ways of improving professional practice.

Chapter 9: Am I on the right track?

Lifelong learning requires self-reflection and self-evaluation. In Chapter 9 we discuss self-evaluation, both of how well evidence is used to inform practice, and of how well evidence-based practices are implemented. In addition, we consider clinical evaluation of the effects of intervention on individual patients.

References

Antman D 1992 A comparison of results of meta-analyses of randomized control trials and recommendations of clinical experts. Treatments for myocardial infarction. JAMA 268(2):240–248

Bury T, Mead J 1998 Evidence-based healthcare: a practical guide for therapists. Butterworth-Heinemann, Oxford

Cherkin DC, Deyo RA, Wheeler K, Ciol MA 1995 Physicians' views about treating low back pain: The results of a national survey. Spine 20:1–10

Coulter A, Entwistle V, Gilbert D 1999 Sharing decisions with patients: is the information good enough? BMJ 318:318–322

Department of Health 1991 Research for health: a research and development strategy for the NHS. Department of Health, London

Edwards A, Elwyn G 2001 Evidence-based patient choice. Oxford University Press, Oxford

Evidence-Based Medicine Working Group 1992 A new approach to teaching the practice of medicine. JAMA 268(17):2420–2425

Gibson B, Martin D 2003 Qualitative research and evidence-based physiotherapy practice. Physiotherapy 89:350–358

Gray JAM 1997 Evidence-based healthcare: how to make policy and management decisions. Churchill Livingstone, Edinburgh

Guyatt GH, Sackett DL, Cook DJ 1994 Users' guides to the medical literature. II. How to use an article about therapy or prevention. B. What are the results and will they help me in caring for my patients? Evidence-Based Medicine Working Group. JAMA 271(1):59–63

Higgs J, Jones M, Edwards I et al 2004 Clinical reasoning and practice knowledge. In: Higgs J, Richardson B, Dahlgren MA (eds) Developing practice knowledge for health professionals. Elsevier, Oxford

Higgs J, Jones M 2000 Clinical reasoning. In: Higgs J, Jones M (eds) Clinical reasoning in health professions. Butterworth-Heinemann, Oxford, pp 3–23

Higgs J, Titchen A 2001 Rethinking the practice–knowledge interface in an uncertain world: a model for practice development. British Journal of Occupational Therapy 64(11):526–533

Jaeschke R, Guyatt GH, Sackett DL 1994 Users' guides to the medical literature. III. How to use an article about a diagnostic test. B. What are the results and will they help me in caring for my patients? Evidence-Based Medicine Working Group. JAMA 271(9):703–707

Koehn D 1994 The ground of professional ethics. Routledge, London

Law M, Cadman D, Rosenbaum P et al 1991 Neurodevelopmental therapy and upper extremity inhibitive casting for children with cerebral palsy. Developmental Medicine and Child Neurology 33(5):379–387

National Institute for Clinical Excellence. Clinical Guidelines – Information for the public. www.nice.org.uk

NHS Executive 2001 The Expert Patient: A new approach to chronic disease management for the 21st century. Department of Health, London

Oxman AD, Sackett DL, Guyatt GH 1993 Users' guides to the medical literature. I. How to get started. The Evidence-Based Medicine Working Group. JAMA 270(17):2093–2095

Richardson B, Higgs J, Dahlgren MA 2004 Recognising practice epistemology in the health professions. In: Higgs J, Richardson B, Dahlgren MA (eds) Developing practice knowledge for health professionals. Elsevier, Oxford

Sackett DL, Straus SE, Richardson WS et al 2000 Evidence-based medicine: how to practice and teach EBM. Churchill Livingstone, Edinburgh

Titchen A, Ersser S 2001 The nature of professional craft knowledge. In: Higgs J, Titchen A (eds) Practice knowledge and expertise in the health professions. Butterworth-Heinemann, Oxford, pp 35–41

Chapter **2**

What do I need to know?

OVERVIEW

The first step in evidence-based practice is to ask relevant clinical questions. In this book we consider questions about the effects of intervention, experiences, prognosis and the accuracy of diagnostic tests. By structuring questions well, relevant evidence can be found more efficiently and easily.

Let us imagine that you are a full time practitioner in an outpatient clinic. One day you are faced with the following patient:

Mr Y is 43 years old. He presents with low back pain of relatively acute onset (about 2 weeks) with pain radiating down his left leg. He has no apparent neurological deficits. The problem has arisen during a period of heavy lifting at work and has become progressively worse over subsequent days. Mr Y's general practitioner prescribed analgesics, anti-inflammatory drugs and bed rest for 5 days, but this brought little improvement. He was then referred to you for treatment to relieve his pain and restore physical functioning.

This scenario will probably make many physiotherapists think how they would manage this patient. Most of us will admit that there is quite a lot we do not know about what the evidence says is the best treatment for patients with back pain. Uncertainty prompts clinical questions, so it is a precondition for evidence-based physiotherapy.

RELEVANT CLINICAL QUESTIONS

A well known saying is that 'the beginning of all wisdom lies not in the answer, but in the question'. The first step in evidence-based practice is to formulate a specific question. The question you have concerning your practice should be formulated so it is possible to find a scientific answer to the question. Posing specific questions relevant to a patient's problem provides a focus to thinking, and it helps in the formulation of search strategies and in the process of critical appraisal of evidence.

Most physiotherapists frequently ask a wide variety of questions during patient encounters. Some information, such as about how the problem affects the patient's day-to-day life, is best obtained by asking the patient. Other information needs are met by practice knowledge that is at our fingertips. But some information needs are best provided by high quality clinical research. This information may be hard to find, and tracking it down is always difficult in the pressurized atmosphere of a busy practice. The intention of this book is to help physiotherapists quickly find important evidence.

In the scenario we have before us, you are faced with the problem of a man with low back pain of relatively acute onset. What questions does this scenario stimulate you to ask? You may have thought of some or all of the following:

- Is heavy lifting the most likely cause of his problem?
- Could this problem, which I frequently see in my practice, be prevented?
- How can I decide if he has nerve root involvement?
- Which tests would be useful to rule out more serious conditions, such as malignancy?
- What is his principal underlying concern about the condition?
- If my aim is to improve his functional capacity, should I advise him to stay active or to rest in bed?
- What does he feel about staying in bed or returning to work?
- What is the probability that the problem will resolve by itself within a month?
- What can I do to relieve his pain during this period?
- Is there anything I can do to speed up his recovery?

All these questions are important. Each is answered with a different kind of evidence. The questions can be categorized as shown in Table 2.1.

The most important clinical questions are those concerning:

- effects of intervention
- patients' experiences
- the course of a condition (prognosis)
- the accuracy of diagnostic tests.

Table 2.1   Categorization of questions

Question	Requires evidence about
■ Could this problem, which I frequently see in my practice, be prevented? ■ If my aim is to improve his functional capacity, should I advise him to stay active or to rest in bed? ■ What can I do to relieve his pain during this period? ■ Is there anything I can do to speed up his recovery?	Effects of intervention
■ What does he feel about staying in bed or returning to work? ■ What is his principal underlying concern about the condition?	Experiences
■ What is the probability that the problem will resolve by itself within a month?	Prognosis
■ How can I decide if he has nerve root involvement? ■ Which tests would be useful to rule out more serious conditions, such as malignancy?	Diagnosis
■ Is heavy lifting the most likely cause of his problem?	Harm or aetiology

Clinical research that answers these sorts of questions is therefore the most important research for clinical practice. In this book we consider how to answer them with high quality clinical research.

We have chosen to start with questions about the effects of intervention because these can be considered the most important sorts of questions for practice. Most of the thinking and concepts in evidence-based physiotherapy have been developed from research on the effects of intervention. Then we will consider questions about patients' experiences because these questions are often complementary to and closely linked with questions about effectiveness. Finally, we consider questions about prognosis and diagnosis.

The separation of clinical questions into those about intervention, experiences, prognosis and accuracy of diagnostic tests is a little contrived. In practice, many clinical questions are complex and require the synthesis of findings of several types of research. A clinical question about whether or not to apply a particular intervention may require information about the effects of that intervention, but it may also need to be informed by studies about prognosis and about patients' experiences. For example, consider a middle-aged man who presents to a physiotherapy department with acute neck pain. He has been told by his general practitioner that a course of cervical mobilization and manipulation will relieve his pain. When deciding how to proceed, his physiotherapist could consider evidence from studies of the effectiveness of mobilization and manipulation, which show a moderate effect on pain and disability (Gross et al 2004), as well as research on the natural course of this condition, which indicates a quite favourable prognosis (Borghouts et al 1998). The physiotherapist might also be interested in what the evidence has to say about patients' expectations of manual therapy, and what it is that most patients hope to be able to achieve with physiotherapy. For the patient, these issues are closely entwined. However, if the physiotherapist is to think clearly about these issues and find relevant research, he or she will do better to break the global question about how to treat into its components concerning effects of intervention, prognosis and experiences.

Our impression is that physiotherapists frequently ask another class of question, about harm or aetiology. (And, in our example we asked about whether heavy lifting is the most likely cause of the patient's problem.) These questions are of great theoretical importance, but they are usually not immediately relevant to practice. To see why, consider the following example. A substantial body of evidence suggests that being overweight exacerbates symptoms of osteoarthritis of the knee (for example, Felson et al 1992, Coggon et al 2001). While that is useful information for researchers, it does not, on its own, indicate that interventions aimed at weight loss are indicated. This is because the causes of most diseases are multifactorial, so intervention that modifies one aetiological factor may have little effect on the course of the disease. Also, interventions aimed at producing weight loss may not have sufficient long term effects to be worthwhile. In general, studies of aetiology suggest interventions but do not confirm their effectiveness. Questions about aetiology could be considered *preclinical* questions. Consequently, we shall not consider questions about aetiology further in this book.

However, there is one type of aetiological research that is of immediate clinical importance: research into unintended harmful effects of intervention. Physiotherapists seldom believe that their treatment could cause harm, but it might be possible for some modalities to do so. Cervical manipulation is one intervention that is known to produce occasional harm (Di Fabio 1999). It causes harm so infrequently that studies of effects of cervical manipulation do not provide a useful estimate of the harm that is caused. The research on harm caused by cervical manipulation is therefore most often of the same type as the traditional aetiological research. In general, evidence of the harmful effects of intervention will often come from aetiological research.

REFINING YOUR QUESTION

Before we begin the hunt for evidence that relates to our clinical questions, we need to spend some time making the questions specific. Structuring and refining the question makes it easier to find an answer. One way to do this is to break the problem into parts. Below we provide some suggestions for breaking questions about effects of intervention, experiences, prognosis and diagnosis into parts. We will use some simple tables to help us formulate well-structured questions.

EFFECTS OF INTERVENTION

We usually break questions about the effects of intervention into four parts (Sackett et al 2000):

- Patient or problem
- Intervention or management strategy
- Comparative intervention
- Outcome.

A useful mnemonic is PICO (Glasziou et al 2003).

The first part identifies the patient or the problem.[1] This involves identifying those characteristics of the patient or problem that are most likely to influence the effects of the intervention. If you specify the patient or problem in a very detailed way you will probably not get an answer, because the evidence is usually not capable of providing very specific answers. (More on this in Chapter 6.) So a compromise has to be reached between specifying enough detail to get a relevant answer, but not too much detail to preclude getting any answer at all.

The second and third parts concern the interventions. Here we specify the intervention that we are interested in and what we want to compare the effect of that intervention to. We may want to compare the effect of an intervention to no intervention, or to a sham intervention (more on sham interventions in Chapter 5) or to another active intervention.

The fourth part of the question specifies what outcomes we are interested in. In some circumstances it may be worth spending some time with the patient to identify precisely what outcomes they are interested in. For example, when considering whether to refer an injured worker to a work-hardening programme it may be important to determine whether the patient is primarily interested in reductions in pain, or reductions in disability, or returning to work, or some other outcome. Traditionally there has been little involvement of patients when it comes to defining the desired outcomes of intervention. There is now an increasing recognition that the patient is the main stakeholder when it comes to choosing outcome measures, and involvement of patients in setting the goals of intervention is an important element in a shared decision-making process.

Let us return to the scenario of the man who presents with acute back pain and ask a question about the effects of intervention. You are considering whether to advise this man to stay in bed or to continue his daily routine as actively as possible. He has been explicit that he wants you to do something to relieve his pain and restore his physical functioning. Consequently, your four-part question is: 'In patients with acute low back pain, does bed rest or advice to stay active produce greater reductions in pain and disability?'

Patient	Intervention	Comparison intervention	Outcome
Adult with acute low back pain	Bed rest	Advice to stay active	Pain and disability

---

[1] The example we use is one of an individual patient. However, health care interventions do not always concern patients. For example, questions related to organizing and funding health services may also be of interest to physiotherapists. This book will, however, focus on problems of individual patients.

EXPERIENCES

Questions about experiences can relate to any aspect of clinical practice. Because such questions are potentially very diverse they must be relatively open. We recommend that, when formulating questions about experiences, you specify the patient or problem and the phenomena of interest.

Returning to our example, you may be interested in your patient's attitudes to his condition. In a similar scenario in your own practice you recently heard a patient expressing concern about whether his complaint might become chronic, or whether he might have a serious illness. You become interested in knowing more about the concerns of patients with acute low back pain. Consequently your two-part question is: 'What are the principal concerns of adults with acute low back pain?'

Patient	Phenomena
Adult with acute low back pain	Principal concerns

PROGNOSIS

When asking questions about prognosis you should specify (again) the patient or problem, and the outcome you are interested in. The question may be about the expected *amount* of the outcome or about the *probability* of the outcome. (We will consider this distinction in more depth in Chapter 6.) Often it is worthwhile specifying the time frame of the outcome as well. In general we can ask questions about the prognosis of people who do not receive treatment (the natural history of the condition) or about the prognosis of people receiving intervention (the clinical course of the condition).

When you discuss different management strategies with your patient he asks you if he is likely to recover within the next 6 weeks, because he has some important things planned at that time. So your first question about prognosis is a broad question about the prognosis in the heterogeneous population of people with acute low back pain. The question is: 'In patients with acute low back pain, what is the probability of being pain-free within 6 weeks?'

Patient	Outcome and time frame
Adult with acute low back pain	Probability of being pain-free within 6 weeks

The patient has previously told you that this is his first-ever spell of low back pain, and you start thinking about whether that is a good or bad indicator for rapid recovery. This is a more detailed question, where you ask about the prognosis for a specific subgroup of patients or the impact of one particular prognostic factor. You try to refine your prognosis by asking: 'In people with first-episode acute low back pain, what is the probability of being pain-free within 6 weeks?'

Patient	Indicator	Outcome and time frame
Adult with acute low back pain	No previous spells of low back pain	Probability of being pain-free at 6 weeks

It is important to understand that questions about prognosis are questions about what will happen in the future, not questions about the causes of what will happen in the future. When we ask questions about the clinical course of a person's condition we want to know what that person's outcome will be, not why it will be what it will be.

DIAGNOSIS

Even the best diagnostic tests occasionally misclassify patients. Misclassification and misdiagnosis are an unavoidable part of professional practice. It is useful to know the probability of misclassification so we can know how much certainty to attach to diagnoses based on a test's findings. The research literature can help us to obtain relatively unbiased estimates of the accuracy of diagnostic tests. When asking questions about diagnostic test accuracy it is useful to specify the patient or problem, the diagnostic test and the diagnosis for which you are testing.

Our patient's general practitioner has told him that he does not have sciatica. You first interpret this to mean there were no neurological deficits, but after the patient describes radiating pain corresponding with the L5 dermatome you are not sure. You are aware that general practitioners often do not examine patients with low back pain very thoroughly so you start thinking about doing further clinical examinations, perhaps using Lasègue's test amongst others, to find out if there is nerve root compromise. So you ask: 'In adults with acute low back pain, how accurate is Lasègue's test as a test for nerve root compromise?'

Patient	Test	Diagnosis
Adult with acute low back pain	Lasègue's test	Nerve root compromise

These four clinical questions are best answered with different types of research. Chapter 3 will describe the sorts of research that best answer each type of question.

References

Borghouts JA, Koes BW, Bouter LM 1998 The clinical course and prognostic factors of non-specific neck pain: a systematic review. Pain 77(1):1–13

Coggon D, Reading I, Croft P et al 2001 Knee osteoarthritis and obesity. International Journal of Obesity and Related Metabolic Disorders 25(5):622–627

Di Fabio RP 1999 Manipulation of the cervical spine: risks and benefits. Physical Therapy 79(1):50–65

Felson DT, Zhang Y, Anthony JM et al 1992 Weight loss reduces the risk for symptomatic knee osteoarthritis in women. The Framingham Study. Annals of Internal Medicine 116(7):535–539

Glasziou P, Del Mav C, Salisbury J 2003 Evidence-based medicine workbook. BMJ Publishing

Gross AR, Hoving JL, Haines TA et al 2004 Cervical overview group. Manipulation and mobilisation for mechanical neck disorders (Cochrane review). In: The Cochrane library, issue 2. Wiley, Chichester

Sackett DL, Straus SE, Richardson WS et al 2000 Evidence-based medicine: how to practice and teach EBM. Churchill Livingstone, Edinburgh

Chapter **3**

What constitutes evidence?

OVERVIEW

Readers looking for evidence of the effects of intervention, experiences, prognosis or accuracy of diagnostic tests should look first for relevant systematic reviews. If relevant systematic reviews cannot be found, the reader can consult reports of individual studies. The best (least biased) evidence of effects of intervention comes from randomized clinical trials. Evidence of experiences can be obtained from qualitative research that typically involves in-depth interviews, observation of behaviours, or focus groups. Evidence of prognosis can be obtained from longitudinal studies. The preferred study type is the prospective cohort study, but sometimes good prognostic information can be obtained from retrospective cohort studies or clinical trials. Evidence of the accuracy of diagnostic tests comes from cross–sectional studies that compare the findings of the test of interest with a reference standard.

WHAT CONSTITUTES EVIDENCE ABOUT EFFECTS OF INTERVENTIONS?

The preceding chapter described four important types of clinical questions: questions about the effects of intervention, experiences, prognosis and diagnostic tests. In this chapter we consider the types of clinical research that can be used to answer these questions.

CLINICAL OBSERVATION

The practice of physiotherapy has always been based, at least in part, on clinical observation.

Day-to-day clinical practice provides physiotherapists with many observations of their patients' conditions. Some physiotherapists supplement their clinical observations with careful measures of outcomes using validated measurement tools. Over time, experienced practitioners accumulate large numbers of such observations. Distillation of clinical observations generates 'practice knowledge' or 'professional craft knowledge' (Higgs et al 2001). The practice knowledge of veteran physiotherapists may be shared with less experienced colleagues in practice or at conferences or workshops.

The simplest way to interpret observations of clinical outcomes is as the effect of intervention. If the condition of most patients improves with intervention then, according to this simple interpretation, the intervention must be effective. Alternatively, if the intervention is designed to prevent adverse outcomes, the observation that most people who receive the intervention do not experience an adverse outcome might be interpreted as indicating that the intervention is effective. The confusion of outcomes and effects of interventions is reinforced by patients. Patients often interpret an improvement in their condition as evidence that intervention was effective, and patients whose condition does not improve may feel dissatisfied with the intervention.

This way of reasoning is attractive but potentially seriously misleading. Many factors determine clinical outcomes.

> It may be incorrect to interpret clinical observations of successful outcomes as evidence of a beneficial effect of intervention because sometimes factors other than the intervention are the primary determinants of outcome.

In epidemiology-speak, the effects of intervention are 'confounded' by 'extraneous factors'. What extraneous factors confound simple cause–effect interpretations of interventions and outcomes?

One important source of confounding is natural recovery. Natural recovery occurs when conditions resolve without intervention. Examples of conditions which can resolve without intervention are acute low back pain and post-surgical respiratory complications. People with these

Figure 3.1   Statistical regression. Patients with episodic disease seek intervention when the severity of the condition exceeds some threshold value. Subsequent fluctuations are more likely to be in the direction of a reduction in disease severity, even if the intervention does not have any effect on the course of the condition.

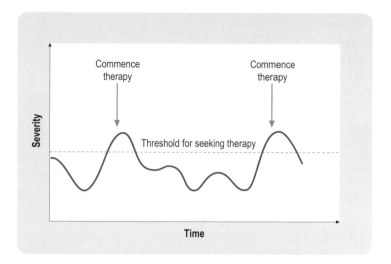

conditions can experience satisfactory outcomes even if they are not given any intervention, or if they are given ineffective interventions. Clinical observations are not always helpful in determining the effects of intervention because it can be difficult, in the course of normal clinical practice, to determine what part of the improvement was due to intervention and what would have occurred without intervention.

Natural recovery may occur because the underlying course of the condition is one of gradual improvement, but it will also tend to occur in chronic conditions that are episodic or that tend to fluctuate in severity. Two common examples of episodic conditions are arthritic pain and respiratory infections. By their very nature, episodic conditions tend to resolve even without intervention, and then they relapse again.

Statisticians consider the spontaneous resolution of episodic disease as an example of a more general phenomenon called statistical regression. The statistical way of thinking about episodic disease is that the disease has a random component to its severity. Sometimes, when the symptoms become particularly bothersome or serious (when random fluctuations are in the direction of worsening of symptoms), patients are driven to seek care. At this stage, when the patient's condition is more severe than usual, still more severe symptoms are relatively unlikely – it is more likely that subsequent random fluctuations will be towards more average symptom levels (see Figure 3.1; Bland & Altman 1994). Consequently conditions of fluctuating intensity, once they become severe, are most likely to resolve, even without intervention.

A third confounder of clinical observations applies when information about outcomes is supplied by the patient rather than directly observed by the physiotherapist. In practice, most useful information about clinical outcomes is obtained in this way.[1] (Two important examples are

---

[1] The real test of most interventions is how they make recipients of the intervention feel. (More on this in Chapter 6.) Consequently the constructs that we most need to know about are intrinsically subjective. The subjectiveness of many clinical outcome measures is a strength, not a weakness, of the measures.

information about pain severity and function, both of which are almost always supplied by the patient.) The only practical way to find out about these types of outcome is to ask patients to tell us whether or not their conditions have improved. But self-reports of outcomes are potentially misleading because patients' responses to questioning about outcomes can be distorted by the social mores that guide interactions between therapists and patients (Kienle & Kiene 1997). Patients understand that most therapists try hard to do their best for their patients, and some patients may find it difficult to report that their condition has not substantially improved. Politeness or a sense of obligation may cause some patients to report improvements that did not occur, or to report exaggerated improvements. In this way, sensitive and polite patients can make intervention look more effective than it truly is. The confounding effect of polite patients is an example of a more general phenomenon, sometimes called the 'Hawthorne effect', which refers to the fact that participants in research may change their behaviours as a result of knowing that their behaviours are under study (Wickstrom & Bendix 2000).

A closely related confounder is the placebo effect (Beecher 1955, Kienle & Kiene 1997, Hrobjartsson & Gotzsche 2003). Placebo effects are improvements in the patient's condition that result from the 'treatment ritual' (Hrobjartsson 2002), as evidenced by effects of inert (sham) interventions. It is widely believed that placebo effects contribute substantially to the benefits of most interventions. For example, a survey showed that many Australian physiotherapists believe that the apparent effects of ultrasound are due largely to placebo effects (Chipchase & Trinkle 2003). Insofar as ultrasound exerts placebo effects, there must be powerful mechanisms that convert the psychological phenomenon of an expectation of effective therapy into the biopsychosocial phenomenon of recovery. But there is considerable controversy surrounding the placebo effect. One point of disagreement is whether placebo effects should be considered confounders or effects of therapy in their own right (Vickers & de Craen 2000). A more radical point of view holds that the placebo effect is an artefact of poorly designed research. We will examine the placebo effect in more detail in Chapter 5.

Interpretations of clinical observations of outcomes may also be confounded by recall bias. Recall bias occurs because the task of keeping track of clinical observations is difficult: experienced physiotherapists who have applied an intervention many times need to maintain an accurate mental ledger of typical outcomes with that therapy. In practice, patients who fared particularly well or particularly badly may feature most prominently in memory. We tend to remember our most successful and most disastrous cases, so our memories of clinical outcomes may be unduly optimistic or unduly pessimistic. Thus accumulation of large numbers of observations of clinical outcomes does not guarantee a reduction in bias.

The preceding paragraphs suggest that simple cause–effect interpretations of clinical observations can be biased (Table 3.1). Most of the biases we have considered act to inflate estimates of effects of interventions; that is, simple cause–effect interpretations of clinical observations tend to

Table 3.1 Summary of major potential causes of bias when using clinical observations to make inferences about effects of intervention

Cause of bias	Effect
Natural recovery	Condition tends to resolve even without intervention
Statistical regression	Patients with episodic disease present for therapy when the condition is severe, but when the condition is severe random fluctuations in severity are likely to be in the direction of a reduction of severity
Polite patients	Polite patients may exaggerate recovery
Placebo effects	The ritual of intervention, rather than the intervention itself, may produce beneficial effects
Recall bias	Extreme cases (successes and disasters) feature most prominently in memory

overestimate effects of interventions. History points to the same conclusion. There are many examples from the history of medicine where clinical observations have suggested that a therapy was effective yet subsequent investigations have shown the therapy to be ineffective or harmful.[2] The simple conclusion is that everyday clinical observations may provide misleading estimates of the effects of interventions.

THEORIES ABOUT MECHANISMS

In some areas of physiotherapy practice the primary justification for intervention is provided not by clinical observations but by theory. The justification is not that the intervention has been observed to be effective but that what we know about the mechanisms of the intervention leads us to believe that intervention should be effective.

There are many examples: physiotherapists began to use ultrasound to treat musculoskeletal lesions back in the 1950s because they believed that ultrasound increased the permeability of cell membranes, which was thought to facilitate healing (Wedlick 1954). The techniques of proprioceptive neuromuscular facilitation (Voss et al 1985), and their successors such as the muscle energy techniques (Chaitow 2001), are based on neurophysiological concepts such as reciprocal inhibition. And many people stretch after sport because they have been told that stretching reduces muscle spasm which causes delayed onset muscle soreness (de Vries 1961).

We need to have theories about the mechanisms of interventions. Properly used, theories about mechanisms can provide hypotheses about which interventions might be effective. Good theories make it possible for us to administer interventions that have the greatest chance of being effective. But theories about mechanisms, on their own, provide very inferior evidence of the effects of intervention. Why?

---

[2] For an extreme example of misleading clinical observations, see Whitehead's description, in 1901, of the use of a tape seton for treatment of migraine. Whitehead treated migraine by passing a dressmaker's tape through an incision in the skin on the back of the neck. He wrote of his experiences with this therapy that: 'During the last five and twenty years I have never failed to treat successfully the most inveterate and severe cases of migraine.'

Physiotherapy involves the application of complex interventions to complex problems, so it should not be surprising that our theories are almost always incomplete. Theories about mechanisms usually have the status of working hypotheses rather than comprehensive and accurate representations of the truth. Theories should be, and usually are, subject to frequent revision. We can rarely know, with any certainty, that theories about intervention are true.

There is another problem with using theory to justify intervention. Theories might tell us about the *direction* of effects of interventions, but they can never tell us about the *size* of effects of interventions. Laboratory studies of the effects of ultrasound might show that insonation of fibroblasts increases their secretion of collagen, or that ultrasound hastens ligament healing, and these findings might suggest that ultrasound will bring about clinically useful effects such as returning subjects to sport faster than would otherwise occur. But how much faster? The theory, even if true, cannot tell us if the application of ultrasound therapy will get patients back to sport one week faster, or one day faster, or one minute faster. We might consider a therapy that gets patients back to sport one week faster is effective, and a therapy that gets patients back to sport just one minute faster than an alternative intervention is ineffective. Theory cannot distinguish between the two. Making rational treatment decisions involves considering the size of treatment effects, and theory cannot tell us about the size of treatment effects.

> Theories of mechanisms can help us develop and refine interventions, but they provide a very poor source of information about the effects of intervention.

We need more than theory.

CLINICAL RESEARCH

Clinical research potentially provides us with a better source of information about the effects of intervention than clinical observation or theories about mechanisms. High quality clinical research is able to prevent ('control for') much of the bias associated with simplistic interpretations of clinical observations and, unlike theories about mechanisms, can provide us with estimates of the size of treatment effects.

> High quality clinical research can provide us with unbiased estimates of the size of the effects of intervention, so it potentially provides us with the best way of assessing effectiveness of interventions.

The systematic and critical use of high quality clinical research in clinical decision-making is what differentiates evidence-based physiotherapy from other models of physiotherapy practice. That is why, in this book, we use the word 'evidence' to mean high quality clinical research.

Unfortunately most clinical research is not of high quality. Surveys of the methodological quality of clinical research have invariably found that most published research does not satisfy basic requirements of good research design (see Chapter 5). One of the consequences is that the findings of many studies cannot be relied upon. It is possible to find studies which purport to demonstrate clinically important effects of particular interventions alongside other studies which draw exactly the opposite conclusions. Undiscriminating readers may find this disconcerting! Readers who have the ability to discriminate between high quality and low quality studies will be more able to make sense of the literature, and should be more able to discern the true effects of interventions. A pre-requisite of evidence-based physiotherapy is the ability to discriminate low quality and high quality clinical research. One of the aims of this book is to provide readers with the skills to discriminate between low and high quality clinical research.

What sorts of clinical research give us the best answers about effects of intervention? There are many ways to design clinical studies of the effec-tiveness of interventions, but some research designs are more suitable than others.

Case series and controlled trials

The simplest studies of the effects of intervention simply involve assess-ing patients presenting with the condition of interest, applying the inter-vention, and determining if, on average, the patients' condition improves. Such studies are sometimes called 'case series'. The simplistic interpret-ation often applied by authors of such studies is that if, on average, patients get better, the intervention is, on average, effective.

These very simple studies just involve systematic recording of normal clinical practice. Like clinical practice they involve the accumulation of observations. And like any clinical observations of the effects of interven-tion they are prone to bias because extraneous factors, other than treat-ment, can masquerade as effective treatment. These sorts of studies are prone to serious bias from natural recovery, statistical regression, placebo effects and polite patients. Therefore they provide very weak evidence of the effects of intervention.

More sophisticated studies compare outcomes in people who do and do not receive the intervention of interest. In such studies the focus is on whether people who receive the intervention of interest have better out-comes than patients who do not receive the intervention. Comparison of outcomes in people who do and do not receive the intervention of inter-est is thought to provide better 'control' of bias than case series, so these studies are called controlled trials.

Controlled trials potentially provide control of bias because both groups (the group that receives the intervention of interest and the group that does not) experience natural recovery and both groups experience statistical regression (and, depending on other features of the design, both groups' outcomes may be influenced by placebo effects or patients' politeness). Therefore, it is reasoned, the *differences* in outcomes of the two groups cannot be due to natural recovery or statistical regression or, in some studies, to placebo effects or polite patients. As these sources of bias have been controlled for, it is more reasonable to attribute differences between the groups' outcomes to the intervention.

A common misunderstanding is the belief that the control group in a controlled trial must receive 'no intervention'. This is not the case. In fact we can distinguish three sorts of controlled studies that differ in the nature of intervention and control:

1. One group receives intervention and the other group receives no intervention.
2. One group receives standard intervention and the other group receives standard intervention plus a new intervention.
3. One group receives a particular intervention and the other group receives a different intervention.[3]

In the rest of this book we will refer, when discussing controlled trials, to the 'intervention group' and 'control group', although we acknowledge that, in the third type of study at least, it may not be clear which group is which.

A common feature of all three designs is that differences in outcomes of the two groups are attributed to differences in the interventions the groups receive. Thus the first sort of study tells us about the effects of intervention over and above no intervention. The second tells about whether there is any benefit in adding the new intervention to standard intervention. The third tells us which of the two interventions is most effective. All three designs tell us something useful, but each tells us something different.

An important assumption of controlled studies is that the two groups are comparable. That is, it is assumed that had the two groups received the same intervention they would experience the same outcomes. When this condition is not met (when the groups consist of subjects that are different in some important way so that they would experience different outcomes even if they received the same intervention) then differences between the groups' outcomes could be attributable, at least in part, to subject characteristics. That is, when the groups are not comparable, differences between outcomes of the two groups cannot be assumed to reflect solely the effects of intervention. (This is called 'allocation bias' or sometimes, less accurately, 'selection bias'. Another way of saying the same thing is to say that the effects of the intervention are confounded by subject characteristics.)

> Controlled studies can only be assumed to provide unbiased estimates of the effects of intervention if the two groups are comparable.

In many studies, groups are self-selected. That is, the grouping occurs naturally, without the intervention of the researcher. For example, in a study of the effects of a movement and swimming programme on respiratory outcomes in children with cerebral palsy, Hutzler and colleagues (1998) compared outcomes of children attending two kindergartens that offered a movement and swimming programme with outcomes of children attending two kindergartens that offered a standard land-based exercise programme. The study found greater improvements in respiratory outcomes among the children receiving the movement and swimming programme. However, this study is unconvincing because it is quite plausible that the

---

[3] In Chapter 5 we shall examine variants of all three designs that involve the provision of sham interventions.

differences in outcomes might be due to different characteristics of the children at the different kindergartens, rather than to the greater effectiveness of the movement and swimming programme. In general, when groups self-select, the groups will not have identical characteristics; some characteristics of the subjects or their experiences causes them to be allocated to one group rather than the other. If those characteristics are related to outcome, the groups will not be comparable. Consequently, controlled trials in which subjects self-select groups are particularly prone to allocation bias.

Randomized trials

How is it possible to assemble two groups of comparable patients? Some researchers try to 'match' subjects in treatment and control groups on characteristics that are thought to be important. For example, in their study of the effects of exercise on lipid profiles in children, Tolfrey and colleagues (1998) matched children undergoing exercise with maturity-matched children not undergoing exercise. Matching on its own is generally unsatisfactory for two reasons. First, there are limitations to the number of variables that can be matched – it is practically impossible to match subjects on more than two or three variables – so the groups may not have equal distributions of other variables that were not matched. Some statistical techniques allow the researchers to statistically match the two groups on many more variables, although these techniques are also limited in the number of variables that can be matched. And, anyhow, it is still necessary to measure all of those variables on all subjects in the study, which may not be practical.[4] Moreover, we usually do not know what all the important prognostic variables are. And if we don't know what is important, we can't match the groups with respect to those variables. In general, the approach of attempting to match groups of patients is generally unsatisfactory because we can never be satisfied that this will produce groups that are comparable in all important respects.

> There is only one way we can assemble intervention and control groups that will give us a high probability of comparable groups, and that is to randomize subjects to groups.

In a randomized trial, subjects agree to be allocated to either the intervention or the control group. Then, when they enter the trial, a random process (sometimes just coin-tossing, but usually a computer-generated random process) allocates each subject to one group or the other.

Random allocation is a marvellous thing. Paradoxically, even though each subject's allocation is indeterminate, the effect of randomizing many subjects is predictable. When many subjects are randomized to groups we can expect that the groups will be comparable. Randomization protects against allocation bias; it prevents confounding of the effects of the intervention by differences between groups.

---

[4] There is another, more technical limitation of these statistical techniques. They can only properly adjust for imbalances in prognostic variables if the prognostic variable is measured without error. In practice most prognostic variables, and almost all prognostic variables measured on a continuous scale, are measured with error. As a consequence, the statistical techniques tend to underadjust. This is called regression dilution bias.

While randomization ensures groups will be comparable, it does not ensure that they will be identical. There will always be small random differences between groups, which means that randomized trials may underestimate or overestimate the true effects of intervention. Herein lies another important benefit of randomization: random processes can be modelled mathematically. This means that it is possible to determine how much uncertainty is associated with estimates of the size of the effects of intervention. We will look at how to ascertain the degree of uncertainty associated with estimates of effects of intervention in Chapter 6.

There are many examples in which randomized and non-randomized trials have examined the effectiveness of the same intervention and have come up with different conclusions. A particularly clear example comes in studies of extracorporeal shock therapy for treatment of plantar fasciitis. Several early but non-randomized studies had shown impressive effects for extracorporeal shock therapy (for example, Chen et al 2001) but subsequent randomized trials found that this therapy had little or no effect (Buchbinder et al 2002, Haake et al 2003). Indeed, some data suggest that this is usually the case: there is a general tendency for randomized trials to be less biased than non-randomized trials. Kunz & Oxman (1998) systematically reviewed studies that had compared estimates from randomized and non-randomized trials of effects of particular interventions and found that non-randomized controlled trials tended to show larger treatment effects than randomized trials. In contrast, systematic reviews of individual trials by Concato et al (2000) and Benson & Hartz (2000) found that studies with non-randomized but contemporaneous controls produced similar estimates of effects to those of randomized trials.

The existing data are, therefore, ambivalent. While there is a substantial body of evidence that suggests non-randomized trials tend to be biased, this has not been unequivocally demonstrated, and there are some examples where non-randomized trials give similar answers to randomized trials. Nonetheless, there is a strong justification for relying on randomized trials for evidence of the effects of intervention.[5] Randomization provides the only mechanism that is *known* to control allocation bias. In our opinion, therefore, randomized trials provide the only way of obtaining estimates of effects of interventions that can be expected to be unbiased. For this reason we should look to randomized trials for evidence of the effects of intervention. There are of course ethical and practical considerations that preclude the conduct of randomized trials in some situations (Box 3.1); in those situations we may have to rely on less rigorous evidence.

Randomized trials come in different flavours and colours. In the simplest designs, subjects are randomly allocated to either a treatment or a control group and outcomes are measured only at the end of the trial. In other trials, measurements may be taken before and after the intervention period, or at several time points during and after the intervention period.

---

[5] Taken to its extreme, the view that only randomized trials can provide unbiased estimates of the effects of therapy is clearly untenable. Some interventions are obviously effective. Smith & Pell (2003) make this case in their systematic review of 'Parachute use to prevent death and major trauma related to gravitational challenge.'

Box 3.1   Ethical and practical impediments to the conduct of randomized trials

It is often said that some randomized trials cannot be carried out because it is not ethical to do so. When is it not ethical to conduct randomized trials of the effects of interventions?

The ethics of randomized trials has been discussed intensely for many decades. One point of view is that it is unethical to randomize subjects to intervention and control conditions unless the clinician is completely ambivalent about which intervention is the better of the two. (This is sometimes called 'equipoise'.) One problem with the requirement of equipoise is that it permits randomization to be vetoed by the clinician, rather than the patient. Arguably, decisions about the acceptability of randomization should be made by properly informed patients, not by clinicians (Lilford 2003). Also, it has been argued that the requirement of equipoise is impractical (clinicians rarely express complete ambivalence), inconsistent with many other apparently ethical behaviours, and not necessarily in the individual patient's best interests (Piantadosi 1997). A more practical and arguably more consistent position is that randomization of properly informed, consenting patients could be considered provided there is not clear evidence that one alternative is superior to the other. In our opinion it only becomes unethical to randomize subjects to groups when it is not plausible that, from an informed patient's perspective, either alternative could be the best available therapy.[6]

There are some situations in which randomized trials cannot practically be conducted (Black 1996). Some interventions, such as the introduction of management strategies, are conducted at the level of organizations. In theory it may be possible to randomize parts of an organization to receive reforms and others not, but in most circumstances this would be logistically impossible. Other circumstances in which randomized trials cannot be conducted are when the intervention involves significant lifestyle modifications, particularly those that must be implemented over long periods of time, or when the outcome of interest is very rare. For example, it may be impossible to use randomized trials to determine if decades of regular exercise increase longevity because few people would be prepared to exercise regularly or not for decades on the basis of random allocation. Also, it could be prohibitively expensive to monitor large numbers of subjects over decades. When the outcome of interest is a rare event it is necessary to study large numbers of subjects, so it is often difficult to use randomized trials to determine the effects of interventions designed to prevent rare events. At the other extreme, it may be wasteful to perform a randomized trial to investigate the effects of a simple, inexpensive and harmless intervention that supplements other therapies, because there may be little to be gained from knowing of the intervention's effects.

[6]There should be systems in place to safeguard the rights, dignity and welfare of people participating in research. The most common mechanism is a Research Ethics Committee (REC) within a hospital or other health care facility. Members of a REC are specially trained in research ethics and often have the sort of experience that will be useful in scrutinizing the ethical aspects of a research proposal. These include patients and members of the public as well as health professionals, academics and people with specific ethical expertise.

Some trials randomly allocate subjects to more than two groups,[7] perhaps a control and two intervention groups. Other trials (called *factorial trials*) examine the effects of more than one intervention by randomly allocating all subjects to receive either one intervention or its control and then randomizing the same subjects to also receive another intervention or its control. (For example, van der Heijden et al (1999) randomized

[7]The groups in a clinical trial are sometimes referred to as 'arms'. Thus a clinical trial that compares three groups might be called a three-armed trial.

subjects with painful shoulders to receive either interferential or sham interferential therapy *and* ultrasound or sham ultrasound therapy. This made it possible to assess the effects of both interferential therapy and ultrasound, and the combination of both in one trial.) In randomized *crossover trials*, all subjects receive both the treatment and control conditions in random order. (For example, Moseley (1997) randomly allocated head-injured patients with plantar flexor contractures to receive either a period of serial casting followed by a period of no casting or a period of no casting followed by a period of casting.) In some types of trial (*cluster randomized trials*), small groups (clusters) of subjects, rather than individual subjects, are randomly allocated to intervention and control conditions. (For example, in their study of over 6000 people with low back pain, Scheel and colleagues (2002) randomized 65 municipalities of subjects to one of two groups.) Although the designs of these studies differ, they all have a common characteristic. All are protected from allocation bias by randomization.

N-of-1 randomized trials

Randomized trials give us probabilistic answers about average effects of interventions: they tell us about the expectation of the effects of intervention.[8] But most patients are uninterested in this technical point. They want to know: 'Will the treatment benefit me?' Unfortunately, randomized trials cannot usually tell us what the effect of intervention will be on any individual patient.

There is, however, one way to determine if a particular treatment is beneficial for an individual patient. This involves conducting a trial on that patient. If the patient receives both the treatment and control condition in random order it is possible to determine if the intervention is more effective than a control condition *for that patient*. To distinguish random effects from real effects, both the treatment and control conditions are administered to the subject several times, or even many times, and a comparison is made between the average outcomes during treated and control conditions. This approach, called the n-of-1 randomized design,[9] has been described in detail (Sackett et al 1991; see also Barlow & Herson 1984).

As with conventional trials, it is necessary to control for potential sources of bias in single-subject trials. If the order of the experimental and control treatment is randomized and the treatment assignment is concealed from the patient and outcome assessor (and perhaps also the therapist), the most important sources of bias are eliminated. We will discuss these features of clinical trials in more detail, in the context of conventional randomized trials, in Chapter 5.

---

[8] We will consider what is meant by 'probabilistic answers about average effects of interventions' in Chapter 6.

[9] There is a long history of n-of-1 trials that precedes their recent discovery in medicine. The methodology was extensively developed by psychologists, notably Herson & Barlow (1984). Psychologists call these studies 'single-case experimental designs'. But the terminology is used inconsistently: the term 'n-of-1 design' is sometimes used inappropriately to describe case series or case studies which do not involve experimental alternation of treatment conditions, and the term 'single-case experimental design' is often used to described studies that are not true experiments because they do not involve random assignment of conditions.

As with cross-over trials, n-of-1 trials are only suitable for certain sorts of conditions and interventions. First, the condition should be chronic, because there is little point in conducting a trial if the condition resolves during the trial. Also, the intervention should be one that produces only transient effects so that when the intervention is withdrawn the condition returns to its baseline level. The beneficial effect should appear relatively quickly when the treatment starts and disappear quickly when the treatment is withdrawn, otherwise the relationship between intervention and outcome will be obscured. As a consequence, n-of-1 trials are most useful for palliative interventions for chronic conditions.

The physiotherapy literature contains many n-of-1 trials, but very few are n-of-1 *randomized* designs. Some examples are trials of orthoses for growing pains in children (Evans 2003) and a trial contrasting effects of graded exposure and graded activity approaches to management of chronic low back pain (Vlaeyen et al 2001).

The strength of n-of-1 trials is also their limitation. N-of-1 trials permit inferences to be made about the effects of intervention on a particular patient, but they provide no logical basis upon which the findings on a single patient can be extrapolated to other patients. Thus n-of-1 trials are of most use for making decisions about that patient, but may be less use for making broader inferences about the effects of an intervention. Some investigators replicate n-of-1 trials on a number of patients, in the belief that this may enable broader inference about the effects of therapy. Replication of n-of-1 trials may enable some degree of generalization.

SYSTEMATIC REVIEWS

A well-designed randomized trial can provide strong evidence of the effects of an intervention. However, readers are entitled to be unconvinced by a single randomized trial. With any single trial there is always the concern that there was some feature of the trial, perhaps a feature that is not apparent in the trial report, that provided aberrant results. For example, there may have been some characteristic of the subjects in the trial that made them unusually responsive or unresponsive to therapy. Alternatively, the intervention may have been administered by an outstanding therapist or, for that matter, a very unskilled therapist. We will consider these issues at greater length in Chapter 6. For now it is sufficient to say that factors that are not easily discerned on reading a trial report may cause an individual trial to unfairly represent the true effects of intervention.

It is reassuring, then, when several trials have investigated the effects of the same intervention and provide data which support the same conclusion. In that case the findings are said to be 'robust'. Conversely, when several trials produce data supporting different conclusions the findings of any one of those trials must be considered less convincing. The combined evidence provided by many clinical trials may provide a truer picture of the effects of intervention than any individual trial. This is one reason why it is best, wherever possible, to use reviews of several trials, rather than individual trials, to answer questions about the effects of interventions.

There is another reason why reviews may provide a better source of information about the effects of intervention than an individual clinical trial. Literature reviews have at their disposal all of the data from all of the trials they review. One of the consequences of having more data is an increase in precision – literature reviews potentially provide more precise estimates of the size of the effects of therapy. This will be considered in more detail in Chapter 6.

We can distinguish two types of review. In the traditional type of review, now called a 'narrative review', an expert in the field locates relevant studies and writes a synthesis of what those studies have to say. Narrative reviews are attractive to readers because they often summarize a vast literature. However, narrative reviews have fallen out of favour because of concerns about bias.

Serious problems with narrative reviews were becoming apparent to psychologists in the late 1970s. By that time the psychological literature had grown to an enormous size and it had become impossible for practising psychologists to read all of the relevant studies pertaining to a particular clinical question; they were forced, instead, to rely on reviews of the literature. But unfortunately there were examples where reviewers had gone to the same literature and come to very different conclusions. For example, Glass and colleagues describe three reviews, completed within about 5 years of each other, that compared effects of drug therapy plus psychotherapy to drug therapy alone. The reviews variously concluded that 'the advantage for combined treatment is striking' and 'there is little difference between psychotherapy plus drug and drug therapy alone' and 'the existing studies by no means permit firm conclusions as to the nature of the interaction between combined psychotherapy and medication' (Glass et al 1981: 18–20).

It is worthwhile contemplating why the different reviewers came up with different conclusions. One explanation is that reviewers had different philosophical orientations that made them see the problems, interventions and outcomes in different ways. Perhaps they were attracted to different parts of the literature and they made different judgements about which studies were and were not important. Unfortunately, the way in which reviewers selected studies and made judgements about study quality was usually not transparent. This is a characteristic of narrative reviews: the process of narrative reviews is usually inscrutable.

The inscrutability of the review process and the inconsistency of review conclusions led to a crisis of confidence. Methodologists began to look for alternatives to narrative reviews. In a short space of time in the late 1970s and early 1980s there was a rapid development of new methods of conducting reviews (Glass et al 1981, Hunter et al 1982, Hedges & Olkin 1985). Soon after, these methods were discovered by medical researchers, and they have since become widely adopted in all areas of health care, including physiotherapy. The new approach to the conduct of reviews is called the 'systematic review' (Egger et al 2001). In systematic reviews the aim is to make the review methodology transparent to the reader and to minimize potential sources of bias.

As their name implies, systematic reviews are conducted using a systematic and explicit methodology. They are usually easily recognizable because, unlike narrative reviews, there is a section of the systematic review which describes the methods used to conduct the review. Typically the Methods section outlines the precise review question and describes criteria used to select studies for inclusion in the review and methods used to assess the quality of those studies, extract data from the studies, and synthesize findings of the studies. As the best studies of effects of intervention are randomized trials, most (but not all) systematic reviews of the effects of interventions only review randomized trials.[10]

> High quality systematic reviews provide comprehensive, transparent and minimally biased overviews of the research literature. Systematic reviews of randomized trials often constitute the best single source of information about the effects of particular interventions.

A particularly important source of systematic reviews of the effects of health interventions is the Cochrane Collaboration, an international network of researchers dedicated to producing systematic reviews of effects of interventions in all areas of health care. Since its inception in 1993, the Collaboration has produced 3440 reviews (Issue 4 of the Cochrane Library 2004). Cochrane reviews tend to be of high quality (Jadad et al 1998), so they are a very useful source of information about the effects of intervention. Where available, relevant Cochrane systematic reviews often provide the best single source of information about effects of particular health interventions.

Systematic reviews, meta-analysis, meta-analysis of individual patient data, and prospective systematic reviews

There is some inconsistency in the terminology used to describe systematic reviews. The first systematic reviews were called 'meta-analyses'. (Another name is 'overviews'.) But over time the term meta-analysis came to mean a class of statistical methods used in systematic reviews (Hedges & Olkin 1985). Now the term meta-analysis is usually reserved to describe certain statistical methods, and the term is no longer used as a synonym for systematic reviews. In contemporary parlance, a meta-analysis is *part of* a review. Meta-analysis can be part of a systematic review or part of a non-systematic (narrative) review. The relationship between systematic reviews, non-systematic reviews and meta-analysis is shown in Figure 3.2.

In the conventional systematic review, published data from randomized trials are used to make inferences about the effects of therapies. Unfortunately, many trial reports provide incomplete data, or present data in an ambiguous way, or present data in a way that is not easily combined with or compared to other studies. To circumvent these problems some reviewers ask the authors of individual trial reports to provide the reviewers with raw data from the original trial. This enables the reviewers to re-analyse the data in an optimal and consistent way. The resulting *systematic reviews of individual patient data* are generally considered more rigorous than conventional systematic reviews. There are, however, very few systematic reviews of individual patient data relevant to physiotherapy. (For an example, see Kelley & Kelley 2004.)

---

[10] In other areas, such as social policy research, most systematic reviews include non-randomized trials.

Figure 3.2 The relationship between systematic reviews and meta-analyses. In contemporary terminology a meta-analysis is a statistical technique used in some reviews. Some, but not all, systematic reviews contain meta-analyses. Meta-analyses can also be found in non-systematic reviews.

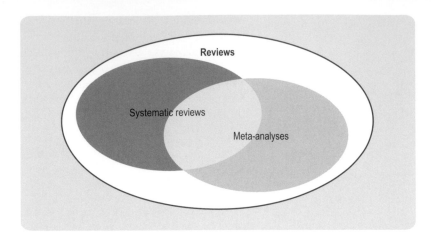

One concern with systematic reviews is that they are usually conducted retrospectively. That is, the review is usually designed and conducted after most of the relevant trials have been conducted. When this is the case it is possible that the reviewers' knowledge of the trials, prior to designing the review, could influence the criteria used to select studies for inclusion in the review, assess the quality of those studies, and extract data. A new kind of systematic review, the *prospective* systematic review, has been designed to control for these kinds of bias (for example, Sacks et al 2000). As the name suggests, prospective reviews are designed prior to the completion of the trials that they review. This ensures that the design of the review cannot be influenced by knowledge of trial results. Prospective reviews of individual patient data from high quality trials potentially provide the strongest possible evidence of effects of an intervention. Unfortunately, prospective systematic reviews tend to be very difficult to perform and take many years to complete, so they are very rare. An example relevant to physiotherapy is the prospective meta-analysis of the FICSIT trials of measures to reduce the risk of falls (Province et al 1995).

SECTION CONCLUSION

In the preceding section we considered a number of sources of information about effects of intervention. It was argued that high quality clinical research usually provides better information about effects of intervention than clinical observations and theory. In general, case series and non-randomized controlled studies do not provide trustworthy sources of information about the effects of therapy so they do not, in our opinion, constitute substantial evidence. The best evidence of effects of interventions is provided by randomized trials or systematic reviews of randomized trials.

There are differing points of view about whether the best evidence of effects of a therapy is provided by a systematic review of relevant trials or by the best individual trial. The answer must be that it depends on how well the review and the best trial were conducted. We encourage physiotherapists seeking answers to clinical questions to first seek systematic reviews relevant to their questions. If the review indicates that there is one trial that is clearly superior to other relevant trials, it may be worthwhile consulting that trial as well.

We conclude this section on evidence of effects of intervention with a comment about a limitation of randomized trials and systematic reviews. The experimental control and lack of bias provided by randomized trials and systematic reviews comes at a cost (Herbert & Higgs 2004). Freedom from bias is achieved by quantifying differences in outcomes of subjects in intervention and control groups. But the act of quantification precludes a deep exploration of subjects' experiences of the intervention (and, for that matter, their experiences of the control condition). Even in trials which examine quality of life or perceptions of the effects of therapy, trials can only provide low-dimensional descriptions of outcomes. A deep understanding of patients' experiences of therapy, and of a number of other clinical phenomena, requires different research approaches. This is the subject of the next section.

WHAT CONSTITUTES EVIDENCE ABOUT EXPERIENCES?

Questions about effects of physiotherapy are crucial in everyday practice. Physiotherapists and patients alike seek information about whether a particular intervention is effective or whether one kind of intervention is better than another. They might also want to know if an intervention causes harmful side-effects. Heads of departments might seek information about cost-effectiveness to help prioritize activities among staff. Where available, evidence of effectiveness and cost-effectiveness from high quality randomized trials should be used to inform decisions about intervention.

But you might have other information needs as well. You might be concerned about how to set up an interdisciplinary team to run an asthma school, how the team should be organized, what opposition you might meet from staff in setting up an interdisciplinary team, or how to handle conflicting views. You may also have questions about which elements of the interventions are the most important and what should be core content. At the same time you might like to know about the experiences of children attending asthma schools, and the experiences of the parents of those children, or how you could motivate families from deprived areas to attend. Most of these questions cannot be answered by clinical trials. Randomized trials and systematic reviews of randomized trials can tell us whether interventions are effective, but not why they are effective, what happened, how it happened or how interventions should be implemented.

Questions such as these, about experiences, attitudes and processes, constitute a separate class of clinical questions. How can we answer these questions? We could start by asking our professional colleagues, or the patients and users of health services, or we could draw on our own observations in practice. Or we could use high quality clinical research designed to answer these questions in a systematic way.

CLINICAL OBSERVATION

You can learn a great deal by asking your patients about their experiences. Skilled physiotherapists develop strategies and skills to ascertain patients' thoughts and values because this information is important for everyday practice. With practice, most physiotherapists become better at understanding how patients regard therapy, and how experiences differ between patients. By talking and listening to patients and observing and reflecting on what happens, skilled physiotherapists learn to better interact and communicate with their patients, and they develop a better understanding of their patients' feelings and perceptions.

However, if you really need to explore a social phenomenon, or dig deep into a question that involves feelings or experiences, there are limitations to what you can find out from clinical observations. Two important limitations are time and resources. Deep exploration of experiences is difficult in the course of everyday clinical practice. An alternative to relying on clinical observations is to look for relevant high quality clinical research.

CLINICAL RESEARCH

Questions about experiences are best answered by qualitative methods.

Qualitative research methods, also called methods of naturalistic inquiry, were developed in the social and human sciences and refer to theories on interpretation (hermeneutics) and human experience (phenomenology) (Malterud 2001). Qualitative methods are useful for the study of human and social experience, communication, thoughts, expectations, meanings, attitudes and processes, especially those related to interaction, relations, development, interpretation, movement and activity (Malterud 2001). Often an aim is to understand the meaning that underpins behaviours.

Qualitative methods can be used to address a diverse spectrum of clinical questions. In this book we refer to those questions as questions about 'experiences'. This term is used as a shorthand for referring to many sorts of questions, including questions about communication, thoughts, expectations, meanings, attitudes and behaviours.

Qualitative research paradigms are rooted in a different philosophical tradition to quantitative research. Consequently, qualitative and quantitative research methods provide complementary ways of understanding the world (Herbert & Higgs 2004). Qualitative research focuses on 'understanding the complex world of lived experience from the point of view of those who live it' (Jones 1995). It is concerned with understanding the views of those being researched. Typically these studies answer questions relating to 'how' and 'why' and 'what is it like'. Answering these sorts of questions requires moving beyond an objective view of the world. Unlike quantitative research, which may aim to find out about 'the' truth, qualitative research aspires to understand a variety of truths. So qualitative and quantitative research methods are based on different ways of knowing, and they produce different types of knowledge (Seers 1999).

The term 'qualitative methods' is an umbrella term for a range of approaches and strategies for collecting, analysing and interpreting

Table 3.2 Research questions and qualitative approaches (Gibson & Martin 2003)

Research question	Qualitative approach	Common methods
What is the meaning attached to this phenomenon?	Phenomenology (philosophy)	In-depth interviews Analysis of personal writings
What is life like for this group?	Ethnography (anthropology)	Participant observation Formal and informal interviews Video or photographic analysis
What is happening? Why is it happening?	Grounded theory (sociology)	In-depth interviews Focus groups
What are they communicating? How are they communicating?	Discourse analysis (sociology, linguistics)	Document analysis

data. Each has its own philosophical perspective and its own methodologies.

Gibson and Martin's useful overview of research questions and qualitative approaches is shown in Table 3.2 (Gibson & Martin 2003). For further reading see Pope & Mays (2000). Data may be collected by use of in-depth interviewing with individuals or groups (focus groups), through observation with or without the participation of the observer, by keeping field notes, by means of open-ended survey questions, or from action research, where data sources are multiple and complex (Malterud 2001).

> Qualitative research can contribute to evidence-based practice in a number of ways. It can challenge taken-for-granted practices, illuminate factors that shape client and clinical behaviour, suggest new interventions based on clients' experiences, identify and evaluate optimal measures of care, enhance understanding of organizational culture and the management of change, and evaluate service delivery (Popay et al 1998).

Common areas of research relevant to clinical practice include the motives, assumptions and perceptions of individuals and groups, and interactions between individuals or between groups. A topic of particular importance is the influence of patient–physiotherapist relationships on health care outcomes. Many studies of patient–physiotherapist relationships have demonstrated the importance of effective communication skills within physiotherapy (Klaber-Mofett & Richardson 1997, Potter et al 2003). Such studies can suggest ways of improving therapeutic relationships.

Another area in which qualitative research methods have been widely used in physiotherapy is in the development of theory. An important part of this research has used qualitative research to inform theories of occupation, particularly about the processes of generating practice knowledge and professional knowledge. We regard this kind of research as important for developing professional practice and clinical expertise but, in the main, this research does not address questions that arise in everyday clinical practice. Physiotherapists in clinical practice will probably find the most immediately useful qualitative research is that which explores patients' health-related perceptions and feelings, particularly those that are a consequence of physiotherapy interventions.

By combining qualitative and quantitative research methods the shortcomings of both approaches can be offset. Consequently it is not surprising that many research projects combine qualitative and quantitative methods. Morgan (1998) classifies combinations of qualitative and quantitative research into four categories: preliminary qualitative methods in a quantitative study, preliminary quantitative methods in a qualitative study, follow-up qualitative methods in a quantitative study and follow-up quantitative methods in a qualitative study. Qualitative research may be conducted prior to quantitative research to set the direction for exploration with quantitative methods, or as follow-up to quantitative studies, where it can aid in interpretation. Researchers frequently use qualitative methods to develop projects, interventions and outcome measures. Before carrying out a survey, qualitative methods are often used to develop a questionnaire, and in-depth interviews can be used to identify attitudes and barriers to phenomena (such as regular exercise) before the development of an intervention that aims to influence it.

Some qualitative research that accompanies quantitative research is not of immediate clinical importance; its primary importance is that it provides insights for researchers into requirements for design and analysis. But other qualitative research is directly relevant to clinical decision-making because it provides insights into the way in which an intervention is experienced by those involved in developing, delivering or receiving the intervention. Qualitative research can also help identify which aspects of the intervention are valued, or not, and why (Cochrane Qualitative Research Methods Group & Campbell Process Implementation Methods Group 2003). So it can be useful to read both a study evaluating the effects of an intervention and a complementary study exploring participants' experiences of the intervention.

Such studies can also help by explaining why some patients do not 'comply' with intervention. This information can be used to tailor interventions to individual needs. For example, researchers evaluating the effectiveness and cost-effectiveness of a progressive exercise programme for patients with low back pain carried out a study that explored associations between factors that influence changes in physical activity and the way individuals perceive and behave with their low back pain, and the impact of those perceptions and behaviours on physical activity (Keen et al 1999). The study found that an aversion to physical activity and fear of pain were the two main factors that hindered increases in physical activity, even though the majority of informants believed strongly that being physically active was beneficial. The study suggests it may be helpful to identify an aversion to physical activity or fear of pain at the earliest stage in order to tailor advice accordingly.

Another example of how qualitative research can complement quantitative research comes from a study of a sports injury prevention programme. The study sought to describe lessons learned from the implementation of a rugby injury prevention programme carried out as a cohort study (Chalmers et al 2004). Qualitative research methods, including informant interviews, participant observation and the scrutiny of written, visual and archival material, were used to describe the process of implementation of the programme. Among the lessons learned were the difficulties in implementing complex interventions, the advantages of a formal agreement between partners in the implementation of a programme, the central role played by coaches in promoting injury prevention strategies, and the value of describing the process of implementation and monitoring injury outcomes and changes in knowledge, attitudes and behaviour. The authors suggested that professionals wishing to develop injury prevention programmes in other sports could learn from these experiences.

Qualitative research can influence how outcomes are measured and interpreted, as in a trial that tested the effect of a package of physiotherapy interventions for patellofemoral osteoarthritis. This study identified discrepancies in outcomes assessed with qualitative in-depth interviews and a quantitative questionnaire (Campbell et al 2003). The lack of agreement between the two measures provided some insights into how interventions benefit patients, how clinicians could measure outcomes of therapy, and the need for patient-centred outcome measures. It is obvious that this knowledge is of importance for researchers and teachers, and for promoting new high quality studies, but it might also be helpful to clinicians by suggesting relevant dimensions of health outcome measures.

There are other areas of qualitative research that are highly relevant to practice. Studies that have as their objective to understand clients' health-related perceptions and explore patients' experiences with therapy can be very useful. For example, a study describing how parents experienced living with a child with asthma uncovered four main themes related to management of asthma (Trollvik & Severinsson 2004). One important finding was that parents felt they were not respected by health professionals and that their competence was questioned. The findings emphasize the importance of a mutual dialogue between health care professionals and parents to enable parents to develop the competence necessary for the care of their children. Another study explored how the process of discharge from physiotherapy following stroke was managed and experienced by patients and physiotherapists (Wiles et al 2004). The study found that patients' expectations and optimism about recovery were not confronted at discharge. The notion of natural recovery that was raised with patients by physiotherapists at discharge, and the information physiotherapists gave about exercise post-discharge, had the effect of maintaining patients' high expectations and hopes for recovery. This might suggest that physiotherapists can make a positive contribution to the process of adaptation and adjustment that stroke survivors experience following discharge.

Qualitative research can also form a basis for developing patient information based on patients' information needs. Much information has been developed over the years based on health professionals' perceptions of patients' needs without asking patients themselves what they perceive their needs to be. By integrating valid and relevant results from research carried out with qualitative methods into clinical practice, physiotherapists may be more able to understand their patients, develop empathy and understanding with them, and convey relevant information to them. Two examples of studies that can inform provision of health information are projects designed to develop patient information for people with low back pain (Skelton et al 1995, Glenton 2002). These studies concluded that patient information should be presented in the user's own language, at several levels of understanding, and should include both evidence-based and experienced-based knowledge.

Importantly, while qualitative research gives insights into attitudes to and experiences of therapy and prevention, this evidence cannot provide definitive answers to questions about effects of interventions. There is a particular danger in using research that is designed to answer 'what' and 'why' questions as justification for a particular intervention. For example, evidence that patients with low back pain enjoy massage should not necessarily be interpreted as indicating that massage should be used to treat back pain. It is often easy to 'jump' directly from information about experiences and attitudes to making inferences about practical interventions. Such interpretations should be made carefully.

SYSTEMATIC REVIEWS

If clinicians are going to use qualitative research in decision-making, the findings of qualitative research need to be accessible and aggregated in a meaningful way. Summaries of existing studies facilitate the dissemination of findings of qualitative research. Gibson & Martin (2003) have called for international collaboration among qualitative researchers to develop methods for meta-synthesis and the translation of evidence into practice. This is difficult because there are many challenges in combining different philosophical approaches in qualitative research syntheses.

There is extensive work going on to integrate studies with qualitative methods into systematic reviews of interventions. The Cochrane Collaboration has established a methods group, the Cochrane Qualitative Methods Group, focusing on the inclusion of evidence from qualitative studies into systematic reviews (Cochrane Qualitative Research Methods Group & Campbell Process Implementation Methods Group 2003). The group argues that studies of qualitative methods can provide insight into 'internal' factors, including aspects of professional, managerial or consumer behaviour, and 'external' factors such as policy developments, which facilitate or hinder successful implementation of a programme or service and how it might need to be adapted for large scale roll-out. Such studies can also generate qualitative data on the outcomes of interventions.

> The findings from qualitative research studies can therefore help to answer questions about the impact, appropriateness and acceptability of interventions and thus enhance the scope, relevance and utility of effectiveness reviews (Cochrane Qualitative Research Methods Group & Campbell Process Implementation Methods Group 2003).

The Cochrane Collaboration's 'sister' organization, the Campbell Collaboration, which aims to prepare systematic reviews of social and educational policies and practices, is currently investigating how to review studies of qualitative methods that have evaluated health programmes and health service delivery. Some organizations have published reports that integrate qualitative research with trials in systematic reviews (Thomas et al 2004). An example is a review of the effects of interventions to promote physical activity among children and young people. The review includes an overview of the barriers and motivators extracted from qualitative research (EPPI-Centre 2003).

WHAT CONSTITUTES EVIDENCE ABOUT PROGNOSIS?

Often our patients ask us when or if or how much their condition will improve. These are questions about prognosis. How can we learn to make accurate prognoses?

In general we can obtain information about prognosis from clinical observation and from clinical research. We consider these in turn.

CLINICAL OBSERVATION

One source of information about prognosis is clinical observation. Experienced clinicians accumulate many observations of patients with a particular condition over the course of their careers. Some therapists may be able to distil their experiences into an accurate statement about typical outcomes. That is, some physiotherapists gain accurate impressions of the prognosis of conditions they see. Astute physiotherapists may go one step further. They may be able to see patterns in the characteristics of patients who subsequently have good outcomes and those who do not. In other words, some physiotherapists may develop the ability to recognize prognostic factors.

Several factors make it difficult for physiotherapists to generate accurate estimates of prognosis or the importance of prognostic factors from their clinical observations. First, we are often particularly interested in long term prognoses, and many physiotherapists do not routinely see patients for long term follow-up. Second, follow-up is usually conducted on a subset of patients, rather than on all patients, and the subset on whom follow-ups are conducted may not be representative, in terms of their prognoses, of all patients initially seen by the physiotherapist. Lastly, in order to obtain reasonably accurate estimates of the prognoses of some conditions, it may be necessary to see several hundred patients with the condition of interest, and, if the condition is not very common, few physiotherapists may ever see enough of the condition to gain accurate impressions of the prognosis (de Bie 2001). For these reasons, deriving prognoses for particular patients or conditions often necessitates supplementing clinical experience with clinical research.

CLINICAL RESEARCH

The requirements of a good study of prognosis are less stringent than the requirements of a good study of the effects of intervention. To generate good information about prognosis, researchers must identify a group of people with the condition of interest and see how those peoples' condition changes over time. Such studies are called longitudinal studies – the term 'longitudinal' implies that observations on any one subject are made at more than one point in time.

The particular type of longitudinal study that involves observing representative samples of people with specific characteristics is called a 'cohort' study. Here the term 'cohort' simply refers to a group of people with some shared characteristics, such as a shared diagnosis. In many, but not all, cohort studies there is more than one cohort. Thus, in most cohort studies the researchers identify two or more groups of people, perhaps with the same diagnosis but differing clinical presentations, and follow them over time. These sorts of studies can provide us with information about prognosis, and may also provide us with information about how we can refine the prognosis based on certain prognostic factors.

Prospective and retrospective cohort studies

If the cohorts are identified before the follow-up data are obtained (that is, if subjects are followed forwards in time) then the study is a 'prospective cohort study'.[11]

> Prospective cohort studies are a particularly useful source of information about prognosis.[12]

In other sorts of cohort studies, follow-up data are obtained before the cohort is identified. For example, outcome data may have been collected in the course of routine clinical care and archived in medical records before the researcher initiated the study. In that case the researcher can extract follow-up data that pre-existed identification of the cohort. Such

---

[11] Some authorities make a slightly different distinction between prospective and retrospective studies. According to Rothman & Greenland (1998), prospective studies are those in which exposure status is measured prior to the onset of disease. We prefer to define prospective studies as those in which the cohort is identified prior to the measurement of outcome because this definition is more broadly applicable: it applies just as well to studies of prognosis (where exposure might be of no interest, and where we may be interested in the evolution of the severity of disease) as it does to studies of aetiology.

[12] Prospective cohort studies are often also the best design for answering another sort of question: questions about aetiology (or 'harm'). Questions about aetiology concern what *causes* disease. (That is, they identify factors that are the last-satisfied component in a series of components necessary for the disease; Rothman & Greenland 1998). Establishing causation is more difficult than describing or predicting outcomes. And although understanding aetiology is important for the development of interventions, it is of less immediate importance to clinical practice than obtaining accurate prognoses. This is because even if we know about risk factors it is not always obvious how to change those risk factors, nor is it necessarily true that changing the risk factors will substantively reduce risk. We will not consider questions about aetiology any further in this book.

studies are called 'retrospective cohort studies'. Sometimes retrospective cohort studies can also provide us with useful prognostic data.

An example of a prospective cohort study was reported by Albert et al (2001). These authors monitored the presence or absence of pelvic pain in 405 women who had pelvic pain at 33 weeks of pregnancy. In this study, each subject was identified as eligible for participation in the study before her outcome measures were obtained, so this was a prospective cohort study. In contrast Shelbourne & Heinrich (2004) performed a retrospective cohort study to determine the prognosis of patients with meniscal tears that were not treated at the time of knee reconstruction for anterior cruciate ligament injury. Outcome data were obtained from a database of clinical outcomes measured over a 13-year period prior to the study. As these data were obtained prior to identification of the cohort, this study was retrospective.

Clinical trials

We can obtain information about prognosis from other sorts of longitudinal studies too. Another sort of longitudinal study design that can provide information about prognosis is the clinical trial. Clinical trials are designed to determine the effects of intervention but they almost always involve longitudinal observation of specific cohorts. Even though the aim of clinical trials is to determine the effects of intervention, they can sometimes generate useful information about prognosis along the way.

The fact that prognostic information exists incidentally in some studies that are designed with a different purpose means that the authors of a clinical trial may not even appreciate that the study contains prognostic information. So prognostic information may be buried, unrecognized and hidden, in reports of clinical trials.[13] This makes finding prognostic information more difficult than finding information about effects of intervention.

Importantly, clinical trials do not have to be *randomized* trials to provide prognostic information. They do not even have to be *controlled* trials. Studies of the effects of intervention must have control groups to distinguish the effects of intervention from the effects of other variables that affect outcomes, but studies of prognosis do not require control groups because the aim of studies of prognosis is not to determine what caused the outcome, just to describe what the outcome is.

An example of a clinical trial that contains useful information about prognosis is a randomized trial of the effects of specific stabilizing exercises for people with first-episode low back pain (Hides et al 2001). The primary aim of this study was to determine the effectiveness of a particular type of exercise, so subjects were randomly allocated to a group which exercised or a group that did not. But because this study followed subjects

---

[13] Another reason that prognostic information may be hard to find is that many researchers are more interested in prognostic factors (factors that are related to prognosis) than in the prognosis itself. Consequently many research reports contain detailed presentations of information about prognostic factors but little or no information about the prognosis.

for 3 years it incidentally provides information about the 3-year prognosis for people with first-episode low back pain.

SYSTEMATIC REVIEWS

Some authors have reviewed the literature on prognosis for particular conditions. As with narrative reviews of effects of interventions, narrative reviews of prognosis are prone to the same sorts of biases as narrative reviews of the effects of intervention. Consequently, over the last decade, methodologists have begun to develop methods for conducting systematic reviews of prognosis. (See, for example, Altman 2001.)[14]

> High quality systematic reviews potentially provide us with a transparent and minimally biased overview of all the best data on the prognosis of a particular condition, so, when they are available, they may constitute the best single source of information about the prognosis for that condition.

Some recent examples of systematic reviews of prognosis are those by Scholten-Peeters et al (2003), on the prognosis of whiplash-associated disorders, and Pengel et al (2003), on the prognosis of acute low back pain.

In summary, we can obtain information about prognosis from prospective and retrospective cohort studies and clinical trials, or from systematic reviews of these studies. Of course, not all such studies provide good information about prognosis. In Chapter 5 we shall examine how to differentiate high quality and low quality information about prognosis.

WHAT CONSTITUTES EVIDENCE ABOUT THE ACCURACY OF DIAGNOSTIC AND SCREENING TESTS?

How can we get good information about the accuracy of diagnostic tests? We could rely on clinical observations or we could consult the research literature.

CLINICAL OBSERVATION

To find out about the accuracy of a diagnostic test we need to apply the test to many people and then see how well the test's findings correspond with what subsequently proves to be the correct diagnosis. It may be possible to do this in routine clinical practice but more often than not circumstances conspire to make it difficult to obtain unbiased estimates of the accuracy of diagnostic tests in the course of routine clinical practice. Why is that so?

In routine clinical practice the true diagnosis may be obtained from subsequent investigations. For example, a clinician's impressions about

---

[14] The chapter by Altman (2001) is primarily concerned with studies of prognostic factors, rather than prognosis itself. Nonetheless much of it is relevant to systematic reviews of prognosis.

the presence of a rotator cuff tear, based on tests such as O'Brien's test, may subsequently be confirmed or refuted by arthroscopy. Usually, however, information about the correct diagnosis is not *routinely* available, because usually not *all* patients are subjected to subsequent investigation. Consequently, clinical observations of the concordance of clinical tests and the true diagnosis are almost always based on a (sometimes small) subset of patients that are tested. Insofar as it is possible that the accuracy of the diagnostic test may be higher or lower in that subgroup, clinical observations of the accuracy of the diagnostic test may underestimate or overestimate the accuracy of the test. This makes it difficult to generate accurate estimates of diagnostic accuracy on the basis of unstructured clinical observations alone.

Better estimate of the accuracy of diagnostic tests may be obtained from high quality clinical research.

CLINICAL RESEARCH
Cross-sectional studies

Like clinical observations, clinical studies of the accuracy of diagnostic tests involve applying the test to many people and then determining how well the test's findings correspond with the correct diagnosis. Such study designs are usually called cross-sectional studies, to distinguish them from longitudinal studies. Studies of the accuracy of diagnostic tests are cross-sectional studies because they are concerned with how accurately a test can determine if a disease or condition is present at the time the test is conducted (Knottnerus 2002).

In cross-sectional studies of diagnostic tests, a group of subjects is subjected to the test of interest. We will call this the clinical test. The same subjects are also tested with some other test that is thought to establish the true diagnosis. The test used to establish the correct diagnosis is often called the 'gold standard' or 'reference standard' test. Reference standards are often tests that are more invasive or more expensive than the clinical test that is the subject of the research. For example, a recent study compared the findings of a range of simple clinical tests for lumbosacral nerve root compression in people with sciatica (questions such as whether pain was worse in the leg than in the back, straight leg raise test, weakness, absence of tendon reflexes, and so on) with the findings of magnetic resonance imaging (MRI; Vroomen et al 2002). In this study, MRI was the reference standard.

Sometimes the reference standard is hindsight, because the true diagnosis only becomes apparent with time. An example is provided by studies of 'red flags' used in the assessment of low back pain (Deyo & Diehl 1988). Red flags such as recent unexplained weight loss may be suggestive of cancer. But there is no satisfactory reference standard for immediate diagnosis of cancer in people presenting with low back pain. It is possible that some sorts of cancer might not be easily detected, even with invasive or expensive diagnostic tools. The diagnosis might only be established some time later when the disease has advanced. In that case the reference standard may involve extended monitoring of patients. The correct diagnosis at the time of the initial test might be considered to be cancer if extended follow-up subsequently detects cancer, and the diagnosis is considered to be something other than cancer if extended follow-up does not detect cancer.[15,16]

Two sorts of cross-sectional studies can be distinguished, based on how the researchers go about recruiting ('sampling') subjects for the study. The most useful sorts of studies seek to sample from the population of subjects suspected of the diagnosis. For example, the study of clinical tests for lumbosacral nerve root compression cited above (Vroomen et al 2002) recruited subjects with back pain radiating into the leg because this is the population in whom the diagnosis of lumbosacral nerve root compression is suspected. As expected, MRI subsequently confirmed nerve root compression in some but not all subjects. The true diagnosis for each subject was not known until after the subject entered the study. Such studies are sometimes called, somewhat confusingly, 'cohort studies'.[17]

In an alternative approach, the researchers recruit two groups of subjects: one group consists of subjects who are thought to have the diagnosis, and the other group consists of subjects thought not to have the diagnosis. For example Bruske et al (2002) investigated the accuracy of Phalen's test for diagnosis of carpal tunnel syndrome by recruiting two groups of subjects: one group had clinically and electromyographically confirmed carpal tunnel syndrome and the other was a group of volunteers who did not complain of any hand symptoms. The researchers sought to determine if Phalen's test could accurately discriminate between the two groups of subjects. Studies such as these are sometimes called 'case–control' studies, although again the terminology is a little confusing. In Chapter 5 we shall see that cohort studies provide a much better source of information about the accuracy of diagnostic tests than case–control studies.

Randomized trials

Theoretically, we could use randomized trials to tell us about diagnostic tests. Trials do not necessarily tell us about the accuracy of diagnostic

---

[15] Technically, such studies are cross-sectional studies and not, as it first appears, longitudinal studies, even though they involve following patients over time (Knottnerus 2002). This is because the focus of the study is the test findings and diagnosis at the time that the initial test was conducted. In studies of diagnostic tests, extended follow-up is intended to provide information about the *diagnosis* at the time of the initial test, not the subsequent *prognosis*.

[16] One problem with diagnostic test studies in which the reference standard involves extended follow-up is that the disease may develop between the time of the initial testing and the follow-up. This would cause the study to be biased in the direction of making the test appear less accurate than it really is.

[17] The application of the terms 'cohort study' and 'case–control study' to cross-sectional studies is confusing because many people think of cohort studies and case–control studies as types of longitudinal studies. Epidemiologists who apply the terms 'cohort study' and 'case–control study' to cross-sectional studies of diagnostic tests argue that the essential characteristic of cohort studies and case–control studies is the method of sampling. In cohort studies the researcher seeks to sample in a representative way from the population about which inferences are to be made. In case–control studies of diagnostic tests the researcher intentionally samples separately from two populations: a population with the diagnosis and a population without the diagnosis.

tests, but they can tell us about the effects of using a diagnostic test on patients' outcomes.

The principle of using randomized trials to investigate the effects of diagnostic tests is simple. Subjects are randomly allocated to groups that either receive or do not receive the diagnostic test of interest[18] and the outcomes of the two groups are compared. If the test provides accurate diagnostic information that supports better decisions about management, this will be reflected in better health outcomes in the group that is tested. On the other hand, if the diagnostic test does not provide accurate information, or if it does provide accurate information but that information does not contribute to better management, the tested group will not have better outcomes.

Several randomized trials have been conducted to determine the value of routine X-rays in primary care of people with low back pain. In the trials by Kerry et al (2000) and Miller P et al (2002), patients presenting to general medical practitioners with low back pain were either routinely referred for X-rays or not, and the outcomes of the two groups (such as disability, subsequent medical consultations and health care costs) were compared.

Screening

We can differentiate two sorts of diagnostic testing. The first is the testing we considered in the preceding section: the test is applied when people present with a particular problem and we use the test to determine a diagnosis to explain that problem. A second sort of test is a screening test. Screening tests are tests that we apply to people who we have no particular reason to suspect of having the diagnosis. The screening may be practice-based (for example, patients presenting with low back pain may be screened for depression; Levy et al 2002) or it may be part of a community-based programme (for example, in some countries adolescent girls are screened for scoliosis in school-based screening programmes; Yawn et al 1999). The potential value of screening is that it makes it possible incidentally to detect disease early. And for some diseases early detection may enable more effective management.

Screening programmes are best evaluated with randomized trials because randomized trials provide information about the end-benefit of screening. The screening test will only produce demonstrable beneficial effects if it is capable of accurately detecting the condition of interest *and* detection occurs significantly earlier than it otherwise would *and* early detection means that intervention can be more effective *and* these beneficial effects are not outweighed by the harm produced by false-positive and false-negative screening tests.

Most of the randomized trials of diagnostic procedures have been trials of medical screening tests. Some important examples are randomized trials of the effects of mammogram screening for breast cancer and PAP smears for cervical cancer (Miller AB et al 2002, Batal et al 2000). Clinical trials of

---

[18] Alternatively, both groups could be tested but the results of the tests made available for only one group.

screening tests usually have to study very large numbers of patients, so they are often very expensive. Consequently there are very few randomized trials of diagnostic or screening tests used by physiotherapists – possibly none! Until randomized trials are conducted, many physiotherapists will continue to screen for a range of conditions in the absence of evidence of a beneficial effect. (An example is the practice, in some countries, of screening first-grade school pupils for clumsiness or minimal cerebral dysfunction.)

As there are very few randomized trials of screening tests in physiotherapy, this book will concentrate on evaluating studies of diagnostic test accuracy, and we will not consider randomized trials of screening tests further. In the next few years we hope to see the publication of randomized trials of screening tests used by physiotherapists.

SYSTEMATIC REVIEWS

In recent years the first systematic reviews of studies of the accuracy of diagnostic tests have been published. Examples are systematic reviews of tests for anterior cruciate ligament injury (Scholten et al 2003), the Ottawa ankle rules (Bachman et al 2003), and tests for carpal tunnel syndrome (d'Arcy et al 2000). Like systematic reviews of studies of the effects of intervention or of prognosis, systematic reviews of studies of the accuracy of diagnostic tests potentially provide transparent and unbiased assessments of studies of diagnostic test accuracy, and some provide precise estimates of test accuracy, so they potentially provide the best single source of information about the accuracy of diagnostic tests. The Cochrane Collaboration has recently established a group to systematically review studies of the accuracy of diagnostic tests.

Enough talk. It's time for some action. Let's find some studies with which to answer our clinical questions.

References

Albert H, Godskesen M, Westergaard J 2001 Prognosis in four syndromes of pregnancy-related pelvic pain. Acta Obstetricia et Gynecologica Scandinavica 80:505–510

Altman DG 2001 Systematic reviews of evaluations of prognostic variables. In: Egger M, Davey Smith G, Altman DG (eds) Systematic reviews in health care. Meta-analysis in context. BMJ Books, London, pp 228–247

Bachmann LM, Kolb E, Koller MT et al 2003 Accuracy of Ottawa ankle rules to exclude fractures of the ankle and mid-foot: systematic review. BMJ 326:417

Barlow DH, Hersen M 1984 Single case experimental designs: strategies for studying behavior change. Allyn and Bacon, Boston

Batal H, Biggerstaff S, Dunn T et al 2000 Cervical cancer screening in the urgent care setting. Journal of General Internal Medicine 15:389–394

Beecher KH 1955 The powerful placebo. JAMA 159:1602–1606

Benson K, Hartz AJ 2000 A comparison of observational studies and randomized, controlled trials. New England Journal of Medicine 342:1878–1886

Black N 1996 Why we need observational studies to evaluate the effectiveness of health care. BMJ 312:1215–1218

Bland JM, Altman DG 1994 Statistics notes: some examples of regression towards the mean. BMJ 309:780

Bruske J, Bednarski M, Grzelec H et al 2002 The usefulness of the Phalen test and the Hoffmann–Tinel sign in the diagnosis of carpal tunnel syndrome. Acta Orthopaedica Belgica 68:141–145

Buchbinder R, Ptasznik R, Gordon J et al 2002 Ultrasound-guided extracorporeal shock wave therapy for plantar fasciitis: a randomized controlled trial. JAMA 288:1364–1372

Campbell R, Quilt B, Dieppe P 2003 Discrepancies between patients' assessments of outcome: qualitative study nested within a randomised controlled trial. BMJ 326:252–253

Chaitow L 2001 Muscle energy techniques. Churchill Livingstone, Edinburgh

Chalmers DJ, Simpson JC, Depree R 2004 Tackling rugby injury: lessons learned from the implementation of a five-year sports injury prevention program. Journal of Science and Medicine in Sports 7:74–84

Chen H-S, Chen L-M, Huang T-W 2001 Treatment of painful heel syndrome with shock waves. Clinical Orthopaedics and Related Research 387:41–46

Chipchase LS, Trinkle D 2003 Therapeutic ultrasound: clinician usage and perception of efficacy. Hong Kong Physiotherapy Journal 21:5–14

Cochrane Qualitative Research Methods Group & Campbell Process Implementation Methods Group 2003. http://mysite.wanadoo-members.co.uk/Cochrane_Qual_Method/index.htm

Concato J, Shah N, Horwitz RI 2000 Randomized controlled trials, observational studies, and the hierarchy of research designs. New England Journal of Medicine 342:1887–1892

d'Arcy CA, McGee S 2000 Does this patient have carpal tunnel syndrome? JAMA 283:3110–3117

de Bie R 2001 Critical appraisal of prognostic studies: an introduction. Physiotherapy Theory and Practice 17:161–171

de Vries HA 1961 Prevention of muscular distress after exercise. Research Quarterly 32:177–185

Deyo R, Diehl A 1988 Cancer as a cause of back pain. Frequency, clinical presentation and diagnostic strategies. Journal of General Internal Medicine 3:230–238

Egger M, Davey Smith G, Altman DG (eds) 2001 Systematic reviews in health care. Meta-analysis in context. BMJ Books, London, pp 228–247

EPPI-Centre 2003 Children and physical activity: a systematic review of research on barriers and facilitators. The Evidence for Policy and Practice Information and Co-ordinating Centre Social Science Research Unit (SSRU), Institute of Education, University of London. http://eppi.ioe.ac.uk/EPPIWeb/home.aspx

Evans AM 2003 Relationship between 'growing pains' and foot posture in children. Journal of the American Podiatric Medical Association 93:111–117

Gibson B, Martin D 2003 Qualitative research and evidence-based physiotherapy practice. Physiotherapy 89:350–358

Glass GV, McGaw B, Smith ML 1981 Meta-analysis in social research. Sage, Beverly Hills

Glenton C 2002 Developing patient-centred information for back pain sufferers. Health Expectations 5:19–29

Haake M, Buch M, Schoellner C et al 2003 Extracorporeal shock wave therapy for plantar fasciitis: randomised controlled multicentre trial. BMJ 327:75

Hedges LV, Olkin I 1985 Statistical methods for meta-analysis. Academic Press, Orlando

Herbert RD, Higgs J 2004 Complementary research paradigms. Australian Journal of Physiotherapy 50:63–64

Herson DH, Barlow M 1984 Single case experimental designs. Strategies for studying behavior change, 2nd edn. Pergamon, New York

Hides J, Jull GA, Richardson CA 2001 Long-term effects of specific stabilizing exercises for first-episode low back pain. Spine 26:E243–E248

Higgs J, Titchen A, Neville 2001 Professional practice and knowledge. In: Higgs J, Titchen A (eds) Practice knowledge and expertise in the health professions. Butterworth-Heinemann, Oxford, pp 3–9

Hrobjartsson A 2002 What are the main methodological problems in the estimation of placebo effects? Journal of Clinical Epidemiology 55:430–435

Hrobjartsson A, Gotzsche PC 2003 Placebo treatment versus no treatment (Cochrane review). In: The Cochrane Library, Issue 2. Wiley, Chichester

Hunter JE, Schmidt FL, Jackson GB 1982 Meta-analysis: cumulating research findings across studies. Sage, Beverly Hills

Hutzler Y, Chacham A, Bergman U et al 1998 Effects of a movement and swimming program on vital capacity and water orientation skills of children with cerebral palsy. Developmental Medicine and Child Neurology 40:176–181

Jadad AR, Cook DJ, Jones A et al 1998 Methodology and reports of systematic reviews and meta-analyses: a comparison of Cochrane reviews with articles published in paper-based journals. JAMA 280:278–280

Jones R 1995 Why do qualitative research? BMJ 311:2

Keen S, Dowell AC, Hurst K et al 1999 Individuals with low back pain: how do they view physical activity? Family Practice 16:39–45

Kelley GA, Kelley KS 2004 Efficacy of resistance exercise on lumbar spine and femoral neck bone mineral density in premenopausal women: a meta-analysis of individual patient data. Journal of Women's Health 13:293–300

Kerry S, Hilton S, Patel S et al 2000 Routine referral for radiography of patients presenting with low back pain: is patients' outcome influenced by GPs' referral for plain radiography? Health Technology Assessment 4:1–119

Kienle GS, Kiene H 1997 The powerful placebo effect: fact or fiction? Journal of Clinical Epidemiology 50:1311–1318

Klaber-Moffett JA, Richardson PH 1997 The influence of the physiotherapist–patient relationship on pain and disability. Physiotherapy Theory and Practice 13:89–96

Knottnerus JA 2002 The evidence base of clinical diagnosis. BMJ Books, London

Kunz R, Oxman AD 1998 The unpredictability paradox: review of empirical comparisons of randomised and nonrandomised clinical trials. BMJ 317:1185–1190

Levy HI, Hanscom B, Boden SD 2002 Three-question depression screener used for lumbar disc herniations and spinal stenosis. Spine 27:1232–1237

Lilford RJ 2003 Ethics of clinical trials from a Bayesian and decision analytic perspective: whose equipoise is it anyway? BMJ 326:980–981

Malterud K 2001 The art and science of clinical knowledge: evidence beyond measures and numbers. Lancet 358:397–399

Miller AB, To T, Baines CJ et al 2002 The Canadian National Breast Screening Study – 1: breast cancer mortality after 11 to 16 years of follow-up. A randomized screening trial of mammography in women age 40 to 49 years. Annals of Internal Medicine 137:305–312

Miller P, Kendrick D, Bentley E et al 2002 Cost-effectiveness of lumbar spine radiography in primary care patients with low back pain. Spine 15:2291–2297

Morgan D 1998 Practical strategies for combining qualitative and quantative methods: applications for health research. Qualitative Health Research 8:362–376

Moseley AM 1997 The effect of casting combined with stretching on passive ankle dorsiflexion in adults with traumatic head injuries. Physical Therapy 77:240–247

Pengel HL 2004 Outcome of recent onset low back pain. PhD thesis, School of Physiotherapy, University of Sydney

Pengel HLM, Herbert RD, Maher CG et al 2003 A systematic review of prognosis of acute low back pain. BMJ 327:323–327

Piantadosi S 1997 Clinical trials: a methodologic perspective. Wiley, New York

Popay J, Rogers A, Williams G 1998 Rationale and standards for the systematic review of qualitative literature in health services research. Qualitative Health Research 3:341–351

Pope C, Mays N (eds) 2000 Qualitative research in health care, 2nd edn. BMJ Books, London

Potter M, Gordon S, Hamer P 2003 The difficult patient in private practice physiotherapy: a qualitative study. Australian Journal of Physiotherapy 49:53–61

Province MA, Hadley EC, Hornbrook MC et al 1995 The effects of exercise on falls in elderly patients. A preplanned meta-analysis of the FICSIT Trials. Frailty and injuries: cooperative studies of intervention techniques. JAMA 273:1381–1383

Rothman KJ, Greenland S 1998 Modern epidemiology. Williams and Wilkins, Philadelphia

Sackett DL, Haynes RB, Guyatt GH et al 1991 Clinical epidemiology. A basic science for clinical medicine. Little, Brown, Boston

Sacks FM, Tonkin AM, Shepherd J et al 2000 Effect of pravastatin on coronary disease events in subgroups defined by coronary risk factors: the Prospective Pravastatin Pooling Project. Circulation 102:1893–1900

Scheel IB, Hagen KB, Herrin J et al 2002 A call for action: a randomized controlled trial of two strategies to implement active sick leave for patients with low back pain. Spine 27:561–566

Scholten RJ, Opstelten W, van der Plas CG et al 2003 Accuracy of physical diagnostic tests for assessing ruptures of the anterior cruciate ligament: a meta-analysis. Journal of Family Practice 52:689–694

Scholten-Peeters GGM, Verhagen AP, Bekkering GE et al 2003 Prognostic factors of whiplash-associated disorders: a systematic review of prospective cohort studies. Pain 104:303–322

Seers K 1999 Qualitative research. In: Dawes M, Davies P, Gray A et al (eds) Evidence-based practice. A primer for health care professionals. Churchill Livingstone, London

Shelbourne KD, Heinrich J 2004 The long-term evaluation of lateral meniscus tears left in situ at the time of anterior cruciate ligament reconstruction. Arthroscopy 20:346–351

Skelton AM, Murphy EA, Murphy RJ et al 1995 Patient education for low back pain in general practice. Patient Education and Counseling 25:329–334

Smith GCS, Pell JP 2003 Parachute use to prevent death and major trauma related to gravitational challenge: systematic review of randomised controlled trials. BMJ 327:1459–1461

Thomas J, Harden A, Oakley A et al 2004 Integrating qualitative research with trials in systematic reviews. BMJ 328:1010–1012

Tolfrey K, Campbell IG, Batterham AM 1998 Exercise training induced alterations in prepubertal children's lipid–lipoprotein profile. Medicine and Science in Sports and Exercise 30:1684–1692

Trollvik A, Severinsson E 2004 Parents' experiences of asthma: process from chaos to coping. Nursing and Health Sciences 6(2):93–99

van der Heijden GJ, Leffers P, Wolters PJ et al 1999 No effect of bipolar interferential electrotherapy and pulsed ultrasound for soft tissue shoulder disorders: a randomised controlled trial. Annals of the Rheumatic Diseases 58:530–540

Vickers AJ, de Craen AJM 2000 Why use placebos in clinical trials? A narrative review of the methodological literature. Journal of Clinical Epidemiology 53:157–161

Vlaeyen JWS, de Jong J, Geilen M et al 2001 Graded exposure in vivo in the treatment of pain-related fear: a replicated single-case experimental design in four patients with chronic low back pain. Behaviour Research and Therapy 39:151–166

Voss DE, Ionta MK, Myers BJ 1985 Proprioceptive neuromuscular facilitation: patterns and techniques, 3rd edn. Harper & Row, Philadelphia

Vroomen PC, de Krom MC, Wilmink JT et al 2002 Diagnostic value of history and physical examination in patients suspected of lumbosacral nerve root compression. Journal of Neurology, Neurosurgery and Psychiatry 72:630–634

Wedlick LT 1954 Ultrasonics. Australian Journal of Physiotherapy 1:28–29

Whitehead W 1901 The surgical treatment of migraine. BMJ i:335

Wickstrom G, Bendix T 2000 The 'Hawthorne effect' – what did the original Hawthorne studies actually show? Scandinavian Journal of Work, Environment and Health 26:363–367

Wiles R, Ashburn A, Payne S et al 2004 Discharge from physiotherapy following stroke: the management of disappointment. Social Science and Medicine 59(6):1263–1273

Yawn BP, Yawn RA, Hodge D et al 1999 A population-based study of school scoliosis screening. JAMA 282:1427–1432

Chapter **4**

Finding the evidence

OVERVIEW

Having formulated a clinical question it is possible to start looking for relevant evidence. This involves searching electronic databases. Searches of the world wide web using generic search engines such as Google or Yahoo will usually fail to find most relevant evidence. Evidence of effects of interventions is best found on PEDro or the Cochrane Library. Evidence of experiences is best found using CINAHL or PubMed. And evidence of prognosis or the accuracy of diagnostic tests is best found using the Clinical Queries function in PubMed. Regardless of what database is searched, it is important to select search terms carefully, and combine search terms in a way that ensures the search is optimally sensitive, specific and efficient.

SEARCH STRATEGIES

In this chapter we explore how to find evidence that can be used to answer questions about the effects of therapy, experiences, prognosis and diagnosis.

Finding evidence involves searching computer databases of the health care literature. The chapter suggests databases to search and search strategies for each database. At the end of the chapter we consider how you can obtain the full text of the studies you have identified.

Databases come and go. And some databases are more accessible than others. We are mindful that suggestions about which database to search can quickly become obsolete, and that some readers will have access to more databases than others. For this reason we have chosen to recommend a small number of widely available databases. Wherever possible we recommend databases that can be accessed without subscription. We also recognize that the ability to access libraries and the internet varies enormously between therapists and across countries. Therefore we suggest a number of mechanisms for obtaining full text. Unfortunately, access will remain difficult for some.

The purpose of this chapter is to help busy clinicians find answers to their clinical questions. It is not intended as a guide for researchers or systematic reviewers. Clinicians need to treat patients, so, unlike systematic reviewers, they do not have the time needed to perform exhaustive searches of the literature. They should perform searches that are efficient, but not comprehensive. Consequently our goal in this chapter will be to identify strategies for finding good evidence that pertains to a clinical question (ideally, the best evidence) in as short a time as possible. We will not try to find *all* relevant evidence.

Efficient searching means performing sensitive and specific searches. By sensitive, we mean that the search finds most of the relevant studies. By specific we mean the search does not return too many irrelevant studies. A sensitive and specific search finds all of the relevant records, but only relevant records; it does not find lots of 'junk'.

You may want to read this chapter with an internet-connected computer at hand. That way you can use databases and search strategies as they are presented. Try using each database and search strategy to search for questions relevant to your clinical practice.

Keep in mind that the aim is to do quick and efficient searches. Sometimes your search will quickly yield what you are looking for. Sometimes you will have to follow a few false leads before finding a gem. And sometimes your search will yield nothing. A temptation, especially for those with more obsessive traits, is to search through screen after screen of many hundreds of studies in the hope of finding something worthwhile. Try to resist the temptation! If your search returns hundreds of hits, refine your search so that you need sift through a smaller number of hits. If you don't find evidence that relates to your question reasonably quickly, give up and resign yourself to the fact that the evidence either does not exist or you were unable to find it without difficulty. It is unproductive and discouraging to search fruitlessly. You can spend a long time looking for something that is not there.

Like all skills, literature searching improves with practice. If you are inexperienced at searching the literature you may find your initial attempts time-consuming and frustrating. (Your searches may be insensitive or non-specific.) Don't be discouraged. With practice you will become quicker and more able to find the best evidence. A reasonable goal to aspire to, at least with a fast internet connection, is to be able to routinely find the best available evidence in 3 minutes.

Some readers will be able to enlist the help of a librarian when searching. If you have this opportunity, take advantage of it. The best way to learn how to conduct efficient searches is to observe a skilled librarian conduct searches and then have the librarian give you feedback on your own search strategies.

THE WORLD WIDE WEB

The world wide web has become an invaluable source of information. It contains information on everything from election results in Paraguay to how to build an atomic bomb. Internet-savvy people, when confronted with almost any question, will open up a web browser and search the world wide web with a search engine like Google or Yahoo.

Google and Yahoo provide a very convenient way to find film reviews and phone numbers, but they are a very poor way of finding high quality clinical research. Most sites containing high quality clinical research cannot be searched by these search engines. Generic search engines such as Google and Yahoo do not provide a useful way of searching for high quality clinical research because they fail to detect most relevant research. If you want to find high quality clinical research you will need, instead, to search specialist databases of health sciences literature. A range of these databases exist, and each is particularly suited to finding evidence pertaining to particular sorts of questions. Later in this chapter we will consider which database should be searched to answer each of our four types of clinical questions, and we will look at database-specific search strategies. But first it is useful to explore some generic issues that apply to searching of all databases.

SELECTING SEARCH TERMS

Regardless of what sort of question you are seeking answers to and what sort of database you search, you will need to select search terms. That is, you will need to specify words that tell the database what you are searching for.

Herein lies the art to efficient searching. Carefully selected search terms will usually find a manageable number of relevant studies. A poorly constructed search may return thousands of studies or none at all, or it may return studies that are irrelevant to your question. Search terms should be selected carefully.

Think through the following steps before typing search terms:

1. First, identify the key elements of your question (see Chapter 2). If the question was 'Does weight-supported training improve walking performance more than unsupported walking training following stroke?', the key elements might be *weight-supported training*, *walking performance* and *stroke*.

2. Now think about which of those key elements are likely to be uniquely answered by the studies you are interested in. There are likely to be

many studies on stroke, and many studies on walking, but few on weight-supported training. Consequently a search looking for studies about weight-supported training is likely to be more specific than a search for studies about stroke or walking.

3. Lastly, think about alternative terms that could be used to describe each of the key elements.

Weight-supported training could be described as 'weight supported training' or 'weight-supported training' (note the hyphen) or 'training with weight support' or 'weight-supported walking' or 'walking with weight support', and so on – these synonyms, and most other alternative terms for weight-supported training, contain the word 'weight', suggesting that 'weight' may be a good search term.

Alternative search terms for walking include 'walking', 'gait', and perhaps 'ambulate', 'ambulation' and 'ambulating'. As at least three distinctly different terms are used to describe walking it is a little more difficult to search for studies using the key element of walking. The same difficulty is found in searches for studies on stroke, because a stroke can also be called a cerebrovascular accident, or cerebro-vascular accident (again, note the hyphen) or CVA. The best search terms are those which have few, quite similar, synonyms.

Sometimes a particular search term is uniquely associated with the search question and has few synonyms. Then the search strategy is obvious. For example, if you wanted to know 'Does the Buteyko technique reduce the incidence of asthma attacks in children?', you could use the term 'Buteyko' because it is likely to be more-or-less uniquely associated with your question; there are few, if any, synonyms for 'Buteyko'.

Wild cards

Most databases have the facility to use wild cards to identify word variants. Wild cards are characters that act as a proxy (or substitute) for a string of characters. For example, PEDro, the Cochrane Library and PubMed all use the asterisk symbol to indicate a wild card. Thus, in these databases, 'lumb*' searches for the words 'lumbar', 'lumbosacral' and 'lumbo-sacral'. Wild cards are particularly useful when it is necessary to find a number of variants of the same word stem.[1]

AND AND OR

All major databases can be searched by explicitly specifying more than one search term. For example, if you were interested in the recurrence of dislocation after primary shoulder dislocation you could search using two terms: 'shoulder' and 'dislocation'. This would result in a more specific search than a search using either search term on its own.

When more than one search term is used it is necessary to specify how the search terms are to be combined. For two search terms we need to

---

[1] Whenever a wild card facility is available you should avoid searching for the plural form of words unless you are only interested in the plural. For example, it is generally better to search for 'knee*' than 'knees', and it is better to search for 'laser*' than 'lasers'.

specify whether we want to find studies that contain *either* of the search terms or (as in the preceding example) *both* of the search terms. For three or more search terms we can specify whether we are interested in studies which contain *any* of the search terms or *all* of the search terms.

To specify that we want to find studies that contain *any* of the search terms, we combine the search terms with OR. For example, if we were interested in studies of lateral epicondylitis we could specify 'epicondylitis OR tennis elbow'.[2,3] Alternatively, to specify that we want to find studies that contain *all* of the search terms we combine the search terms with AND. For example, if we were interested in studies of effects of the use of ultrasound for ankle sprain we could specify 'ultrasound AND ankle'.[4]

In general, we specify OR when we want to broaden a search by looking for alternative key terms or synonyms for key terms. We specify AND when we want to narrow a search by mandating more than one key term. The appropriate use of ANDs and ORs can greatly increase the sensitivity and specificity of database searches. In most (not all) databases it is possible to combine multiple search terms mixing both ANDs and ORs. Box 4.1 illustrates how AND and OR can be combined in a single search.

In the rest of this chapter we shall consider specifically how to find evidence of the effects of interventions, experiences, prognosis and accuracy of diagnostic tests. We will depart from the order that we use in most of this book and consider searching for evidence of experiences last, because it is convenient first to discuss issues regarding searches for prognosis and accuracy.

---

[2] In some databases, such as PubMed, we actually type in the word OR, just as shown. In other databases, such as PEDro, we indicate that we want to combine search terms with OR by clicking on the OR button at the bottom of the screen. (If, in PEDro, you typed 'epicondylitis or tennis elbow', and the AND button was checked (as is the default) then PEDro would go looking for studies that contain all four words, including the word 'or'!) We consider how to specify ANDs and ORs for specific databases later in this chapter.

[3] Wild cards and OR have a similar function: both enable you to search for word variants. Wild cards are efficient in the sense that they don't require as much typing, and they don't even require that you think of the possible variants of a particular word stem. But wild cards are not as flexible as OR. OR makes it possible to find variants of a word with different stems (such as 'neck' and 'cervical').

[4] Note that the search specified 'ultrasound and ankle', not 'ultrasound AND ankle sprain'. The term 'ankle' is likely to be more sensitive than ankle sprain, because some studies will talk about 'sprains of the ankle' or 'sprained ankles' rather than 'ankle sprains'. The search term 'ankle' will capture either, but the search term 'ankle sprain' might not capture studies which refer to 'sprains of the ankle' or 'sprained ankles'. (Some databases, such as PubMed and the simple search in PEDro will capture either instance with the search term 'ankle sprain'.) Of course the search term 'ankle' will be far less specific than 'ankle sprain', so the best approach might be to combine all three search terms using AND. The search 'ultrasound AND ankle AND sprain' is likely to be both sensitive and specific.

Box 4.1   Using AND and OR

In general, AND is used to mandate more than one search term, and OR is used to search for word variants or synonyms. We can illustrate how ANDs and ORs are combined using a table such as the following:

	Key term 1	AND	Key term 2	AND ...
Synonym 1				
OR				
Synonym 2				
OR ...				

To perform a search for a question about the effects of ultrasound for lateral epicondylitis we might consider two key terms, one pertaining to ultrasound and the other pertaining to epicondylitis. There are no obvious synonyms for ultrasound, but a common synonym for 'epicondylitis' is 'tennis elbow'. Also, epicondylitis is occasionally referred to as epicondylalgia. Hence:

	Key term 1	AND	Key term 2
Synonym 1	ultrasound		epicondyl*
OR			
Synonym 2			tennis elbow

Thus our search would be 'ultrasound AND (epicondyl* OR tennis elbow)'.[5]

---

[5] Note the use of brackets. When mixing ANDs and ORs there is potential for ambiguity, and the brackets remove the ambiguity. Can you see the difference between 'ultrasound AND (epicondyl* OR tennis elbow)' and '(ultrasound AND epicondyl*) OR tennis elbow'?

FINDING EVIDENCE OF EFFECTS OF INTERVENTIONS

In Chapter 3 we saw that the best evidence of effects of interventions comes from randomized trials or systematic reviews of randomized trials.

Contrary to popular belief, there is an extensive literature of randomized trials and systematic reviews in physiotherapy. At the time of writing (July 2004) there are at least 4100 randomized trials and 780 systematic reviews. (For a description of the trials, see Moseley et al 2002.) The rate of production of trials and systematic reviews has accelerated rapidly (Figure 4.1) so that more than one-third of all trials and nearly two-thirds of all systematic reviews have been published in the preceding 5 years. At the time of writing, about seven new randomized trials and two new systematic reviews in physiotherapy are published each week.

Figure 4.1   Number of randomized trials and systematic reviews archived on the PEDro database, by year of publication. (Data extracted July 2004.) The first trial on the database was published in 1929 (not shown on the graph), and the first systematic review was published in 1982. Since then, the number and rate of publication has increased exponentially with time. Updated and redrawn from Moseley et al 2002.

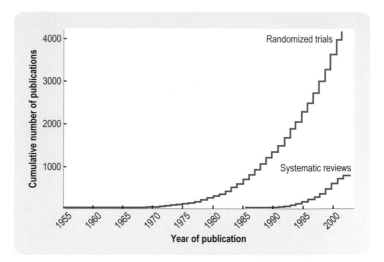

PEDro

Perhaps the first place to go looking for evidence of the effects of physiotherapy interventions is PEDro.[6] PEDro is a database of randomized trials, systematic reviews and evidence-based clinical practice guidelines in physiotherapy. The database is freely available on the world wide web at www.pedro.fhs.usyd.edu.au. Parts of the PEDro web site have been translated into Arabic, French, German, Italian, Korean, Portuguese and Spanish.

The most useful parts of the web site are the two search pages. PEDro offers two search facilities: *Simple Search* and *Advanced Search*. We will begin by looking at the *Simple Search* page.

Simple search

Let's use the *Simple Search* to find evidence about the effects of pulsed ultrasound for reducing pain and disability associated with lateral epicondylitis. (The *Simple Search* page is shown in Figure 4.2.) Click on *Search* in the menu bar, and then *Simple Search*. The *Simple Search* page contains just one box in which you can type words that tell PEDro the topic of your search. When you enter a search term or multiple search terms in this box, PEDro searches for studies that contain those search terms.[7] If you enter more than one search term, PEDro will only find records that contain *all* the search terms you entered. (That is, the *Simple Search* always combines search terms with ANDs.)

In the text box type 'ultrasound epicondylitis'[8] and click on *Start Search* (or just hit enter). PEDro returns a list of titles of all the records on the database that contain both the words 'ultrasound' and 'epicondylitis'. The search results are shown in Figure 4.3.

---

[6] PEDro stands for **P**hysiotherapy **E**vidence **D**atabase. The 'ro' at the end just gives it a more catchy name.

[7] For each study, PEDro stores a range of information in containers called 'fields'. Fields include authors' names, the title and abstract, journal name and other bibliographic details and, importantly, subject headings. Subject headings will be discussed in more detail later in this chapter. The PEDro *Simple Search* looks for records that contain all the search terms in any fields.

[8] Note that, in the PEDro *Simple Search*, the AND is assumed. Do not type AND.

Figure 4.2 PEDro: Simple Search page.

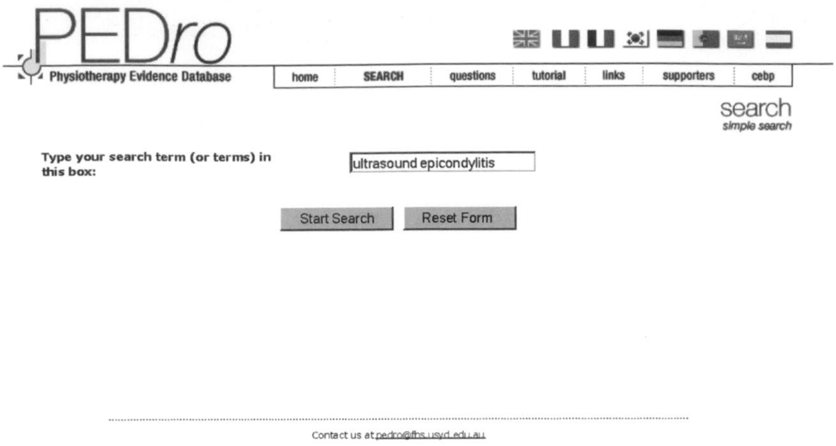

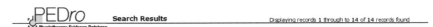

Figure 4.3 PEDro: Simple Search results page.

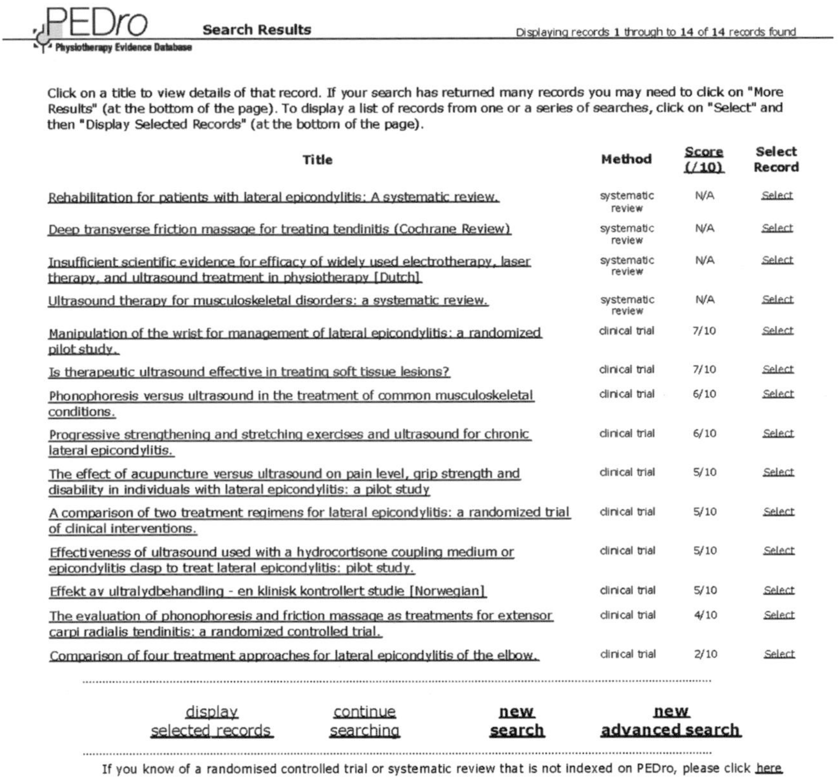

PEDro Physiotherapy Evidence Database **Search Results** Displaying records 1 through to 14 of 14 records found

Click on a title to view details of that record. If your search has returned many records you may need to click on "More Results" (at the bottom of the page). To display a list of records from one or a series of searches, click on "Select" and then "Display Selected Records" (at the bottom of the page).

Title	Method	Score (/10)	Select Record
Rehabilitation for patients with lateral epicondylitis: A systematic review.	systematic review	N/A	Select
Deep transverse friction massage for treating tendinitis (Cochrane Review)	systematic review	N/A	Select
Insufficient scientific evidence for efficacy of widely used electrotherapy, laser therapy, and ultrasound treatment in physiotherapy [Dutch]	systematic review	N/A	Select
Ultrasound therapy for musculoskeletal disorders: a systematic review.	systematic review	N/A	Select
Manipulation of the wrist for management of lateral epicondylitis: a randomized pilot study.	clinical trial	7/10	Select
Is therapeutic ultrasound effective in treating soft tissue lesions?	clinical trial	7/10	Select
Phonophoresis versus ultrasound in the treatment of common musculoskeletal conditions.	clinical trial	6/10	Select
Progressive strengthening and stretching exercises and ultrasound for chronic lateral epicondylitis.	clinical trial	6/10	Select
The effect of acupuncture versus ultrasound on pain level, grip strength and disability in individuals with lateral epicondylitis: a pilot study	clinical trial	5/10	Select
A comparison of two treatment regimens for lateral epicondylitis: a randomized trial of clinical interventions.	clinical trial	5/10	Select
Effectiveness of ultrasound used with a hydrocortisone coupling medium or epicondylitis clasp to treat lateral epicondylitis: pilot study.	clinical trial	5/10	Select
Effekt av ultralydbehandling - en klinisk kontrollert studie [Norwegian]	clinical trial	5/10	Select
The evaluation of phonophoresis and friction massage as treatments for extensor carpi radialis tendinitis: a randomized controlled trial.	clinical trial	4/10	Select
Comparison of four treatment approaches for lateral epicondylitis of the elbow.	clinical trial	2/10	Select

display selected records | continue searching | **new search** | **new advanced search**

If you know of a randomised controlled trial or systematic review that is not indexed on PEDro, please click here

You can see that in the top right-hand corner PEDro indicates there were 14 'hits'.[9] (By 'hits' we mean records that satisfy the search criteria.) Underneath there is a list of the titles of the records that satisfied the search criteria, an indication of whether the record is a randomized trial, systematic review or practice guideline, a methodological quality score, and a column for selecting items. Titles of systematic reviews are listed first, then titles of clinical practice guidelines, then randomized trials. The randomized trials

[9] If you are doing this search yourself you may find you get more hits. That is because new records are continually being added to the database.

Figure 4.4 PEDro: Detailed
Search Results page.

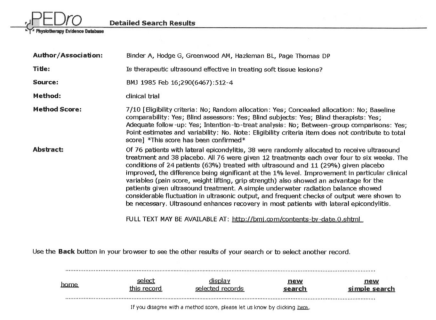

PEDro Physiotherapy Evidence Database **Detailed Search Results**

Author/Association:	Binder A, Hodge G, Greenwood AM, Hazleman BL, Page Thomas DP
Title:	Is therapeutic ultrasound effective in treating soft tissue lesions?
Source:	BMJ 1985 Feb 16;290(6467):512-4
Method:	clinical trial
Method Score:	7/10 [Eligibility criteria: No; Random allocation: Yes; Concealed allocation: No; Baseline comparability: Yes; Blind assessors: Yes; Blind subjects: Yes; Blind therapists: Yes; Adequate follow-up: Yes; Intention-to-treat analysis: No; Between-group comparisons: Yes; Point estimates and variability: No. Note: Eligibility criteria item does not contribute to total score] *This score has been confirmed*
Abstract:	Of 76 patients with lateral epicondylitis, 38 were randomly allocated to receive ultrasound treatment and 38 placebo. All 76 were given 12 treatments each over four to six weeks. The conditions of 24 patients (63%) treated with ultrasound and 11 (29%) given placebo improved, the difference being significant at the 1% level. Improvement in particular clinical variables (pain score, weight lifting, grip strength) also showed an advantage for the patients given ultrasound treatment. A simple underwater radiation balance showed considerable fluctuation in ultrasonic output, and frequent checks of output were shown to be necessary. Ultrasound enhances recovery in most patients with lateral epicondylitis.

FULL TEXT MAY BE AVAILABLE AT: http://bmj.com/contents-by-date.0.shtml

Use the **Back** button in your browser to see the other results of your search or to select another record.

home	select this record	display selected records	new search	new simple search

If you disagree with a method score, please let us know by clicking here.

are listed in order of descending quality scores. So, to a rough approximation, the most useful evidence will tend to be towards the top of the list.

It is a simple matter to scroll through the list of titles looking for those that appear to be most relevant. Clicking on a title links to a *Detailed Search Results* page (Figure 4.4), which displays bibliographic details, abstracts (where available) and details of how the methodological quality score was determined (for randomized trials only). You can select articles that look relevant by clicking on the *Select* button (in the right-hand column of the *Search Results* page, or at the bottom of a *Detailed Search Results* page). This saves the record to a 'shopping basket'. You can return to your shopping basket of selected search results at any time by clicking on *Display Search Results* at the bottom of the page.[10]

It is useful to understand that PEDro searches for words in a special way. If your search terms include a particular word, PEDro will search for records containing that word or any word that starts with the same word stem as the full search term. For example, if you specify the word 'work' in your search, PEDro will return records that contain the words 'work', 'worker', 'workplace' and 'work-place'. You can exploit this function when searching (see footnote 1). For example, instead of typing 'ultrasound epicondylitis' in the *Simple Search* box, we could have typed 'ultrasound epicondyl', as this will also return studies that refer to epicondylalgia.

The *Simple Search* is useful because it is easy to use, but it has some significant limitations: you need to think of the relevant text words, and they must be combined with AND. For some questions, like 'Does spinal manipulative therapy reduce pain and increase function in people with acute neck pain?', this is problematic. There are many clinical trials on necks, and many more

---

[10] The shopping basket is emptied when you click on *New Search* or *New Advanced Search*. If you want to continue searching without emptying the shopping basket, click on *Continue Search*.

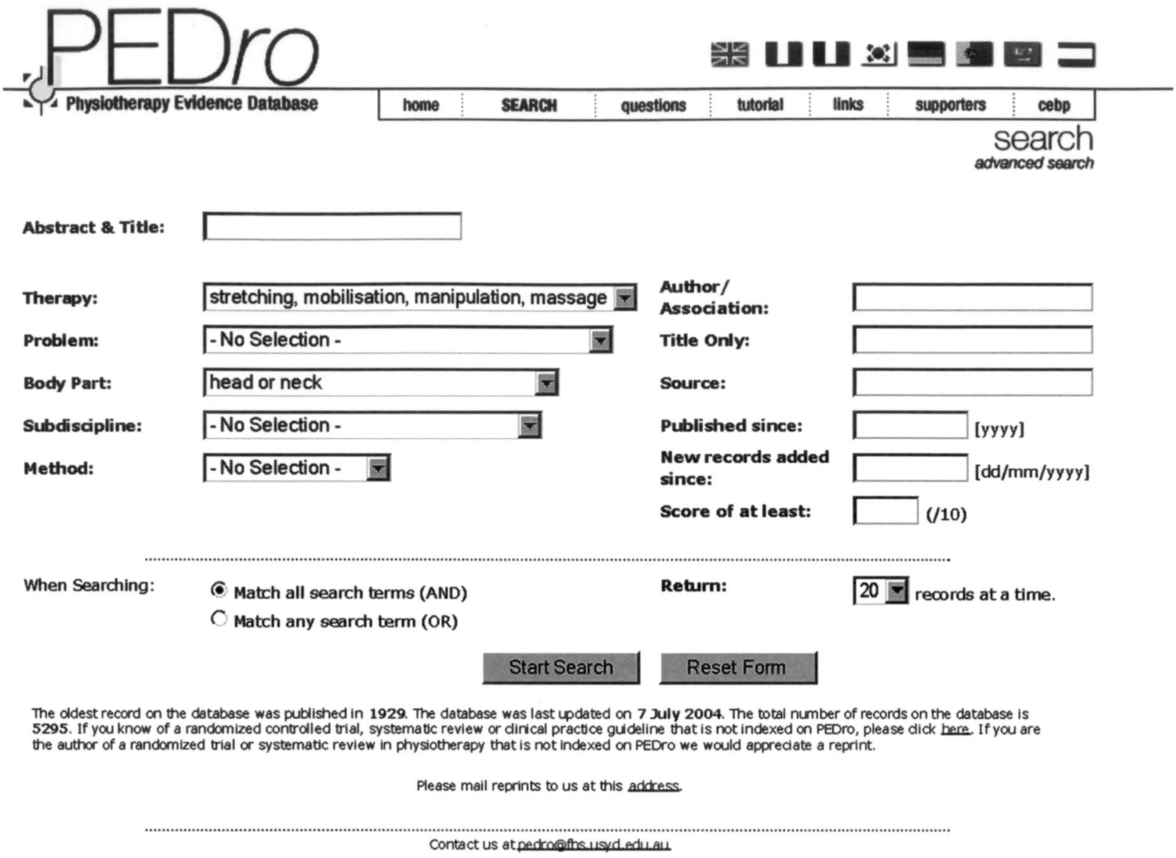

Figure 4.5   PEDro: Advanced Search page.

on manipulative therapy, so we really need to combine both neck-related terms and manipulative therapy-related terms in a single search to be efficient. And there are at least two important synonyms for 'neck' ('neck and cervical') and several more for 'manipulative therapy' ('manipulative therapy', 'manual therapy', 'manipulation', 'mobilization', 'adjustment', and so on). The *Simple Search* mode doesn't enable us to deal with this level of complexity. The *Advanced Search* mode gives us more flexibility.

Advanced Search

To use the *Advanced Search*, click first on *Search* in the menu bar and then on *Advanced Search*. You will be taken to the *Advanced Search* page, which is shown in Figure 4.5. The *Advanced Search* page contains 12 search fields, any of which can be used to search the database. At the top left is the *Abstract & Title* field. Entering text into this field instructs PEDro to search for the search terms in the titles or abstracts of all records on the database. In addition, if you know what study you are looking for you can search by the *Author/Association*, *Title* or *Source* of the record.[11] You can also select

---

[11] The '*Source*' refers to where the article can be found. Most of the articles on PEDro are published in journals, so the source is usually a reference to a particular journal article. But PEDro also contains clinical practice guidelines, some of which are published on the world wide web. In that case the source is a web address.

subject headings from pull-down menus of the *Therapy*, the *Problem* or *Body Part* being treated, or the *Subdiscipline* of practice. Finally, you can limit the search just to one *Study Type* (randomized trials, systematic reviews or evidence-based clinical practice guidelines), to those *Published Since or Added Since* a specific date, or (for randomized trials only) for trials of greater than a specified *Quality Score*. In *Advanced Search* mode you can search by simultaneously specifying as few or as many of these search criteria as you wish.

For our particular question on the effects of spinal manipulative therapy for neck pain we can take advantage of the subject headings to specify *Therapy* as 'stretching, mobilization, manipulation, massage' and *Body Part* as 'head or neck'. Then we combine these search criteria with an AND by checking the button at the bottom left of the screen, and we click on *Start Search*. PEDro returns 150 records. This is too many titles to scroll through, so we could select 'systematic reviews' under *Method*. This returns 31 systematic reviews, most of which appear to be relevant to our question.[12] We could further narrow the search by specifying that the review must have been published since 2003, which returns just three systematic reviews. One is a Cochrane systematic review, and that would be a good place to start reading!

This example illustrates one of the strengths of the *Advanced Search*: subject headings can be used as a substitute for two or more synonyms. In fact you can combine any number of subject headings and you can combine a subject heading with search terms entered as text. (So you could, if you wished, combine the text 'ultrasound' in the *Title & Abstract* field with the subject heading 'forearm and elbow' in the *Body Part* field). However, you can only select one subject heading from each menu. (So you couldn't select both 'lower leg or knee' and 'foot or ankle' from the *Body Part* menu.)

PEDro has one significant limitation: either all search criteria must be combined with ANDs or they must all be combined with ORs. It is not generally possible, in PEDro, to perform searches with combinations of ANDs and ORs. (Proficient users of PEDro might like to consult Box 4.2 for some suggestions on how to trick PEDro into effectively combining AND and OR searches.) A consequence is that, in PEDro at least, it is good policy to resist the temptation to use many search terms. Searches that employ many search terms will tend either to return many irrelevant records (when OR is used), or no records at all (when AND is used). In general the best search strategies have few search terms. It is often possible to use just one carefully selected search term, and it is rarely necessary to use more than three.

THE COCHRANE LIBRARY

The Cochrane Library is a remarkable resource. It is a collection of databases, the most important of which are the Cochrane Database of Systematic Reviews, the Database of Abstracts of Reviews of Effects (DARE) and the Cochrane Central Register of Controlled Trials (CENTRAL).

---

[12] The first six titles are clinical practice guidelines, even though we selected 'systematic reviews'. PEDro is able to identify those clinical practice guidelines which contain systematic reviews and it returns these titles in searches for systematic reviews.

> **Box 4.2   Three Tips for PEDro Power Users**
>
> 1. **Backdoor ANDs and ORs I: Perform multiple searches.** PEDro won't allow you to mix ANDs and ORs. However, you can get around this problem by performing a search using AND, selecting the records that are of interest, and then repeating the search using alternative terms. For example, to search effectively for 'cystic fibrosis' AND ('flutter' OR 'PEP'), you could search for 'cystic fibrosis' and 'flutter', combining these terms with the AND button, and select the relevant records by clicking on *Select*. Then repeat the search, this time for 'cystic fibrosis' and 'PEP', again combining these terms with the AND button, and again select the relevant records. All of the records selected from both searches can be retrieved by clicking on *Display Selected Records*.
>
> 2. **Backdoor ANDs and ORs II: Specify strings with inverted commas.** Normally PEDro treats a word string (like 'continuous passive motion') as independent words. If the whole search string is of interest, you can make PEDro treat the string as a single word by enclosing the string in inverted commas. By typing 'continuous passive motion' in inverted commas, PEDro will look for records that only contain these three words in that order, and it will ignore studies which use the words 'continuous' and 'passive' and 'motion' in any other way. This makes it unnecessary to combine the words in the string with AND, so you could, for example, combine the terms 'continuous passive motion' and 'CPM' with the OR button.
>
> 3. **Searching for ranges.** Sometimes it is handy to be able to search the *Published Since* or *Score of at Least* fields using ranges. This is done by separating the upper and lower limit of the range by '..'. For example, if you can remember a paper was published in the early 1990s you could enter '1990..1995' in the *Published Since* field. (You will need to combine this with other search criteria!) Or, to find all randomized trials published before 1950, type '0..1950'.

We have already come across the Cochrane Database of Systematic Reviews in Chapter 3. This database contains the full text of all of the systematic reviews produced by the Cochrane Collaboration. DARE, on the other hand, is produced by the Centre for Reviews and Dissemination at the University of York. It contains structured abstracts of systematic reviews published in the medical literature. Each abstract contains a commentary that indicates the quality of the reviews. And the third part of the trinity, CENTRAL, is indisputably the world's largest database of clinical trials. It contains bibliographic details of over 400 000 clinical trials.[13]

Most of the physiotherapy-relevant randomized trials and systematic reviews in the Cochrane Library are also indexed in PEDro. In fact

---

[13] Most but not all of these are *randomized* trials. If, however, we take this as a rough estimate of the number of randomized trials in health care (~400 000), and we take the number of randomized trials on PEDro as an estimate of the number of randomized trials in physiotherapy (~4000), we can estimate that approximately 1% of all randomized trials in health care are trials of physiotherapy.

the developers of the PEDro database regularly search the Cochrane Library to find randomized trials and systematic reviews in physiotherapy, and PEDro and the Cochrane Collaboration have a reciprocal agreement to exchange data. This means that a search of PEDro will yield most physiotherapy-relevant contents of the Cochrane Library. Nonetheless, we will describe how to search the Cochrane Library because, unlike PEDro, the Cochrane Library contains the full text of Cochrane systematic reviews. Also, unlike PEDro, the Cochrane Library indexes randomized trials and systematic reviews in all areas of health care. Physiotherapists who are interested in the effects of medical or surgical interventions, or interventions provided by other allied health professions, will find the Cochrane Library contains a wealth of useful information.

Access to the full text of the Cochrane Library is by subscription only. Nonetheless, it is widely available. If you are a student or employee of a university or hospital you may find you can access the Cochrane Library on-line at www.thecochranelibrary.com with a password. Alternatively your nearest medical library may provide you access from a library computer. Many countries have negotiated free on-line access to the Cochrane Library for all their citizens, or for all health professionals. Free access is provided for people from most developing countries. (From the Cochrane Library homepage, click on 'Do you already have access' for a list of countries that have free access to the Cochrane Library.) People who do not have free full text access can perform limited searches and view abstracts (not full text) of the Cochrane Database of Systematic Reviews.

When you arrive at the Cochrane Library homepage you will see a link to the *Cochrane Advanced Search* in the right column. Clicking on this link takes you to the *Advanced Search* facility (Figure 4.6).[14]

Let's see what happens if we repeat our earlier search for studies of the effects of pulsed ultrasound for reducing pain and disability associated with lateral epicondylitis. Advanced searches are conducted by typing search terms into one or more of the text boxes in the left frame. The search strategy we use is similar to the strategy we used earlier in PEDro except that we type in the AND. That is, we type 'ultrasound AND epicondyl*' in the first text box. (The default option is to 'Search All Text', which is appropriate here.)

Clicking on *Search* runs a search of the Cochrane Database of Systematic Reviews, as well as of the DARE and CENTRAL databases. A summary of the search results appears under the *Search Results* box. Altogether there were 32 hits.[15] Of these, 9 were in the Cochrane Database of Systematic Reviews; the titles of these records are displayed in a list. Eight of the nine are completed reviews (indicated by the letter "R" in a dark blue circle), but the titles do not look exactly relevant to our question. If any of the titles looked more relevant we could click on *Record* and we would

---

[14] We will use the Cochrane Library's native "front-end". Other front-ends are available, notably the one produced by Ovid. The other front-ends look very different, and may differ in their search syntax.

[15] If you replicate this search you may get different results, because new records are continually being added to the databases, and because protocols eventually become reviews.

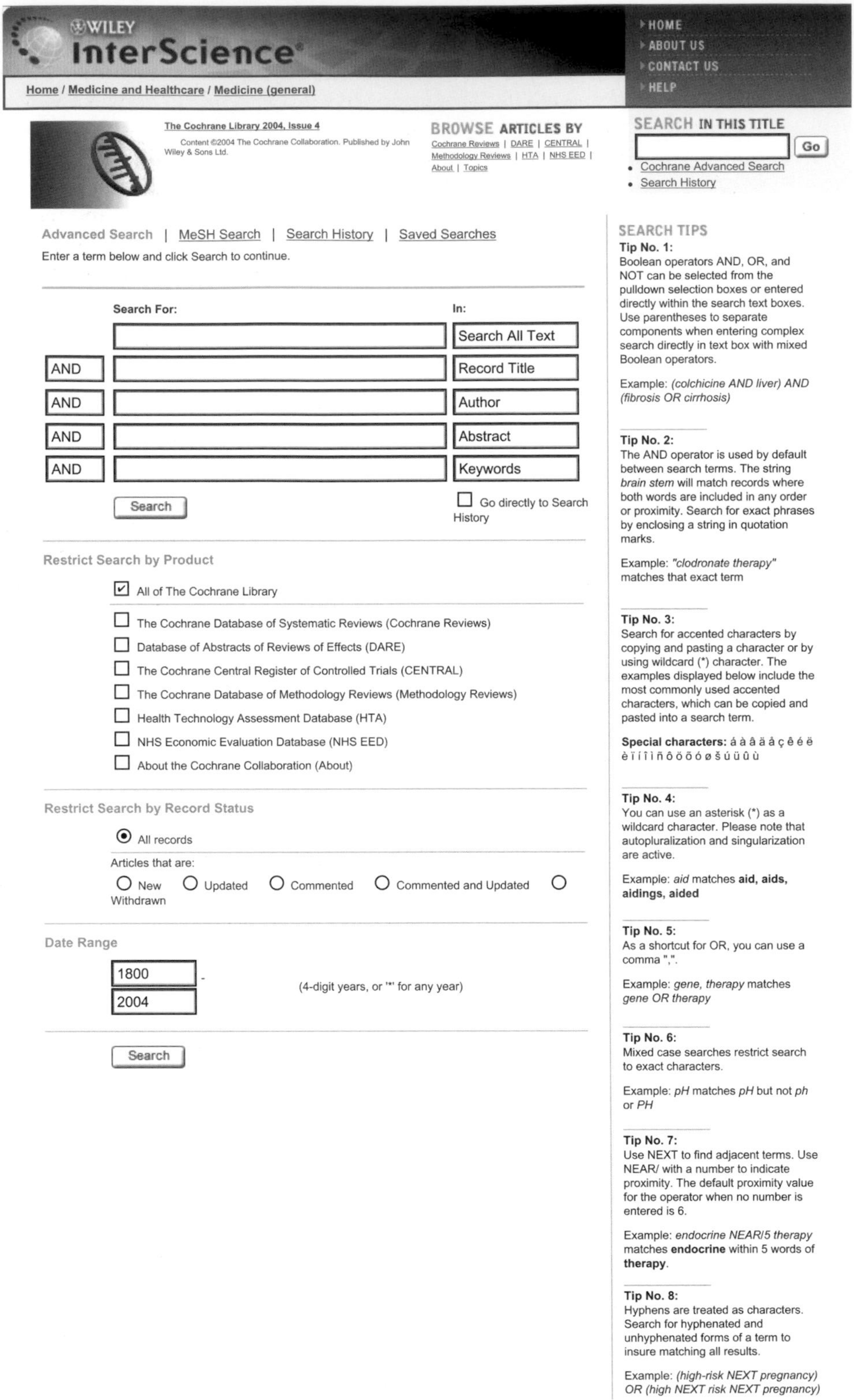

WILEY InterScience®

HOME
ABOUT US
CONTACT US
HELP

Home / Medicine and Healthcare / Medicine (general)

The Cochrane Library 2004, Issue 4
Content ©2004 The Cochrane Collaboration. Published by John Wiley & Sons Ltd.

BROWSE ARTICLES BY
Cochrane Reviews | DARE | CENTRAL
Methodology Reviews | HTA | NHS EED
About | Topics

SEARCH IN THIS TITLE
[   ] Go
- Cochrane Advanced Search
- Search History

Advanced Search | MeSH Search | Search History | Saved Searches

Enter a term below and click Search to continue.

	Search For:		In:
	[ ]		Search All Text
AND	[ ]		Record Title
AND	[ ]		Author
AND	[ ]		Abstract
AND	[ ]		Keywords

[Search]   ☐ Go directly to Search History

Restrict Search by Product

☑ All of The Cochrane Library

☐ The Cochrane Database of Systematic Reviews (Cochrane Reviews)
☐ Database of Abstracts of Reviews of Effects (DARE)
☐ The Cochrane Central Register of Controlled Trials (CENTRAL)
☐ The Cochrane Database of Methodology Reviews (Methodology Reviews)
☐ Health Technology Assessment Database (HTA)
☐ NHS Economic Evaluation Database (NHS EED)
☐ About the Cochrane Collaboration (About)

Restrict Search by Record Status

⦿ All records

Articles that are:
○ New   ○ Updated   ○ Commented   ○ Commented and Updated   ○ Withdrawn

Date Range

[1800] - [2004]   (4-digit years, or '*' for any year)

[Search]

SEARCH TIPS

Tip No. 1:
Boolean operators AND, OR, and NOT can be selected from the pulldown selection boxes or entered directly within the search text boxes. Use parentheses to separate components when entering complex search directly in text box with mixed Boolean operators.

Example: *(colchicine AND liver) AND (fibrosis OR cirrhosis)*

Tip No. 2:
The AND operator is used by default between search terms. The string *brain stem* will match records where both words are included in any order or proximity. Search for exact phrases by enclosing a string in quotation marks.

Example: *"clodronate therapy"* matches that exact term

Tip No. 3:
Search for accented characters by copying and pasting a character or by using wildcard (*) character. The examples displayed below include the most commonly used accented characters, which can be copied and pasted into a search term.

Special characters: á à â ä å ç é ë è ï í î ñ ô ö ó ø š ú ü û ù

Tip No. 4:
You can use an asterisk (*) as a wildcard character. Please note that autopluralization and singularization are active.

Example: *aid* matches **aid, aids, aidings, aided**

Tip No. 5:
As a shortcut for OR, you can use a comma ",".

Example: *gene, therapy* matches *gene OR therapy*

Tip No. 6:
Mixed case searches restrict search to exact characters.

Example: *pH* matches *pH* but not *ph* or *PH*

Tip No. 7:
Use NEXT to find adjacent terms. Use NEAR/ with a number to indicate proximity. The default proximity value for the operator when no number is entered is 6.

Example: *endocrine NEAR/5 therapy* matches **endocrine** within 5 words of **therapy**.

Tip No. 8:
Hyphens are treated as characters. Search for hyphenated and unhyphenated forms of a term to insure matching all results.

Example: *(high-risk NEXT pregnancy) OR (high NEXT risk NEXT pregnancy)*

Figure 4.6   The Cochrane Library home page.

see the full text of the review. Very handy indeed! One further hit is a protocol (indicated by the letter "P" in a light blue circle), titled "Physiotherapy and physiotherapeutical modalities for lateral epicondylitis" (Smidt et al 2004). This looks very relevant. Protocols are reviews that are not yet completed. They sometimes contain some useful information (for example, they may provide the results of a literature search), but they are not as helpful as completed reviews.

At the top of the page, under the *Search Results* heading, you can also see that DARE has four relevant systematic reviews and, by clicking on the DARE heading, we find that all four appear relevant to our question,

---

Box 4.3   Tips for searching the Cochrane Library

1. **Use subject headings.** Subject headings (called MeSH terms) are assigned to every systematic review on the database. Often it is more efficient to search for records with specific MeSH headings than it is to search for records containing specific text words. To search by MeSH headings, click on *MeSH Search* immediately above the text box. This brings up a text box, and you are instructed to enter a MeSH term. Type in a key search term (say, 'epicondylitis') and then click on *Thesaurus*. The search engine will search the dictionary of MeSH terms and, if there is a relevant MeSH term, it will indicate below the text box what the relevant MeSH heading is. (In our example it indicates that the relevant MeSH heading is 'tennis elbow'.) Clicking on the MeSH heading takes you to a further dialogue in which you can refine how you use the MeSH heading,[16] and then clicking on *Go* applies the refined MeSH search.

2. **Use the History function to construct complex searches.** When you perform a search in the Cochrane Library, details of that search are kept in the search history. If you perform a search using the text words 'ultrasound' and then perform a second search with the MeSH term 'Tennis elbow', and then click on the *Search History* symbol in the top right corner, you will see your search history:

    #1. ultrasound in All Fields, from 1800 to 2004 in
         all products   3972
    #2. MeSH descriptor Tennis Elbow explode tree 1 in MeSH
         products   102

    (The exact wording may be a little different, depending on how you qualified MeSH headings.) You can then combine searches. For example, you could combine these two searches by typing #1 AND #2. This yield 13 hits.

---

[16] In this dialogue you can add qualifiers to narrow the search. Also, you can indicate how related MeSH headings are used. MeSH terms are arranged in hierarchies (trees). Clicking on the *Explode* text box tells the search engine to look for any record that contains that MeSH term or any MeSH term located further up the tree. Clicking on *Search this term only* tells the search engine to look for any record that contains that MeSH term, but to ignore MeSH terms further down the tree. *Explode all terms* is always more sensitive; *Search this term only* is more specific.

although at the time of writing one is eight years old – probably too old to be useful now. But the most recent review, titled "Effectiveness of physiotherapy for lateral epicondylitis: a systematic review", looks relevant (Smidt et al 2003), and would probably be the first choice of evidence on this topic. We can view a structured abstract of this review, with commentary, by clicking on the title.

If we had not found a relevant and recent systematic review in DARE, we could have looked at the CENTRAL register of clinical trials. We do that by clicking on the link to CENTRAL under the *Search Results* heading. There are 16 trials on CENTRAL that satisfied our search criteria. Again, we could scan the titles and, if a title looked interesting, we could click on Record and see bibliographic details.

The search strategy we used in this example was quite simple. But the Cochrane Library supports quite sophisticated searching. Some tips for searching the Cochrane Library are given in Box 4.3. More tips are given on the Cochrane web site.

FINDING EVIDENCE OF PROGNOSIS AND DIAGNOSTIC TESTS

In Chapter 3 we saw that best evidence of prognosis is obtained from longitudinal studies, particularly prospective cohort studies. The best evidence of the accuracy of diagnostic tests is provided by cross-sectional studies that compare the findings of the test of interest with a high quality reference standard. Although these two sorts of question are answered by different sorts of studies, the strategies for finding studies of prognosis and diagnostic tests are very similar so we will deal with them together.

Finding studies of prognosis and diagnosis of physiotherapy-related questions can be difficult. A general problem with questions about prognosis is that prognostic information is sometimes buried inside clinical trials that were intended to test the effects of an intervention. The authors may not have flagged (or even appreciated) that the study contains prognostic information. Finding studies of diagnostic tests used by physiotherapists may be difficult for a different reason: there are relatively few studies. Searches for studies of diagnostic tests used by physiotherapists may be frustrated by the fact that relevant studies do not exist.

At the time of writing there is no database dedicated to archiving studies of prognosis or diagnostic tests in physiotherapy.[17] Thus it is necessary to search general medical databases for this information. The most useful databases are Medline (PubMed), Embase, CINAHL and PsycINFO. Unlike PEDro and the Cochrane Library, these databases do not restrict their focus to studies of the effects of intervention. Instead they index enormously diverse literatures. The Box 4.4 indicates how these databases differ.

Ideally it would be possible to simultaneously search Medline, Embase, CINAHL and PsycINFO. In fact some vendors (such as Ovid) provide a

---

[17] Note that a search of PEDro is likely to miss many studies of prognosis, and almost all studies of diagnostic test accuracy. Do not use PEDro to search for studies of prognosis or diagnosis.

Box 4.4   Databases of the health literature

Medline is the largest database of the medical literature. It archives about 12 million records from 4800 thousand journals published since 1966. Although it is the largest medical literature database, it contains few physiotherapy-specific journals.[18] It is likely that Medline currently indexes only a small proportion of all studies on prognosis and diagnostic tests relevant to physiotherapy.[19] Only two of the top five journals identified by Maher et al (2001) as core journals exclusively in physiotherapy are indexed on Medline. One of the best characteristics of Medline is that it has been made freely available on the web, where it is called PubMed. The PubMed URL is http://www4.ncbi.nlm.nih.gov/PubMed/.

    Embase is nearly as big as Medline. It contains about 10 million records published since 1974 in 4600 journals. There is surprisingly little overlap between Embase and Medline. Embase has relatively good coverage of physiotherapy-specific journals; it indexes 4 of 5 exclusively physiotherapy core journals. The biggest limitation of Embase is that it is available only by subscription.

    CINAHL is the smallest of the four databases. It contains less than 1 million records published since 1982 in about 1200 journals. Although smaller than Medline and Embase, CINAHL is 'richer' because it contains many enhancements, including the full text of articles and other materials such as clinical practice guidelines, comments, book reviews and patient education (McKibbon 1999). The greatest strength of CINAHL, from a physiotherapist's perspective at least, is that it has a specific focus on nursing and allied health journals. It indexes most physiotherapy journals and all core physiotherapy journals. Unfortunately CINAHL, like Embase, is only available by subscription.

    PsycINFO is a large database of the psychological literature. It contains nearly 8 million records published since 1872 in about 1900 journals. PsycINFO is an excellent place for evidence of psychological interventions, but it too is available only by subscription.

[18] The journals whose titles indicate they are specifically related to physiotherapy are the *Australian Journal of Physiotherapy, Journal of Orthopaedic and Sports Physical Therapy, Physical Therapy, Physiotherapy Research International,* and *Physical and Occupational Therapy in Pediatrics.*

[19] This statement is not supported by strong data. However, Medline indexes only a small proportion of the randomized trials on PEDro. It is likely that a similar proportion of physiotherapy-relevant studies of prognosis and diagnostic accuracy are indexed on Medline.

service that enables such searches. However, the capacity to search across the four databases is available by subscription only and not widely available so we will not consider this further. Instead, we will focus on using PubMed to search the Medline database. PubMed has two major advantages: it is freely available to anyone who has access to the internet, and it has an excellent search engine that makes searching for studies of prognosis and diagnostic test accuracy relatively straightforward.

Figure 4.7   PubMed Clinical
Queries home page. Source:
National Center for
Biotechnology Information
(NCBI).

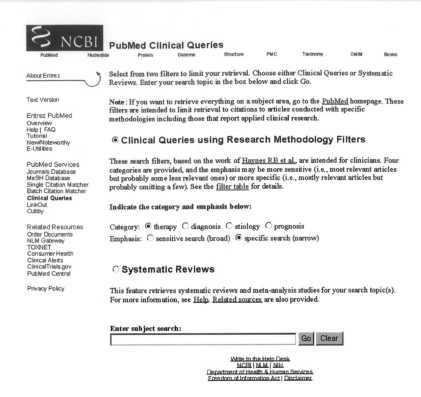

Many people use the main PubMed search interface to search for studies of prognosis and diagnostic accuracy. This is suboptimal. A part of PubMed, called Clinical Queries, is designed to assist people searching for such studies. Clinical Queries automatically applies search strategies that have been designed for sensitive and specific searching.[20] If you want to conduct quick searches for studies of prognosis or diagnostic tests then you should use Clinical Queries rather than the main PubMed search page. You can find Clinical Queries by following the link from the PubMed homepage, or by going directly to http://www.ncbi.nlm.nih.gov/entrez/query/static/clinical.html

A reproduction of the Clinical Queries home page is shown in Figure 4.7. You can see that there are a series of buttons that allow you to search specifically for studies of therapy, prognosis, diagnosis or aetiology. We will use Clinical Queries to search for studies of prognosis and diagnostic tests.

You can tell Clinical Queries that you want to search specifically for studies of prognosis or diagnosis by clicking on the prognosis or diagnosis button. Then you need only type in search terms to specify the particular question you are interested in and Clinical Queries will search for studies of the type you have indicated that include your search terms.[21]

---

[20] We have not used PubMed Clinical Queries to search for studies of the effects of intervention because such searches are better conducted using PEDro or the Cochrane Library. PEDro and the Cochrane Library index many randomized trials that are not on PubMed.
[21] The search terms used by PubMed Clinical Queries have been subjected to extensive testing and have been shown to have a high sensitivity and specificity (Haynes & Wilczynski 2004, Wilczynski & Haynes 2004).

Clinical Queries provides another option: you can also choose to search only for systematic reviews. (These can be systematic reviews of studies of prognosis, or of studies of diagnostic tests or, for that matter, of studies of therapy or aetiology.) However, there are so few systematic reviews of prognosis and diagnostic tests that a search for them is usually fruitless. For routine searching we recommend that you don't search specifically for systematic reviews; if a relevant systematic review exists it will be turned up with a search that does not specifically specify systematic reviews.

One final decision needs to be made. We need to decide whether we want to conduct a sensitive search or a specific search. Of course we would like both, but we need to tell Clinical Queries whether we are more concerned with getting every possible relevant study (emphasis on sensitivity) or with minimizing the number of irrelevant search results (emphasis on specificity). Medline is a huge database, and sensitive searches often yield unmanageable numbers of hits, so we recommend that you begin by specifying a specific search. If, subsequently, you find that a specific search yields no hits you might then try conducting a sensitive search. (Alternatively you might consider trying a different set of search terms, or you might decide to give up and have a cup of coffee instead.)

Let's imagine that we are seeking an answer to the following question about prognosis: 'In a young male who has just experienced his first shoulder dislocation, what is the risk of re-dislocating within one year?'

In Clinical Queries we could specify 'prognosis' and 'specific' search, and then type in 'shoulder AND dislocat*'. Note that in Clinical Queries, as in the Cochrane Library but unlike PEDro, the AND is typed in explicitly. Also, as in the Cochrane Library, we need to specify explicitly that we want to look at all words using the root 'dislocat' ('dislocat*' = 'dislocated OR dislocation OR dislocate OR dislocating'). A very nice feature of Clinical Queries is that it automatically looks for related MeSH terms and includes them in the search.[22]

This search returns 95 hits. A quick scroll through the results identifies several promising looking titles, including one titled 'Prognosis of primary anterior shoulder dislocation in young adults' (Hoelen et al 1990). Clicking on the title displays the detailed search result. In general, you will need to screen search results by reading titles and, if the titles look relevant, by skimming the abstracts. (At the same time you could also screen for methodological quality; more on this in Chapter 5.) The abstract of the paper with the promising looking title confirms this is a very relevant study.

Sometimes you will find a study that looks to be relevant but which, for one reason or another, turns out not to be. Or it may be that the study is relevant, but it is from an obscure journal and it is not possible to get a copy of the full paper. In that case you could click on *Related Articles* at the right-hand margin of the search results screen. This brings up a list of studies that are similar in content to the first. Once you have identified one study that is relevant to your search question, the *Related Studies* facility provides a quick and easy way to find more relevant studies.

---

[22] You can see the exact search terms that Clinical Queries has applied by clicking on *Details* underneath the text box.

The question we have just asked, on prognosis after primary shoulder dislocation, is quite a simple one because there are relatively few synonyms for the key search terms of shoulder and dislocation.[23] A more difficult question might be: 'How much return of hand function can we expect 6 months after a completely flaccid hemiparetic stroke?' This question is difficult because there are a number of synonyms for stroke (CVA, hemiparesis, cerebrovascular accident, etc.) and for hand function (upper limb function, manual dexterity, etc.). Clinical Queries allows us to combine many search terms using both ANDs and ORs in a single search. This allows us to simultaneously deal with synonyms (by using OR) and require the presence of multiple key terms (using AND). For example, we could click on the prognosis button and the specificity button and then type:

(Stroke OR CVA OR cerebro-vascular OR cerebrovascular OR hemipare*) AND (hand OR upper limb OR manual).[24]

In this example we have used brackets to remove the ambiguity that otherwise potentially arises when we mix ANDs and ORs in a single search.[25,26] The search returns 230 hits, too many to screen quickly. So the search was refined by adding 'AND (flaccid* OR paralys*)'. This reduced the number of hits to 14, and the first on the list was titled 'Probability of regaining dexterity in the flaccid upper limb: impact of severity of paresis and time since onset in acute stroke' (Kwakkel et al 2003). Bingo!

We shall look at one more example, this time of a search for studies of accuracy of a diagnostic test. Our question is: 'In nursing home patients, how accurate is auscultation for diagnosis of pneumonia?' The initial search strategy in PubMed Clinical Queries is to conduct a specific search for studies of diagnosis using the terms 'auscultation AND pneumonia'. This returns nine hits of which one, titled 'Diagnosing pneumonia by physical examination: relevant or relic?' (Wipf et al 1999), looks nearly relevant but does not pertain specifically to nursing home patients. Clicking on *Related Articles* yields 244 hits. This was narrowed by combining with 'AND (nursing home OR aged care)'. (This requires use of the History function, which we introduce below under the heading of Searching PubMed for qualitative studies.) The narrower search yielded 27 hits, of which one, titled 'Clinical findings associated with radiographic pneumonia in nursing home residents' (Mehr et al 2001), looks very relevant.

---

[23] It is true that synonyms for shoulder could be 'gleno-humeral joint' or 'glenohumeral joint', and synonyms for dislocation could be 'subluxation' or 'instability'. Nonetheless, the synonyms are used relatively infrequently in this context, which means that a search for 'shoulder AND dislocation' is likely to be quite sensitive.

[24] Note that none of the search terms pertain to the time window we are interested in (6 months). This is because, while our question concerns a specific time window, we would usually be happy to take studies with any similar time window. In general, search terms relating to time hugely reduce search sensitivity, so in general they should not be used.

[25] Can you see the problem if brackets are not used? When we type 'X AND Y OR Z' it may not be clear whether we mean '(X AND Y) OR Z' or 'X AND (Y OR Z)'. In fact there is no real ambiguity because Clinical Queries has a rule for how to deal with such apparent ambiguities. Nonetheless, the use of brackets makes it much easier to ensure that ANDs and ORs are combined in the correct way.

[26] It is also possible to use brackets in the same way in search queries of the Cochrane Library.

FINDING EVIDENCE OF EXPERIENCES

If you want to find evidence about how people feel or experience certain situations, or what attitudes they have towards a phenomenon, you should look for studies that use qualitative methods. Unfortunately finding studies of experiences is very difficult.

One of the problems is that qualitative research is indexed in many different ways. For example, it may be identifiable as qualitative research only by the method used to collect data (e.g. in-depth interviews, focus groups or observation) or only by the type of qualitative research (e.g. phenomenology, grounded theory, ethnographic research). Another problem is that the popularity of qualitative research approaches is relatively new in the health care literature and, consequently, methodological 'hedges' (search strategies used to locate particular types of studies) have not yet been developed, and databases do not yet have qualitative research-related index terms. There is not a button in PubMed Clinical Queries for locating qualitative study designs, nor is there a specific PEDro-like database that indexes only qualitative research. This makes it hard to find high quality studies relating to experiences. Consequently you may need to read many studies to identify the 'best' or most relevant study to your question.

Here we make some suggestions on how you can find studies of experiences with CINAHL (if you are able to access this database) or PubMed. We consider CINAHL, even though it has the disadvantage of being available by subscription only, because it is one of the best databases for locating studies of attitudes and experiences. And we consider PubMed because it also contains many relevant studies, and it is freely available.

Both CINAHL and PubMed can be searched by 'text words'. Text words are the words provided by the authors in the titles and abstracts of the original study report; these are entered into the database just as they were printed in the journals. Alternatively, the databases can be searched by subject headings. Every study on these databases is assigned subject headings that have been derived from a standardized vocabulary developed by the database producers. Each database has slightly different subject headings (for example, bedsores are indexed as pressure sores in CINAHL, as decubitus ulcers in PubMed, and as decubitus in Embase. PsycINFO does not have a term for bedsores). Both text words and subject headings are used in effective searching.

Unfortunately, when you go looking for studies of experiences, meanings or processes you will find there are very few index terms in PubMed that relate to qualitative research. The exception is that, in 2003, the National Library of Medicine (makers of PubMed) introduced a new MeSH term: 'Qualitative research'. This will make searching for studies of experiences much more straightforward. But beware, there is no retrospective indexing, meaning you will not be able to find qualitative studies published before 2003 using this term. The situation is even worse in Embase, because Embase has no subject heading that is relevant to studies of experiences (McKibbon 1999). In contrast, CINAHL has many index terms related to qualitative study designs. This makes CINAHL one of the most useful databases for identifying qualitative studies.

The Social Sciences Citation Index is another resource that might be relevant for finding qualitative research, although again it is available by subscription only. This database provides a multidisciplinary index to the journal literature of the social sciences. It fully indexes more than 1725 journals across 50 social sciences disciplines, and it indexes individually selected, relevant items from over 3300 leading scientific and technical journals. It provides access to current information and retrospective data from 1956 onward. More information can be found at www.isinet.com/products/citation/ssci/.

CINAHL

Now let's consider how you could structure a search of the CINAHL database for evidence about experiences.

An efficient search might have two parts. The first part could specify the subject you are interested in and the second part could specify qualitative research and methodology. The two parts are combined with AND. This helps you find qualitative studies that are potentially relevant to your question. Both parts could contain text words or subject headings. Box 4.5 lists headings and text words relevant to qualitative research that could be used for CINAHL searches (McKibbon 1999).

Databases such as Medline, CINAHL, Embase, PsycINFO and Social Sciences Citation Index have a number of different 'front-ends'. That is, each database may be queried using any of a number of interfaces, each

---

Box 4.5   Search terms for finding qualitative research in CINAHL (McKibbon 1999)

Subject headings
Qualitative studies
Ethnological research
Ethnonursing research
Focus groups
Grounded theory
Phenomenological research
Qualitative validity
Purposive sample
Theoretical sample
Semi-structured interview
Phenomenology
Ethnography
Observational methods
   Non-participant observation
   Participant observation

Text words
Lived experience
Narrative analysis
Hermeneutic

of which looks different on the screen and uses slightly different ways of entering and combining search terms. In the following example we will describe how to use the widely used Ovid front-end to search CINAHL. Other front-ends (such as Silver Platter) can be searched using similar but not identical strategies.

An example of searching CINAHL is shown in Table 4.1. The question is: 'What are immigrants' attitudes and experiences towards exercise?' Each line of the table shows a new search that introduces new search terms or combines searches from previous lines. The first column shows the number corresponding to each search, the second column shows the search terms, and the third column shows the number of hits from each search. In this search, search terms (both text words and subject headings) for 'exercise' and 'immigrants' are combined, yielding 39 citations. Normally you then would have to combine this result with the search terms for qualitative studies selected from those shown in Box 4.5 (both subject headings and text words), but since this search only gave 39 hits you might merely browse through titles or abstracts to identify relevant studies.

PubMed

When searching PubMed for qualitative research you will need to base your search on text words because, as mentioned above, PubMed has few subject headings relevant to qualitative research. Relevant text words for identifying qualitative research are shown in Box 4.6.

Table 4.1 Strategy for searching CINAHL with the Ovid front-end for answers to the question 'What are immigrants' attitudes and experiences towards exercise?'

Search	Terms	Hits
#1	exercise/	6 903
#2	exercis$.tw.	23 674
#3	physical activ$.tw.	3 864
#4	1 or 2 or 3	25 662
#5	immigrants/	1 313
#6	emigra$.tw.	54
#7	immigra$.tw.	1 296
#8	5 or 6 or 7	1 977
#9	4 and 8	39

/ = subject heading; tw = text word; $ = 'wild card' (any combination of characters).

Box 4.6   Search terms (text words) for finding qualitative studies in PubMed

Qualitative research
Ethnon*
Hermeneutic
Focus group
Lived experience
Life experience
Ethnography

Table 4.2 Combining the terms for exercise and immigrants

Search	Terms	Hits
#1	'exercise'[MeSH]	28 808
#2	exercis*	140 182
#3	physical activ*	17 766
#4	#1 OR #2 OR #3	149 551
#5	'emigration and immigration'[MeSH]	15 744
#6	emigra*	18 561
#7	immigra*	20 708
#8	#5 OR #6 OR #7	23 151
#9	#4 AND #8	166

[MeSH] = subject heading; * = wild card.

Table 4.3 Combining exercise and immigrant terms with terms for qualitative research

Search	Terms	Hits
#1	'exercise'[MeSH]	28 808
#2	exercis*	140 182
#3	physical activ*	17 766
#4	#1 OR #2 OR #3	149 551
#5	'emigration and immigration'[MeSH]	15 744
#6	emigra*	18 561
#7	immigra*	20 708
#8	#5 OR #6 OR #7	23 151
#9	#4 AND #8	166
#10	qualitative research	2976
#11	ethnon*	68
#12	hermeneutic	523
#13	focus group	5013
#14	life experience	10 686
#15	lived experience	1136
#16	ethnography	56 177
#17	#10 OR #11 OR #12 OR #13 OR #14 OR #15 OR #16	74 682
#18	#9 AND #17	25

Strategies for searching PubMed for studies of immigrant attitudes and experiences towards exercise are shown in Tables 4.2 and 4.3. Table 4.2 outlines the first part of the search combining the terms for exercise and immigrants.

The search strategies we will use here are a little more complex than the ones we used in the earlier section where we searched PubMed Clinical Queries for studies of prognosis and accuracy of diagnostic tests. This means that it becomes awkward fitting the search terms on to one line. To be able to perform multiline searches in PubMed you have to use the *History* button. (This button is found immediately underneath the text box.) When searching this way you should search each term individually before combining them. Terms are combined by referring to the line number of the search. Thus '#1' refers to the search on line number 1, and '#2 AND #6' combines the results of searches on lines 2 and 6 with AND.

The search in Table 4.2 yields 166 studies; perhaps too many to screen efficiently. So, to narrow your search, you can combine the result with text words for qualitative studies using the *History* button (Box 4.6) as shown in Table 4.3. This yields 25 studies. You can easily screen through the 25 titles to see if there are any relevant studies.

Note that it will not generally be useful to search using the text word 'phenomenology' in PubMed, because many articles use the term 'phenomenology' to mean the description or classification of things, and not to refer to the qualitative design or methodology of phenomenology (McKibbon 1999).

GETTING FULL TEXT

A search of the literature will yield the titles, bibliographic details and abstracts of relevant research reports. But this is usually not sufficient for critical appraisal. It is almost always better to have at hand the full report of the study.

Obtaining the full text of a report can be difficult, and for some physiotherapists this can be a major impediment to evidence-based practice. How can full reports be obtained?

The best way to obtain full text is electronically. Physiotherapists affiliated with large institutions (such as hospitals or universities) may have full text electronic access to a selection of subscription-only journals by virtue of their affiliation with that institution. This makes it possible to download the selected paper to any computer that is connected to the internet.

Even physiotherapists who do not have access to subscription-only journals can access a wide range of journals electronically. Some journals are made freely available on the internet. (Notably, at the time of writing, the full text of the *BMJ* is free at www.bmj.com, although there are plans to restrict access to non-subscribers.) Many journals make back issues (typically, issues more than 1 year old) freely available on the web. A very useful hub that provides access to all such journals is FreeMedicalJournals.com at http://www.freemedicaljournals.com/. Some professional associations provide members access to free full text. For example, the Australian Physiotherapy Association provides its members access to approximately 450 journals through the APA Library, which members access through a members-only part of the association's web site. And at the time of writing several other associations are in the process of setting up similar facilities for their members. Finally, some countries provide full text access to the Cochrane Library for all their citizens, or to all health professionals. (See http://www.update-software.com/cochrane/provisions.htm for a list of countries that provide such access.) Other countries provide full access to a range of electronic journals for health workers. Examples are the National Electronic Library for Health (http://www.nelh.nhs.uk/) in England, and state-based sites in Australia (New South Wales, http://www.clininfo.health.nsw.gov.au/; Queensland, http://ckn.health.qld.gov.au/; Victoria,

Table 4.4 Which database should I use? Summary of recommendations

Question is about	Recommended database	Comments
Effects of therapy	PEDro	Physiotherapy interventions only
	Cochrane Library	Subscription only*
Experiences	CINAHL	Subscription only
	PubMed	
Prognosis	PubMed	Use Clinical Queries
Diagnostic tests	PubMed	Use Clinical Queries

*Many countries provide free access to the Cochrane Library. See http://www.update-software.com/cochrane/provisions.htm for details.

http://www.clinicians.vic.gov.au; Western Australia, http://www.ciao.health.wa.gov.au/; South Australia, http://www.salus.sa.gov.au/).

Of course many journals are not available as electronic full text. In that case it may be possible to obtain a copy of the paper from a local library. For some (especially physiotherapists in teaching hospitals in developed countries) this may be straightforward, albeit a little time-consuming. But other physiotherapists will not have access to a well-stocked local library, or they may find that travel to the library is too time-consuming, or their library does not hold the particular journals that are needed. The unfortunate reality is that many physiotherapists still find it difficult to access reports of the full text of high quality clinical research.

In this chapter we have looked at how to find evidence to answer questions about effects of interventions, experiences, prognosis and accuracy of diagnostic tests. Table 4.4 provides a simple summary of our recommendations concerning which databases to consult for particular questions.

FINDING EVIDENCE OF ADVANCES IN CLINICAL PRACTICE (BROWSING)

The preceding sections have described search strategies for finding answers to specific questions about the effects of intervention, experiences, prognosis and diagnosis. It is useful to supplement the process of seeking answers to specific clinical questions with 'browsing'. Browsing is reading that is not targeted at specific clinical questions. Browsing provides a mechanism by which we can keep abreast of new developments in professional practice that might otherwise pass us by.

Until recently there have been few mechanisms for efficient browsing. Physiotherapists who wished to stay up-to-date with research may have stumbled across important papers while browsing recent issues of journals in the New Issues shelves at a library, or they may have exchanged key papers with colleagues. But, by and large, keeping up-to-date was a hit and miss affair.

A number of relatively new resources have greatly increased the efficiency of browsing. One example is 'pre-appraised' papers, such as those published in journals like *Evidence-Based Medicine*, *Evidence-Based Nursing* and the *Australian Journal of Physiotherapy* (where they are called 'Critically Appraised

Critically Appraised Paper

Spinal manipulative therapy for low back pain is effective only when compared to sham or ineffective treatments

Synopsis

Summary of Assendelft WJJ, Morton SC, Yu EI, Suttorp MJ and Shekelle PG (2003): Spinal manipulative therapy for low back pain: A meta-analysis of effectiveness relative to other therapies. *Annals of Internal Medicine* 138: 871–882. [Prepared by Gro Jamtvedt, Norwegian Health Services Research Centre, and Kåre Birger Hagen, Norwegian Directorate for Health and Social Services.]

Question: Is spinal manipulative therapy (SMT) an effective treatment for low back pain (LBP)?

Data sources: MEDLINE, EMBASE, CINAHL, the Cochrane Controlled Trials Register and previous systematic reviews.

Study selection: Randomised controlled trials of patients with LBP that evaluated SMT with at least 1 day follow up and one clinically relevant outcome measure.

Data extraction: Two reviewers extracted data independently. SMT was compared with the following categories of other therapies: a) sham, b) conventional general practitioner care and analgesics, c) physical therapy and exercises, d) therapies considered to lack evidence of benefit or have evidence of harm, and e) back school.

Main results: 39 studies (5468 participants) were included. For patients with acute LBP, SMT was better than sham therapy in short term pain improvement, 10 mm difference (95% CI 2 to 17 mm) on a 0–100 scale, and back specific function 2.8 point difference (95% CI -0.1 to 5.6 point) on a 0–24 scale. Compared to the other therapies, no clinically important differences were found. For patients with chronic LBP, SMT was better than sham therapy in short term pain improvement, 10 mm difference (95% CI 3 to 17 mm), long term pain improvement, 19 mm difference (95% CI 3 to 35 mm), and back specific function 3.3 points difference (95% CI 0.6 to 6.6 points). Compared to therapies considered to lack evidence of benefit or to have evidence of harm, clinically important differences in favour of manipulative therapy were found for pain and functional status. Study quality, profession of manipulator, and use of manipulation alone or in combination with other therapies did not affect these results.

Conclusion: SMT had clinically significant benefits when it was compared with sham treatment or therapies judged to be ineffective or harmful. Compared with other commonly used therapies, SMT had no clinically significant benefits.

Commentary

Three extensive reviews of SMT for the treatment of LBP were published in 2003 (Assendelft et al 2003, Cherkin et al 2003, Ferreira et al 2003). Each review concluded that SMT is only effective when compared to sham or ineffective treatments and has no significant benefits over other conservative treatments for low back pain. The present study is the most extensive, and includes a methodologically rigorous meta-analysis of treatment effect. It should, however, be noted that the meta-analysis did not distinguish between patients with and without the presence of leg pain. In the light of the different prognosis in patients with and without radiating symptoms, this may have influenced the results.

Meta-analysis allows precise comparison of the effect sizes of one type of therapy with different kinds of control groups. Establishing the effect size provides perhaps the most important clinical implication of the present work. The effect size compared to no therapy was statistically significant and lies within recommendations both from the Cochrane Back Editorial Board and Roland and Fairbank (2000) of what should be judged as a clinically important difference. Despite this, the authors state that SMT is very unlikely to be a particularly effective therapy for any group of patients with LBP, a statement that appears to be somewhat exaggerated.

On the other hand, the authors correctly point out that the effect size is modest and probably smaller than former reviews may have suggested.

Another important clinical implication of the present meta-analysis is the conclusion that SMT, physiotherapy care (conventional physiotherapy, exercise, back school), and GP care (included medication) appear to produce similar outcomes in patients with LBP. Hence, cost-effectiveness should be a focus of future clinical trials.

Kjersti Storheim
Norwegian Centre for Active Rehabilitation, Oslo, Norway

References

Assendelft WJJ et al (2003): *Annals of Internal Medicine* 138: 871–881.

Cherkin DC et al (2003): *Annals of Internal Medicine* 138: 898–906.

Ferreira ML et al (2003): *Journal of Manipulative and Physiological Therapeutics* 26: 593-601.

Roland & Fairbank (2000): *Spine* 25: 3115–3124.

Figure 4.8 A critically appraised paper (CAP). Reproduced with permission from the *Australian Journal of Physiotherapy.*

Paper', or CAPs for short). A common characteristic is that they provide easily read, short summaries of high quality, clinically relevant research.

A CAP from the *Australian Journal of Physiotherapy* has been reproduced in Figure 4.8. The CAP describes Assendelft and colleagues' systematic review of spinal manipulative therapy for low back pain (Assendelft et al 2003). This study, like others that are described in CAPs, was chosen by the CAP Editors because it was considered to be a high quality study of importance to the practice of physiotherapy. The CAP has a declarative title that gives the main findings of the study, a short, structured abstract that describes how the study was conducted and what it found, and a commentary from an expert in the field giving the commentators opinion of the implications of the study for clinical practice.

The CAPs in the *Australian Journal of Physiotherapy*, and similar features in *Evidence-Based Medicine* and *Evidence-Based Nursing*, provide a simple way that physiotherapists can keep up-to-date. All three are available by subscription, but CAPs in past issues of the *Australian Journal of Physiotherapy* are freely available at www.physiotherapy.asn.au/AJP.

References

Assendelft WJJ, Morton SC, Yu EI et al 2003 Spinal manipulative therapy for low back pain: a meta-analysis of effectiveness relative to other therapies. Annals of Internal Medicine 138:871–882

Haynes RB, Wilczynski NL 2004 Optimal search strategies for retrieving scientifically strong studies of diagnosis from Medline: analytical survey. BMJ 328:1040

Hoelen MA, Burgers AM, Rozing PM 1990 Prognosis of primary anterior shoulder dislocation in young adults. Archives of Orthopaedic and Trauma Surgery 110:51–54

Kwakkel G, Kollen BJ, van der Grond J et al 2003 Probability of regaining dexterity in the flaccid upper limb: impact of severity of paresis and time since onset in acute stroke. Stroke 34:2181–2186

McKibbon A 1999 PDQ. Evidence-based principles and practice. Decker BC, Ontario

Maher C, Moseley A, Sherrington C et al 2001 Core journals of evidence-based physiotherapy practice. Physiotherapy Theory and Practice 17:143–151

Mehr DR, Binder EF, Kruse RL et al 2001 Clinical findings associated with radiographic pneumonia in nursing home residents. Journal of Family Practice 50: 931–937

Moseley AM, Herbert RD, Sherrington C et al 2002 Evidence for physiotherapy practice: a survey of the Physiotherapy Evidence Database (PEDro). Australian Journal of Physiotherapy 48:43–49

Robertson VJ, Baker KG 2001 A review of therapeutic ultrasound: effectiveness studies. Physical Therapy 81: 1339–1350

Smidt N, Assendelft WJ, Arola H et al 2003 Effectiveness of physiotherapy for lateral epicondylitis: a systematic review. Annals of Medicine 35:51–62

Smidt N, Assendelft WJJ, Arola H et al 2004 Physiotherapy and physiotherapeutical modalities for lateral epicondylitis (protocol for a Cochrane review). In: The Cochrane Library, Issue 2. Wiley, Chichester

Wilczynski NL, Haynes RB 2004 Developing optimal search strategies for detecting clinically sound prognostic studies in MEDLINE: an analytic survey. BMC Medicine 2:23

Wipf JE, Lipsky BA, Hirschmann JV et al 1999 Diagnosing pneumonia by physical examination: relevant or relic? Archives of Internal Medicine 24:1082–1087

Chapter **5**

Can I trust this evidence?

OVERVIEW

Well-designed research can produce relatively
unbiased answers to clinical questions. Poorly
designed research can generate biased answers.
Readers of the clinical research literature need to be
able to discriminate between well-designed and
poorly designed research. This is best done by asking
simple questions about key methodological features
of the study. When reading clinical trials you should

consider if treated and control groups were comparable, if there was complete or near-complete follow-up, and if there was blinding of patients and assessors. For studies of experiences you should consider if the sampling strategy was appropriate, if the data collection procedures were sufficient to capture the phenomenon of interest, and if the data were analysed in a rigorous way. For studies of prognosis you should consider if there was representative sampling from a well-defined population at a uniform point in the course of the condition. And for studies of diagnostic tests you should consider if there was blind comparison of the test with a rigorous reference standard on subjects in whom there was diagnostic suspicion. For systematic reviews on any type of question you should consider if it was clear which studies were to be reviewed, if there was an adequate literature search, and if the quality of individual studies was taken into account when drawing conclusions.

As discussed in the previous chapter, ideally the search for evidence will yield a small number of studies. If you have systematically sought out studies of the type needed to answer your question then you can begin the process of critical appraisal that we describe below. If you have happened upon a study incidentally (for example, if you were given a copy from a friend), you will first need to confirm that the study has the right sort of design to answer your question (see Chapter 2).

The studies you find may or may not be well designed and executed, so they may or may not be of sufficient quality to be useful for clinical decision-making. In this chapter we consider how to decide if a study is of sufficient quality that its findings are likely to be valid.[1] We begin with a general discussion of approaches to appraising validity and then describe specific methods for appraising validity of studies of the effects of interventions, experiences, prognosis and the accuracy of diagnostic tests.

A PROCESS FOR CRITICAL APPRAISAL OF EVIDENCE

Many physiotherapists experience a common frustration. When they consult the research literature for answers to clinical questions they are confronted by a range of studies with very different conclusions. Consider, for example, the findings that confront a physiotherapist who would like to know whether acupuncture protects against exercise-induced asthma. One study, by Fung et al (1986) concluded 'acupuncture provided better protection against exercise-induced asthma than did

---

[1] There are several dimensions to validity. (For enlightening discussions of aspects of validity in experimental research, see the classic texts by Campbell & Stanley (1963) and Cook & Campbell (1979).) In this chapter we look at some aspects of study validity when we consider aspects of study design (as distinct from aspects of the analysis, or of the selection of subjects, implementation of interventions and measurements of outcomes) that can control for bias. In studies of the effects of interventions, we could say our concern is with what Campbell and Stanley call 'internal validity', but the term internal validity is not easily applied to studies of prognosis of diagnostic tests. Other aspects of validity will be considered in Chapter 6.

sham acupuncture'. On the other hand, Gruber et al (2002) concluded 'acupuncture treatment offers no protection against exercise-induced bronchoconstriction'. These conclusions appear inconsistent. It seems implausible that both could be true. Situations like this, where similar studies draw contradictory conclusions, often arise.

Why is the literature apparently so inconsistent? There are several possible explanations. First, there may be important differences between studies in the type of patients included, the way in which the intervention was administered, and the way in which outcomes were measured. Simple conclusions may obscure important details about patients, interventions and outcomes. However, as we shall see later, it may be difficult to draw more precise conclusions from clinical research.

Another important cause of inconsistency is bias. Many studies are poorly designed and may therefore have seriously biased conclusions. The findings of poorly designed studies and well-controlled studies of the same interventions can differ very markedly. Of the two studies of acupuncture for exercise-induced asthma cited above, only the study by Gruber et al (2002) blinded the subjects and assessors of outcomes. The inconsistency of the conclusions of these studies may arise because the study by Gruber et al provides a relatively unbiased estimate of the effects of acupuncture, while the study by Fung et al (1986) may have been subject to a range of biases.

How much of the published research is of high quality? How much research provides us with findings that we can be confident is not distorted by bias? Methodologists have conducted numerous surveys of the quality of published research and the conclusion has almost always been that much of the published research is of poor quality (see, for example, Anyanwu & Treasure 2004, Kjaergard et al 2002, Dickinson et al 2000). Systematic reviewers typically conclude the same: inspection of the abstracts of a sample of 20 systematic reviews randomly selected from the PEDro database found that 8 (40%) explicitly mentioned problems with trial quality in their conclusions. There is, however, some evidence that the quality of the research literature is slowly improving (Kjaergard et al 2002, Moher et al 2002, Moseley et al 2002, Quinones et al 2003).

Many people who are not familiar with the research process find it difficult to believe that much of the published research is potentially seriously biased. They imagine that research is usually carried out by experts, that research reports are peer-reviewed by people with methodological expertise, and that research papers are therefore usually of a high standard. The reality is that much of the clinical research we read in journals is conducted by people who have little or no training in research design. Some researchers are intent on proving a point of view rather than objectively testing hypotheses. And even informed and well-intentioned researchers may be unable to conduct high quality research because they are thwarted by practical impediments, such as difficulty recruiting adequate numbers of subjects for the research. Research reports, particularly those in lower quality journals, may be peer-reviewed by people who have little better understanding of research design than the people who conducted the research. And journal editors

Figure 5.1   Distribution of quality scores of randomized trials in physiotherapy (2297 trials). Reproduced with permission from Moseley et al (2002).

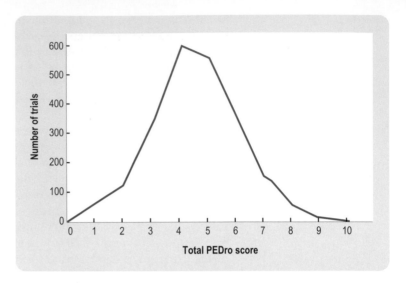

may be forced to publish reports of poorly designed studies to fill the pages of their journals.

These and other factors conspire to make a substantial proportion of published research potentially seriously biased.

A quantitative estimate of the quality of randomized trials in physiotherapy is provided by the PEDro database. All trials on the database are assessed according to ten methodological criteria. A methodological quality score is generated by counting the number of criteria that are satisfied. Figure 5.1 shows that most trials on the database satisfy some but not all of the key methodological characteristics. The typical trial satisfies 5 of the 10 criteria. (In many trials it is not possible to satisfy the criteria of blinding patients or therapists; in such trials the maximum possible score is effectively 8.) Thus a small proportion of trials are of very high quality, the typical trial is of moderate quality, and there are many trials of low quality. There are few data on the quality of typical studies of experiences and processes, prognosis, or diagnosis, but our impression is that the quality of such studies tends to be somewhat lower than that of clinical trials.

If it is true that a substantial proportion of the clinical research published in journals is poorly designed and potentially misleading, readers of clinical research must be able to distinguish between high quality studies that potentially provide useful information for clinical decision-making and low quality clinical research which is potentially misleading. Readers who are unable to make that distinction will be unable to make sense of the apparently contradictory clinical research literature.

This might appear to be too much to ask of readers. Surely, if many researchers and journals reviewers cannot distinguish between high quality and low quality research, it is unreasonable to expect readers of clinical trials to be able to do so. In fact, as the pioneers of evidence-based medicine recognized (Department of Clinical Epidemiology and Biostatistics 1981), it is probably possible to use very simple checklists to distinguish coarsely between high quality research and research that is likely to be biased. The assumption is that a few carefully chosen criteria can be used to discriminate between studies that are likely to produce relatively unbiased answers to clinical questions and those that are potentially seriously biased. The value of this approach is that it puts the assessment of the quality of clinical research within the reach of readers who do not necessarily have research expertise themselves. A little bit of training (or just reading this chapter) is all that is needed to be able to discriminate coarsely between low quality and high quality clinical research.

What criteria should be used to discriminate between high quality and low quality research? How should these quality criteria be developed? The most common approach is to seek the opinions of experts. In fact there are now numerous sets of criteria based on expert opinion that have been used to assess the quality of studies of effects of intervention, and several sets of criteria based on expert opinion that have been used to assess the quality of studies of experiences, prognosis or the accuracy of diagnostic tests. One set of criteria that is of particular interest is the Delphi list of criteria for assessing the quality of clinical trials, developed by Verhagen and colleagues (Verhagen et al 1998a). These researchers asked experts to nominate criteria they felt were important and then used a formal method (the 'Delphi technique') to achieve a consensus. The Delphi list forms the basis of the PEDro scale that was introduced in Chapter 4.[2]

In this chapter we will use the approach to critical appraisal popularized in the *JAMA* Users' Guides (Guyatt & Rennie 1993) and refined by

---

[2] An alternative approach is more empirical and less subjective. This approach bases the selection of quality criteria on findings of research into characteristics of research designs that minimize bias. Most of this research has been directed at assessing the quality of studies of the effects of intervention, rather than studies of prognosis or accuracy of diagnostic tests, and the approach cannot easily be applied to studies of experiences. The usual approach with studies of the effects of intervention is to assemble large numbers of clinical trials and extract from each an estimate of the effect of intervention. Then statistical techniques are used to determine which study characteristics correlate best with estimates of effects of intervention. Study characteristics that correlate strongly with effects of intervention are thought to be those that are indicative of bias. Thus, if studies without a particular characteristic (such as concealment of allocation) tend to show larger effects of interventions, this is thought to be evidence the characteristic (concealment) reduces bias.

While this approach is less subjective and more transparent than seeking expert opinion, it relies on the questionable assumption that study characteristics which correlate strongly with effects of intervention are indicative of bias. The design of these studies does not provide rigorous control of confounding, so it may be that this approach identifies spurious quality criteria or fails to identify important quality criteria. It is reassuring, then, that several studies have produced more or less consistent findings. The available evidence suggests that control of bias is provided by randomization (particularly concealed randomization), blinding and adequate follow-up (Chalmers et al 1983, Colditz et al 1989, Schulz et al 1995, Kunz & Oxman 1998, Moher et al 1998).

A smaller number of studies have used a similar approach in an attempt to identify characteristics that control for bias in studies of diagnostic tests (Lijmer et al 1999). To our knowledge there have not yet been similar investigations of studies of prognosis.

Sackett et al (2000). This approach involves first asking a small number of key questions about study design in order to distinguish between low quality and high quality studies, before proceeding to interpret study findings. Such questions have been called 'methodological filters' because they can be used to 'filter out' studies of low methodological quality. Most (not all) of the methodological filters we will describe are the same as those described by others.

We have made the case that readers of clinical research need to be careful to discriminate between high quality research, which can be used for clinical decision-making, and low quality research, which is potentially biased. But we do not wish to encourage excessively critical attitudes. Inexperienced readers of clinical research may be inclined to be very dismissive of imperfect research and apply methodological filters harshly. However, no research is perfect, so the highly critical reader will find very little research trustworthy.

> We should not demand perfection from clinical research because it is not generally attainable. Instead, we should look for studies that are *good enough* for clinical decision-making.

That is, we need to identify studies that are sufficiently well designed to give us more certainty than we could otherwise have. Usually we need to be prepared to accept the findings of good but not excellent studies because they give us the best information we can get.

In the following sections we consider how to assess the validity of studies of effects of interventions, experiences, prognosis and accuracy of diagnostic tests.

CRITICAL APPRAISAL OF EVIDENCE ABOUT THE EFFECTS OF INTERVENTION

In Chapter 3 it was argued that the preferred source of evidence of the effects of a therapy is usually a recent systematic review. But for some questions there are no relevant, recent systematic reviews, in which case it becomes necessary to consult individual randomized trials.

We first consider how to assess the validity of randomized trials, even though the reader is encouraged to look first for systematic reviews, because it is easier to understand critical appraisal of systematic reviews after having first contemplated critical appraisal of randomized trials.

RANDOMIZED TRIALS

Readers of clinical trials can ask three questions to discriminate coarsely between those trials that are likely to be valid and those that are potentially seriously biased.

Were treated and control groups comparable?

In Chapter 3 it was argued that we only expect to obtain unbiased estimates of the effects of intervention from studies that compare outcomes in treated and untreated groups. It is essential that the groups are comparable, and comparability can only be assured by randomly assigning subjects to groups. 'Matching' of subjects in the treatment and control groups cannot, on its own, ensure that the groups are comparable, regardless of how diligently the matching is carried out. The only way to ensure comparability is to randomize subjects to treatment and control groups.

Randomization is best achieved by using a computer to generate an allocation schedule. Alternatively, random allocation schedules can be generated by effectively random processes like coin-tossing or the drawing of lots. Sometimes quasi-random allocation procedures are used: subjects may be allocated to groups on the basis of their birth dates (for example, subjects with even-numbered birth dates could be assigned to the treatment group and subjects with odd-numbered birth dates assigned to the control group), or medical record numbers, or the date of entry into the trial. It is likely that, if carried out carefully, all of these procedures could assign subjects to groups in a way that is effectively random in the sense that all the procedures could generate comparable groups. That is not to say that coin-tossing and drawing of lots is optimal (see the discussion of concealment of allocation later in this section), but it may be adequate.

Some studies match subjects *and* randomly allocate subjects to groups. The technical term for this is stratified random allocation. Stratification of allocation has the effect of constraining chance. It ensures that there is an even greater comparability of groups than could be achieved by simple random allocation alone. For example, a randomized trial that compared home-made and commercially available spacers in metered-dose inhalers for children with asthma (Zar et al 1999) allocated subjects to one of four groups after stratifying for severity of airways obstruction (mild or moderate/severe). The researchers constrained randomization to ensure that within each stratum of severity of airways obstruction equal numbers of subjects were allocated to each group. By separately randomizing strata with and without moderate/severe airways obstruction it was possible to ensure that the two groups were 'balanced' with respect to the proportion of subjects with moderate/severe airways obstruction.[3]

In general, stratified random allocation ensures more similarity between groups, but usually only slightly more similarity, than would occur with simple randomization. For readers of clinical trials the important point is that it is the randomization, not the stratification, that ensures comparability of groups. Stratified random allocation ensures comparability of

---

[3] Usually, if allocation is to one of two groups the stratum is even numbered in size; if allocation is to one of three groups the size of the stratum is a multiple of three, etc. Random allocation is then conducted in a way that ensures subjects in each stratum are allocated to equally sized groups. (The equally sized groups are called 'blocks'; blocked random allocation is analogous to randomly drawing lots without replacement). Stratification without blocking does not ensure greater comparability of groups than simple randomization alone (Lavori et al 1983).

groups because it involves randomization. But randomization on its own is adequate.[4]

It is usually a very easy matter to determine if a clinical trial was randomized or not. Reports of randomized trials will usually explain that subjects were 'randomly allocated to groups'.[5] This might appear in the title of the paper, or in the abstract, or in the Methods section.

One concern is that particularly naïve authors may refer to 'random allocation' when describing *haphazard* allocation to groups. These authors might believe that if they made no particular effort to ensure that subjects were in one group or the other (for example, if subjects or their therapists, but not the researchers, determined whether the treatment or control condition was received) then they could call the allocation process 'random'. This, of course, is potentially seriously misleading, because there is no guarantee in such trials that the groups are comparable in the sense that they differ only by chance; these sorts of processes should not be referred to as random allocation. The term 'random allocation' should be strictly reserved for allocation procedures that use random number generators or, perhaps, random processes such as coin-tossing or the drawing of lots. As there is always the concern that the term 'random allocation' has been used in an inappropriate way, it is reassuring if the trial report describes the randomization procedure, so that the reader can know that the allocation procedure was truly random rather than just haphazard. An example of a clear description of the randomization is provided in the report of a trial of community-based physiotherapy for people with chronic stroke (Green et al 2002). The authors reported that: 'Randomization was achieved by numbered, sealed, opaque envelopes prepared from random number tables …'.

True randomization can only be ensured if randomization is concealed.[6] This means that the researcher is not aware, at the time a decision is made about eligibility of a person to participate in the trial, if that person would subsequently be randomized to the treatment or control group. Concealment is important because, even though most trials specify inclusion and exclusion criteria that determine who is and who is not eligible to participate in the trial, there is sometimes uncertainty about

---

[4] At this stage some readers may want to object to the assertion that randomization ensures comparability. They might argue that randomization ensures comparability only when sample sizes are sufficiently large. In one sense that is true; the groups will be more similar, on average, when the sample size is large. The consequence is that trials with larger samples provide more precise estimates of effects of intervention; we will consider precision at more length later in this chapter. But there is another way of looking at comparability. Comparability can also be thought of as a lack of bias. In so far as 'bias' refers to a *long-run tendency* to overestimate or underestimate the true value of a parameter, randomization removes bias regardless of sample size.

[5] Some studies will state that subjects were 'randomly *selected*' for treatment or control groups, when they really mean subjects were randomly *allocated* to treatment or control groups. The term 'selection' is best reserved for describing the methods used to determine who participated in the trial, not which groups subjects were allocated to.

[6] Concealment of allocation is commonly misunderstood to mean blinding. Blinding and concealment are quite different features of clinical trials. It would probably be clearer if concealment of allocation was called concealment of recruitment.

whether a particular patient satisfies those criteria, and often the researcher responsible for entering new patients into the trial has some latitude in such decisions. It could seriously bias the trial's findings if the researcher's decision about who was and was not entered into the trial was influenced by knowledge of which group patients would subsequently be assigned to. For example, a researcher who favoured the hypothesis that intervention was effective might be reluctant to admit patients with particularly severe cases if he or she knew that the next patient entered into the trial was to be allocated to the control group. (This might occur if the researcher did not claim equipoise, and was concerned that this patient received the best possible treatment.) In that case, allocation would no longer be random even if the allocation sequence itself was truly random, because subjects with the most severe cases could only be allocated to the treatment group. Consequently the groups would not differ only by chance, and they would no longer be 'comparable'. Similar reasons necessitate that potential *subjects* are not aware, at the time they decide whether to participate in the trial, whether they would subsequently be randomized to treatment or control groups. Foreknowledge about which group they are to be allocated could influence the patient's decision about whether to participate in the trial, potentially producing serious allocation bias. Lack of concealment potentially leads to non-random allocation.

How can the allocation be concealed? The simplest way is for a person not otherwise involved in entering subjects into the trial to draw up the random allocation schedule. Then each subject's allocation is placed in a sealed envelope. The allocation schedule is concealed from the researcher who enters subjects into the trial, and from potential subjects, so that neither the researcher nor potential subject knows, at the time a decision is made about participation in the trial, which group the subject would subsequently be allocated to. Then, when the researcher is satisfied that the subject has met the criteria for participation in the trial and the subject has given informed consent to participate, the envelope corresponding to that subject's number is opened and the allocation is revealed. Once the envelope is opened the subject is considered to have entered the trial. This simple procedure ensures that allocation is concealed.

An alternative procedure involves holding the allocation schedule off-site. Then, when the researcher is satisfied a patient is eligible to participate in the trial and the patient has given informed consent, the researcher contacts the holder of the allocation schedule and asks for the allocation. Again, once the researcher is informed of the allocation, the patient is considered to have entered the trial. This procedure also ensures concealment of allocation.

There are other, less satisfactory ways to conceal random allocation. Allocation could be concealed if, once the researcher was satisfied that a patient was eligible to enter a trial and had given informed consent, allocation was determined by the toss of a coin ('heads' = treatment group, 'tails' = control group) or by the drawing of lots. Theoretically this would provide an allocation schedule that is both effectively random and concealed. The problem with coin-tossing and the drawing of lots is that the process is easily corrupted.[7] For example, the researcher could toss the coin or draw lots *before* making a final decision about the patient's eligibility for the trial. Alternatively, if either the patient or researcher was unhappy with the coin toss or the lot that was drawn it might be tempting to repeat the toss or draw lots again until the preferred allocation is achieved. The benefit of using sealed envelopes or contacting a central allocation registry is that the randomization process can be audited, and corruption of the allocation schedule is more difficult.

Some reports of clinical trials will explicitly state that allocation was concealed. Usually statements about concealment of allocation are made in the part of the Methods section that describes the allocation procedures. More often, trial reports do not explicitly state that allocation was concealed, but they describe methods such as the use of sealed envelopes or contacting a central registry that probably ensured concealment. Unfortunately, most trials do not either explicitly state that allocation was concealed or describe methods that would have ensured concealment. Some (perhaps most) of these trials may have used concealed allocation (Soares et al 2004), but we cannot know which trials did.[8]

Was there complete or near complete follow-up?

Doing clinical trials is hard and often mundane work. One of the difficulties is ensuring that the trial protocol is adhered to. And one of the hardest parts of the trial protocol to adhere to is the planned measurement of outcomes ('follow-up').

Most clinical trials involve interventions that are implemented over days or weeks or months. Usually outcomes are assessed at the end of the intervention, and they are often also assessed at one or several times after the intervention has ceased. Trials of chronic conditions may assess outcomes several years after the intervention period has ceased.

A problem that arises in most trials is that it is not always possible to obtain outcome measures as planned. Occasionally subjects die. Others become too sick to measure, or they move out of town, or go on long holidays. Some may lose interest in participating in the study or simply be too busy to attend for follow-up appointments. For these and a myriad of other reasons it may be impossible for the researchers to obtain outcome measures from all subjects as planned, no matter how hard the researchers try to obtain follow-up measures from all patients. This phenomenon of real-life clinical trials is termed 'loss to follow-up'. Subjects lost to follow-up are sometimes called 'dropouts'.[9]

Loss to follow-up would be of little concern if it occurred at random. But in practice loss to follow-up may be non-random, and this can produce bias. Bias occurs when dropouts from one group differ systematically, in

---

[7] Schulz & Grimes (2002) argue that unless mechanisms are put in place to prevent corruption of allocation schedules, corruption of allocation is likely to occur.

[8] Systematic reviewers often write to the authors of papers to seek clarification of the exact methods used in the study. But this is not usually practical for readers of trials. Consequently, it is often not possible for readers of clinical trials to determine whether there was concealed allocation or not.

[9] Note that a subject is *not* a dropout if he or she discontinues therapy, or does not comply with the allocated intervention, provided that follow-up data are available for that subject.

terms of their outcomes, from dropouts in the other group. When this occurs, differences between groups are no longer attributable just to the intervention and chance. Randomization is undone. Estimates of the effect of treatment become contaminated by differences between groups due to loss to follow-up.

It is quite plausible that dropouts from one group will differ systematically from dropouts in the other group. This is because it is quite plausible that subjects' experiences of the intervention or its outcomes will influence whether they attend for follow-up.[10] Imagine a hypothetical trial of treatment for cervical headache. The trial compares the effect of six sessions of manual therapy to a no-intervention control condition, and outcomes in both groups are assessed 2 weeks after randomization. Some subjects in the control group may experience little resolution of their symptoms. Understandably, these subjects may become dissatisfied with participation in the trial and may be reluctant to return for outcome assessment after not having received any intervention. The consequence is that there may be a tendency for those subjects in the control group with the worst outcomes to be lost to follow-up, more so than in the treated group. In that case, estimates of the effects of intervention (the difference between the outcomes of treated and control groups) are likely to be biased and the treatment will appear less effective than it really is.

We could imagine many such scenarios that would illustrate that loss to follow-up can bias estimates of the effects of intervention in either direction. Unfortunately, while statistical techniques have been formulated to try to reduce the bias associated with loss to follow-up (Raghunathan 2004), none are completely satisfactory. All involve estimating, in one way or another, values of missing data. But because the missing data are not available it is never possible to check how accurate these estimates are. Ultimately it will always be true that trials with missing data are potentially biased.

The potential for bias is low if few subjects dropout. When only a small percentage of subjects are lost to follow-up, the findings of the trial can depend relatively little on the pattern of loss to follow-up in such subjects. On the other hand, large numbers of dropouts can seriously bias the findings of a study. The more subjects lost to follow-up, the greater the potential for bias.

How much loss to follow-up is required to seriously threaten the validity of a study's findings? Many statisticians would not be seriously concerned with dropouts of as much as 10% of the sample. On the other hand, if more than 20% of the sample was lost to follow-up there would be grounds for concern about the possibility of serious bias. A rough rule of thumb might be that, if greater than 15% of the sample is lost to follow-up then the findings of the trial could be considered to be in doubt. (This is an arbitrary threshold. Some experts recommend a threshold of 20%; van Tulder et al 2003. However, a threshold of 10% might also be reasonable.) Of course this 'rule' ought to be applied judiciously: where trialists can

---

[10] In some trials it may be *others'* experiences of the intervention or its outcomes that influence loss to follow-up. For example, if the subject is dependent on a carer and the subject's carer is unhappy with therapy, the carer may be reluctant to attend follow-up and the subject may be lost to follow-up.

provide data to show that losses to follow up of greater than 15% were largely due to factors that were clearly not related to intervention, we may be prepared to accept the findings of the trial. On the other hand, where loss to follow-up is much greater in one group than in the other (clear evidence that loss to follow-up is due to intervention), or where loss to follow-up is clearly dependent on the intervention, we may be suspicious of the findings of trials that have loss to follow-up of less than 15%.

In some trials, particularly trials of the management of chronic conditions, the outcomes of most interest are those at long term follow-up. But follow-up becomes progressively more difficult with time, so long term follow-ups are often plagued by large losses to follow-up. Consequently, many studies have adequate short term follow-up but inadequate long term follow-up. Such studies may provide strong evidence of short term effects of intervention but weak evidence of long term effects.

Some clinical trial reports clearly describe loss to follow-up. It is particularly helpful when the trial report provides a flow diagram (as recommended in the CONSORT statement, Moher et al 2001) that describes the number of subjects randomized to each group and the number of subjects from whom outcomes could be obtained at each occasion of follow-up. An example is shown in Figure 5.2. Flow diagrams such as this make it relatively easy for the reader to assess whether follow-up was adequate.

Figure 5.2   An example of a flow diagram, showing how subjects progress through the trial or are lost to follow-up. Redrawn from Hinman et al (2003), with permission from BMJ publishers.

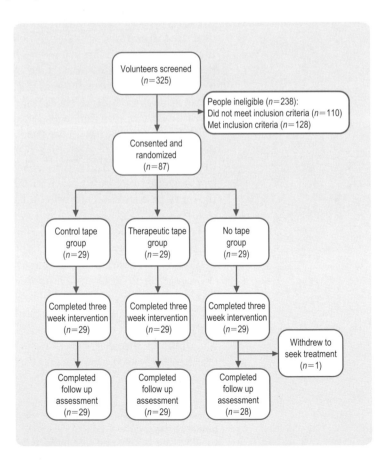

More often, trial reports do not explicitly supply data on loss to follow-up. In that case the reader must calculate loss to follow-up from the data that are supplied. Two pieces of information are required. It is necessary to know both the number of subjects randomized to groups (i.e. the number of subjects in the trial) and the number of subjects from whom outcome measures are available at each time point. These numbers are sometimes given in the text. Alternatively, it may be possible to find these data in tables of results, or in summaries of statistical analyses.[11] A degree of detective work is sometimes required to extract these data. Calculation of loss to follow-up is straightforward: the percentage lost to follow-up = 100 × number lost to follow-up/number randomized.

Some trial reports commit a special crime: they provide no clues about loss to follow-up, even for the most cunning detective. In such studies there may, of course, have been no loss to follow-up. But it is unusual to have no loss to follow-up. The more likely explanation, particularly in trials with long follow-up periods, is that loss to follow-up occurred but was not reported.

> Studies which do not provide data on loss to follow-up and which do not explicitly state that there was no loss to follow-up should be considered potentially biased.

A problem that is closely related to loss to follow-up is the problem of protocol violation. Protocol violations occur when the trial is not carried out as planned. In trials of physiotherapy interventions, the most common protocol violation is the failure of subjects to receive the intended intervention. For example, subjects in a trial of exercise may be allocated to an exercise group but may fail to do their exercises, or fail to exercise according to the protocol (this is sometimes called 'non-compliance' or 'non-adherence'), or subjects allocated to the control condition may take up exercise. Other sorts of protocol violations occur when subjects who do not satisfy criteria for inclusion in the trial are mistakenly admitted to the trial and randomized to groups, or when outcome measures cannot be taken at the time that it was intended they be taken. Protocol violations are undesirable, but usually some degree of protocol violations cannot be avoided. Usually they present less of a problem than loss to follow-up. How would we prefer that data from clinical trials with protocol violations are analysed?

One alternative would be to discard data from subjects for whom there were protocol violations. Readers should be suspicious of studies that

---

[11] A good place to look is the column headers in tables of results. These often give '$n = X$'. (Even then, it may not be clear if the X is the number of subjects that entered the trial or the number of subjects followed up). When outcomes of dichotomous measures are expressed as the number *and* percentage of subjects experiencing some outcome then the total number of subjects followed up can easily be calculated (number followed up = 100 × number experiencing event/percentage experiencing the event). (Dichotomous outcomes are those with one of two possible outcomes, like lived or died. We will consider dichotomous outcomes further in Chapter 6.) Readers with a good understanding of tests based on t, F or χ^2 distributions may be able to determine the number of subjects followed up from quoted degrees of freedom of t, F or χ^2 statistics.

discard data because, insofar as protocol violations are influenced by the intervention, discarding data biases results. (This is because, once a subject's data are discarded, that subject effectively is, as far as interpretation is concerned, lost to follow-up). Another unsatisfactory 'solution' is sometimes applied when there has been non-compliance with intervention. Some trialists will analyse data from non-complying intervention group subjects as if these subjects had been allocated to the control group. This is sometimes called a 'per protocol' analysis. Per protocol analyses potentially produce even greater bias than discarding data of non-compliant subjects.[12] The most satisfactory solution is the least obvious one. It involves ignoring the protocol violations and analysing the data of all subjects in the groups to which they were allocated. This is called 'analysis by intention to treat'.[13]

Analysis by intention to treat has properties that make it better than other approaches to dealing with protocol violations. Most importantly,

analysis by intention to treat preserves the benefits of randomization

it maintains the comparability of groups. Also, from a pragmatic point of view, analysis by intention to treat provides the most meaningful estimates of effects of intervention. This is because, pragmatically speaking, interventions can only be effective if patients comply.[14] When analysis is by intention to treat, non-compliance reduces estimates of the magnitude of treatment effects. To the pragmatist, this is as it should be. We consider the issue of pragmatic interpretation of clinical trials in more detail later in this chapter.

It will usually only be apparent that a trial has analysed by intention to treat if the authors of the trial report refer explicitly to 'analysis by intention to treat'. However, analysis by intention to treat is often not reported, even when the trial was analysed by intention to treat (Soares et al 2004).[15]

Was there blinding to allocation of patients and assessors?

There is reason to prefer that, in clinical trials, subjects are unaware of whether they received the intervention or control condition. This is called blinding of subjects.[16] Blinding of subjects is considered important because it provides a means of controlling for placebo effects.

---

[12] In trials with equally sized groups, the bias produced by crossing non-compliant intervention group subjects over to the control group is twice that produced by omitting data of non-compliant subjects.

[13] With the intention to treat approach, protocol violations are ignored in both the conduct and analysis of the trial. Follow-up measurements are obtained from all subjects, wherever possible, even if there were serious protocol violations. For example, subjects are followed up, wherever possible, even if they were incorrectly admitted to the trial, or even if as soon as they were randomized they decided not to participate further in the study. In trials that do not use an intention to treat approach, these subjects may not be followed up, in which case they become lost to follow-up. So the intention to treat approach has two benefits: it minimizes loss to follow-up and provides a coherent method for dealing with protocol violations.

[14] This assumes that the response to exercise continues to increase with the amount of exercise, at least up to the amount of exercise that is prescribed.

[15] Occasionally the opposite is true: some trials may state they analysed by intention to treat even though the description of their methods indicated they did not.

[16] Sometimes 'blinding' is referred to as 'masking'.

In the following paragraphs we define placebo effects and we discuss in more detail why and how blinding of subjects is used. Then we present an alternative point of view which holds that blinding of subjects may be relatively unimportant.

Placebo effects are effects of intervention attributable to patients' expectations of a beneficial effect of therapy. The placebo effect is demonstrated when patients benefit from interventions that could have no direct physiological effects, such as detuned ultrasound. Although the mechanisms are unknown, some have speculated that expectation or conditioning could trigger beneficial biochemical responses (Brody 2000). Placebo effects of one kind or another are widely believed to accompany most interventions. The effects, it is thought, can be very large – placebo can be more effective than many established interventions. Many good clinicians seek to exploit the placebo effect by maximizing the credibility of interventions in the belief that this will give the best possible outcomes for their patients.

A goal of many trials is to determine what effects intervention has over and above those effects due to placebo. Clinical trials that blind subjects can provide just this information. Blinding means that subjects in intervention and control groups do not know which group they were allocated to. Blinded subjects can only guess whether they received the intervention or control condition. In the absence of any information about which group they were in, the guesses of subjects in treated and control groups will be, on average, similar. Consequently,

> Blinding of subjects ensures that estimates of the effects of intervention (the difference between outcomes of treated and control groups) cannot be due to placebo effects.

How is it possible to blind patients to allocation? How can subjects not know if they received the intervention or control? The general approach involves giving a 'sham' intervention to the control group. Sham interventions are those that look, feel, sound, smell and taste like the intervention but could not effect the presumed mechanism of the intervention. The clearest examples in physiotherapy come from studies of electrotherapies. Several clinical trials (for example, McLachlan et al 1991, Ebenbichler et al 1999, van der Heijden et al 1999) have used sham interventions in studies of pulsed ultrasound. In these studies the ultrasound machine is adapted so that it either emits pulsed ultrasound (the intervention) or does not (the sham intervention). In the study by McLachlan et al (1991), the sham ultrasound transducer was designed to become warm when turned on, so the patient was unable to distinguish between intervention and sham. The intervention and sham could not be distinguished by the patient, and yet the sham could not effect the presumed mechanisms of ultrasound therapy because no ultrasound was emitted. Consequently this is a near-perfect sham. Other near-perfect shams used in clinical trials of physiotherapy interventions include the use of coloured light as sham low-level laser therapy (for example, de Bie et al 1998), and the use of specially constructed collapsing needles in studies of acupuncture (Kleinhenz et al 1999).

Often it is not possible to apply sham interventions that are truly indistinguishable from the intervention. It is hard to imagine, for example, how one might apply a convincing sham stretch for ankle plantarflexor contractures, or sham gait training for people with Parkinson's disease, or a community-based rehabilitation programme after stroke. In these circumstances the highest degree of control is supplied by a quasi-sham intervention that is similar to the intervention (rather than indistinguishable from the intervention) yet has no direct therapeutic effect. One example comes from a study of motor training of sitting balance after stroke. Dean & Shepherd (1997) trained subjects in the intervention group by asking them to perform challenging reaching tasks in sitting; subjects in the sham control group performed similar tasks but did not reach beyond arm's length. Another example comes from a recent trial of advice for management of low back pain. Subjects in the intervention ('advice') group received specific advice on self-management strategies from physiotherapists, whereas subjects in the control ('ventilation') group talked to a physiotherapist who refrained from providing specific advice (Pengel 2004). In these examples the sham control is similar to but distinguishable from the intervention; nonetheless the sham probably provides quite a high degree of control for potential placebo effects.

In many physiotherapy trials there is no real possibility of applying a sham intervention because it is not possible to construct an ineffective therapy that even moderately resembles the true intervention. In that case, some control of placebo effects may be achieved by providing a control intervention which, like a sham, has no direct therapeutic effect, but which, unlike a sham, does not resemble the true intervention at all. In this case, as the control condition does not resemble the true intervention, it probably should not be called a sham. It may, nonetheless, still provide some control of placebo effects. This strategy has been used in trials of manipulative physiotherapy. It is difficult to apply sham manipulative therapy, so several trials have compared the effects of manipulative physiotherapy with de-tuned ultrasound (for example, Schiller 2001). De-tuned ultrasound has no direct therapeutic effects, but it does not resemble manipulative therapy. These *partially* blinded trials may provide some control for placebo effects[17] but they provide less control than studies which use true shams.

We have seen that some studies employ true shams that are indistinguishable from the true intervention. And other studies employ shams that are similar to but not indistinguishable from the true intervention, or use control interventions that do not have direct therapeutic effects but do not resemble the true intervention. Some studies compare two active therapies, and yet other studies compare an active therapy to no-treatment

---

[17] In some studies the sham therapy may be very unconvincing to patients. That is, the sham may be an obviously ineffective therapy. It is possible that such studies accentuate, rather than control for, placebo effects. It is reassuring, in clinical trials employing sham therapies, to read that subjects were asked if they believed they received the experimental or sham therapy. If the sham was convincing, similar proportions of subjects in the treated and sham groups should say they thought they were given the experimental intervention.

controls. These latter studies are exposed to potential bias from placebo effects. We will consider the seriousness of this bias further below.

Although the purpose of applying sham interventions is usually to control for placebo effects, there is a potentially useful secondary effect. In Chapter 3 we introduced the idea that polite patients can make interventions appear more effective than they truly are. When outcomes in clinical trials are self-reported, subjects in the intervention group may exaggerate perceived improvements in outcome because they feel that is the socially appropriate thing to do, and patients in the control group may provide pessimistic reports of outcomes because they perceive that is what the investigators want to hear. Blinding of subjects means that subjects in intervention and control groups should have similar beliefs about whether they received intervention or control conditions, so trials with blinded subjects cannot be biased by polite patients.

The preceding paragraphs have presented a conventional view of the value of blinding of subjects in randomized trials. But there is another point of view that says blinding of subjects may not be necessary.

The first argument against the need for blinding subjects is that, from a pragmatic view, it does not matter if the effects of therapy are direct effects of therapy or effects of placebo (Vickers & de Craen 2000). In this pragmatic view, the purpose of clinical trials is to help therapists determine which of two alternatives (intervention or control conditions) produces the better outcome. The intervention that produces the better clinical outcomes is the better choice, even if its effects are due only to placebo. Therefore, it is argued, therapists need not be concerned whether an effect of intervention is due to placebo. They need only determine whether the intervention produces better outcomes. (Box 5.2, at the end of this section, summarizes the differences between pragmatic and explanatory perspectives of clinical trials.)

This point of view has some merit, but is not without problems. Perhaps the strongest counterargument is that it could be considered unethical to administer interventions whose only effects are placebo effects, because administration of placebo interventions would usually involve some sort of deception. The administration or endorsement of the intervention by a health professional might imply, either implicitly or explicitly, that there was some effect other than a placebo effect.[18] Another problem with applying interventions whose only effects are due to placebo is that this may stall the development of alternative interventions that have more scope for becoming more effective therapies.

A more radical argument against the need for blinding of subjects in clinical trials is that the placebo effect may not exist. Why is there a widespread belief in the powerful effects of placebo?

Belief of the existence of placebo effects must have existed long before modern times because some of the earliest clinical trials used sham controls. In modern times, an early stimulus for the now near-universal belief in the placebo effect was a literature review by Beecher (1955),

---

[18] It would be very interesting to know what patients receiving the intervention thought of this issue.

aptly titled 'The powerful placebo'. Beecher summarized the results of 15 'illustrative' studies of a total of 1082 patients in which sham drugs (usually saline or lactose) were used to treat a range of conditions, including wound pain, angina pain, headache and cough. He concluded that 'placebos are found to have an average significant effectiveness of $35.2 \pm 2.2\%$'. Until recently Beecher's methods have not been seriously challenged and his conclusions became widely accepted as true.

But Beecher's data do not provide strong support for the existence of a placebo effect because they are based on an inappropriate methodology (Keinle & Kiene 1997). Beecher focused on the magnitude of the reduction in pain experienced by people receiving placebo analgesia. Even though these data have been extracted from randomized trials, they do not involve comparison with a control condition. The effects observed in patients treated with placebo analgesia may have been partly due to placebo, but any such effects were almost certainly confounded by natural recovery, statistical regression,[19] polite patients and other biases. It is unremarkable to observe that many patients who receive placebo therapy experience recovery, because the recovery may not have been due to the placebo.

To determine the effects of placebo we need to examine randomized controlled studies that compare outcomes of people treated with sham interventions to outcomes of people who receive no intervention. In fact such comparisons are often made incidentally in clinical trials. This is because there are many randomized trials that compare intervention, sham control and no-intervention control. These trials provide estimates of the total effects of therapy (the difference between outcomes of the intervention and no-intervention groups), and also allow for the total effect of therapy to be partitioned into direct effects of therapy (the difference between outcomes of the intervention and sham intervention groups) and effects of placebo and polite patients (the difference between outcomes of the sham intervention and no-intervention groups).

In a landmark study, Hrobjartsson & Götsche (2001) systematically reviewed the evidence for effects of placebo. They found 114 randomized trials, distributed across all areas of health care, comparing intervention, sham intervention and no-intervention groups. To ascertain the effects of placebo they conducted a meta-analysis of the difference in outcomes of sham intervention and no-intervention groups. They found little or no effect of placebo on binary outcomes.[20] However, there was evidence of a small effect of placebo on continuous outcomes.[21] (The magnitude of this effect was about one-quarter of one standard deviation[22] of the outcomes.)

---

[19] The concept of statistical regression, as it pertains to clinical trials, is explained in Chapter 3.

[20] Binary outcomes are events (like lived/died, or returned to work/did not return to work). Typically binary outcomes are relatively 'hard' (objective) outcomes. We will look at examples of binary outcomes in more detail in Chapter 6.

[21] Continuous outcomes are those that have a measurable magnitude, such as pain intensity or degree of disability. We will look at examples of continuous outcomes in more detail in Chapter 6.

[22] The standard deviation is a measure of variability of a set of scores. It is calculated by taking the square root of the average squared deviation of the scores from the mean.

Subgroup analyses found the effect was apparent in trials which measured subjective outcomes but not in trials which measured objective outcomes.[23] The 27 trials which employed pain as an outcome showed a small effect (again, the magnitude was about one-quarter of one standard deviation; this corresponds to a pain reduction of 6.5 mm on a 100 mm visual analogue scale). The magnitude of this effect was less in trials with larger sample sizes, suggesting that the effect could be inflated by bias in small trials. An important limitation of the review is that it included trials which had imperfect shams; consequently it provides an assessment of the value of attempting to blind subjects, but not necessarily of the effect of blinding subjects. These findings are provocative because they suggest that placebo effects may have been exaggerated, and that the concept of the powerful placebo is a myth built on the artefact of poorly designed research. Incidentally, the review's findings also indicate that, in the typical randomized trial, bias caused by polite patients is small or negligible. The implication of Hrobjartsson and Götsche's fascinating study is that it is not important to blind subjects in randomized trials.

While the need for blinding of *subjects* is, therefore, arguable, there are compelling reasons to want to see blinding of *assessors* in randomized trials.

> Wherever possible, assessors (the people who measure outcomes in clinical trials) should be unaware, at the time they take each measurement of outcome, whether the measurement is being made on someone who received the intervention or control condition.

This is because blinding of assessors protects against measurement bias. In the context of clinical trials, measurement bias is the tendency for measurements to be influenced by allocation. For example, measurements obtained from subjects in the intervention group might tend to be slightly optimistic, or measures obtained from subjects in the control group might tend to be slightly pessimistic, or both. This would bias (inflate) estimates of the effect of intervention.

Potential for measurement bias occurs whenever the measurement procedures are subjective. In practice there are very few clinical measurement procedures that do not involve some subjectivity. (By subjectivity we mean operator-dependency.) Even measurement procedures that look quite objective, such as measurements of range of motion, strength or exercise capacity, probably involve some subjectivity. Indeed, the history of scientific research suggests that even relatively objective measures are prone to measurement bias.[24] Fortunately, measurement bias is often easily prevented by asking a blinded assessor to measure outcomes. In the words of Leland Wilkinson and the American Psychological Association's Task Force on Statistical Inference (1999), 'An author's self-awareness, experience, or resolve does not eliminate experimenter bias. In short,

---

[23] We shall see, later in this chapter, that subgroup analyses are potentially misleading and ought to be interpreted cautiously.
[24] For an excellent example, and a ripping good read, see Steven Jay Gould's account of nineteenth century craniometry (Gould 1997).

there are no valid excuses, financial or otherwise, for avoiding an opportunity to double-blind.'

This statement might imply that blinding of assessors is easier than it really is. There *is* one circumstance which often prevents the use of blind assessors: in many trials outcomes are self-reported. In that case the assessor is the subject, and assessors are only blinded if subjects are blinded. This is often overlooked by readers of clinical trials. The trial may employ blinded assessors to measure some outcomes, but self-reported outcomes cannot be considered assessor blinded unless the subjects themselves are blinded. An example is the trial by Powell et al (2002) that examined if a community-based rehabilitation programme could reduce disability of patients with severe head injury. The authors ensured that, as far as possible, the researcher performing assessments was blinded to allocation.[25] However, one of the primary outcomes was assessed 'by the research assessor based on a combination of limited observation and interview with the client and, if applicable, carers'. The other outcome, a questionnaire, was completed 'by patients who were able to do so without assistance [or] on their behalf by a primary carer (where applicable)'. Consequently this trial was not assessor-blinded because patients and carers were not blinded.

There are other participants in clinical trials who we would also like to be blind to allocation. Ideally, the providers of care (physiotherapists or anyone else involved in the delivery of the intervention) are also blinded, because care providers may find it difficult to administer experimental and control therapies with equal enthusiasm, and care providers' enthusiasm may influence outcomes. We would prefer that the effects of therapy were not confounded by differences in the degree of enthusiasm offered by care providers when treating experimental and control groups. Unfortunately, it is even harder to blind care providers than it is to blind patients. Thus only a small proportion of trials, notably those investigating the effects of some electrotherapeutic modalities such as low energy laser or pulsed ultrasound, are able to blind care providers. An example is the randomized trial, by de Bie and colleagues (1998), of low-level laser therapy for treatment of ankle sprains. In this trial, people with ankle sprains were treated with either laser therapy or sham laser therapy. The output of the machines was controlled by inputting a code that was concealed from patients and physiotherapists so both patients and physiotherapists were blind to allocation.[26] In most trials, blinding of

---

[25] The authors mention that 'Inevitably, however, some patients who had been treated by outreach, despite being instructed not to do so, inadvertently gave information [about their allocation] to the assessor during the interview assessment.' This is a common experience of clinical trialists!

[26] The authors reported that 'The additional 904 nm [laser therapy] was similar in all three groups except for the dose ... Laser dose at skin level was $0.5\,J/cm^2$ in the low-dose group, $5\,J/cm^2$ in the high-dose group, and $0\,J/cm^2$ in the placebo group ... Blinding of the treatment setting was ensured by randomizing the three settings (high, low or placebo) over 21 treatment codes (7 for each group) ... Both the patient and therapist were fully blinded. In all three groups, the laser apparatus produced a soft sound and the display read 'Warning: laser beam active!', Both patients and therapists also wore protective glasses. In addition, 904-nm laser light is invisible to the human eye.'

Box 5.1   Assessing validity of clinical trials of effects of intervention

Were treated and control groups comparable?
Look for evidence that subjects were assigned to groups using a concealed random allocation procedure.

Was there complete or near-complete follow-up?
Look for information about the proportion of subjects for whom follow-up data were available at key time points. You may need to calculate loss to follow-up yourself from numbers of subjects randomized and numbers followed up.

Was there blinding to allocation of patients and assessors?
Look for evidence of the use of a sham therapy (blinding of patients or therapists) and an explicit statement of blinding of assessors. Remember that when outcomes are self-reported, blinding of assessors requires blinding of subjects.

---

care providers is not possible, so readers have to accept that many trials may be biased to some degree by care provider effects.[27]

Some trials also blind the statistician who analyses the results of the trial. This is because the methods used to analyse most trials cannot usually be completely specified prior to the conduct of the trial; some decisions can only be made after inspection of the data. It is preferable that decisions about methods of analysis are made without regard to the effect they would have on the conclusions of the trial. This can be achieved by blinding the statistician. Statisticians can easily be blinded by presenting them with coded data – the statistician is given a spreadsheet that indicates subjects are in the Apple group and the Orange group, rather than experimental and control group. Blinding of statisticians is rarely done, but it is easily done, and arguably should be routine practice.

Reports of clinical trials frequently refer to 'double-blinding'. This is a source of some confusion because, as we have seen, there are several parties who could be blinded in clinical trials (subjects, the person recruiting subjects, therapists, assessors and statisticians). For this reason the term 'double-blind' is often uninformative.[28]

To summarize this section, readers of clinical trials should routinely appraise the trial validity. This can be done quickly and efficiently by considering whether treatment and control groups were comparable (that is, if there was concealed random allocation), if there was sufficiently complete follow up, and if patients and assessors were blinded (Box 5.1).

---

[27] Moseley and colleagues (2002) found that only 5% of all trials on the PEDro database used blinded therapists.

[28] This leads to an obvious recommendation for authors of reports of clinical trials: avoid reference to double-blind and instead refer explicitly to blind subjects, blind therapists, blind assessors and blind statisticians.

Box 5.2   Pragmatic and explanatory trials

The distinction between 'explanatory' and 'pragmatic' clinical trials, first made by Schwartz & Lellouch (1967), is subtle but important, and it is the source of much confusion amongst readers of clinical trials.[29] (An accessible and contemporary interpretation of the distinction between explanatory and pragmatic trials is given by McMahon (2002)). An example might illustrate the distinction between the two approaches.

Imagine you are a clinical trialist who has decided to investigate whether a programme of exercise reduces pain and increases function in patients with subacute non-specific neck pain. You could adopt a pragmatic or an explanatory approach.

If your primary interest was about the *effects of the exercise* you would adopt the explanatory approach. You would carefully select from the pool of potential subjects those subjects expected to comply with the exercise programme,[30] reasoning that it will only be possible to learn of the effects of exercise if the subjects actually do their exercises. You are fastidious about ensuring the exercises are carried out exactly according to the protocol because your aim is to find out about the effects of precisely that exercise protocol. You design the trial so that subjects in the control group perform sham exercise, and you ensure that control group subjects do exercises of a kind that could not be considered to have therapeutic effects, and that they exercise as frequently and as intensely as subjects in the experimental group. In this way you can determine specifically the effects of the exercise over and above the effects (such as placebo effects) of the ritual of intervention. If there were protocol deviations then you would be tempted, when analysing the data, to

analyse on a per protocol basis. You seek to verify subjective outcomes with objective measures wherever possible.

Alternatively, your interest could be in the more clinical decision about *whether prescription of an exercise programme produces better clinical outcomes*, in which case you could adopt a more relaxed, pragmatic approach. Instead of recruiting only those subjects expected to comply with the intervention, you recruit those subjects who might reasonably be treated with this intervention in the course of normal clinical practice. As a pragmatist you are less choosy about who participates in the trial because your aim is to learn of the effects of prescribing exercise for the clinical spectrum that might reasonably be treated with this intervention, not on a subset of patients carefully selected because they comply unusually well. Even pragmatists like to see the exercise protocol complied with (all clinicians do), but as a pragmatist you see no point in going to unusual ends to ensure compliance – you want to know what the effects of exercise are when it is administered in the way it would be administered in everyday clinical practice. You specify that the control group receives no treatment, rather than a sham treatment, because you reason that this is the appropriate comparison group when the aim is to know if people will fare better when given exercise than if they are not given exercise. (You are not interested in determining whether better outcomes in exercised subjects are due to the exercise itself or to placebo effects; either way, from your perspective, you have achieved what you want to achieve.) And as a pragmatist you will always analyse the data by intention to treat

---

[29] Some authors refer to 'efficacy' trials and 'effectiveness' trials (e.g. Nathan et al 2000). The distinction between efficacy and effectiveness trials is similar to the distinction between explanatory and pragmatic trials. Efficacy refers to the effects of an intervention under idealized conditions (as determined by trials with carefully selected patients, carefully supervised protocols, and per protocol analysis) and effectiveness refers to the effects of an intervention under 'real-world' clinical conditions (as determined by trials with subjects from a typical clinical spectrum, clinical levels of protocol supervision, and intention to treat analysis). Thus efficacy trials have much in common with

explanatory trials and effectiveness trials have much in common with pragmatic trials. It would appear that the most logical sequence would be for efficacy trials to be performed before effectiveness trials. If efficacy trials demonstrate an intervention *can* have clinically worthwhile effects, effectiveness trials can be conducted to determine if the intervention *does* have clinically worthwhile effects.

[30] A common practice, in explanatory trials, is to have a 'run-in' period prior to randomization. Only subjects who comply with the trial protocol in the run-in period are subsequently randomized. (That is, only subjects who comply are given the opportunity to participate in the trial.)

Box 5.2   (*Contd*)

because you want to know the effects of therapy on the people to whom it is applied, not the effects of therapy on the selected group who comply. In your pragmatic view, a therapy cannot be effective if most people do not comply with it. You are happy to base your conclusions on patients' perceptions of outcomes because your view is that the role of intervention is to make patients perceive that their condition has improved.

This example shows just some of the critical differences between explanatory and pragmatic approaches to clinical trials. The important point is that both perspectives, explanatory and pragmatic, are useful.[31] Both can tell us something worth knowing about. Nonetheless, readers of clinical trials often come to the literature with an interest in either an explanatory question or a pragmatic question. In that case they should look for trials with designs that are consistent with their focus. This is not always easy, because often the authors themselves are not clear on whether the trial has an explanatory or pragmatic focus, and often trials mix features of explanatory and pragmatic designs.

---

[31] But explanatory trials are hard; explanatory trialists have gastric ulcers and high blood pressure.

SYSTEMATIC REVIEWS OF RANDOMIZED TRIALS

If a systematic review is to produce valid conclusions it must identify most of the relevant studies that exist and produce a balanced synthesis of their findings. To determine if this goal has been achieved, readers can ask three questions.

Was it clear which trials were to be reviewed?

When we read systematic reviews we need to be satisfied that the reviewer has not selectively reviewed those trials which support his or her own point of view. One of the strengths of properly conducted systematic reviews is that the possibility of selective reviewing is reduced.

To reduce the possibility of selective reviewing, reviewers should clearly define the scope of the review prior to undertaking a search for relevant trials. The best way to do this is to clearly describe criteria that are used to decide what sorts of trials will be included in the review, and perhaps also which trials will not. The inclusion and exclusion criteria usually refer to the population, interventions and outcomes of interest.

An example of a systematic review which provides clear inclusion and exclusion criteria is the review by Green et al (1998) of interventions for shoulder pain. In their review the authors indicated that they 'identified trials independently according to predetermined criteria (that the trial be randomized, that the outcome assessment be blinded, and that the intervention was one of those under review). Randomized controlled trials which investigated common interventions for shoulder pain in adults (age greater than or equal to 18 years) were included provided that there was a blinded assessment of outcome.' Systematic reviews which specify clear inclusion and exclusion criteria provide stronger evidence of effects of therapy than those that do not.

Were most relevant studies reviewed?

Well-conducted reviews identify most trials relevant to the review question. There are two reasons why it is important that reviews identify most relevant trials. First, if the review does not identify all relevant trials it

> **Box 5.3   An optimized search strategy for finding randomized trials in PubMed (Robinson & Dickersin 2002).**
>
> These search terms would be combined with subject-specific search terms to complete the search strategy for a particular systematic review:
>
> (randomized controlled trial [pt] OR controlled clinical trial [pt] OR randomized controlled trials [mh] OR random allocation [mh] OR double-blind method [mh] OR single-blind method [mh] OR clinical trial [pt] OR clinical trials [mh] OR ('clinical trial' [tw]) OR ((singl* [tw] OR doubl* [tw] OR trebl* [tw] OR tripl* [tw]) AND (mask* [tw] OR blind* [tw])) OR ('latin square' [tw]) OR placebos [mh] OR placebo* [tw] OR random* [tw] OR research design [mh:noexp] OR comparative study [mh] OR evaluation studies [mh] OR follow-up studies [mh] OR prospective studies [mh] OR cross-over studies [mh] OR control* [tw] OR prospectiv* [tw] OR volunteer* [tw]) NOT (animal [mh] NOT human [mh])

may conclude that there is less evidence than there really is.[32] More seriously, when not all relevant trials are found there is the possibility that those trials that were not found had systematically different conclusions from those included in the review. In that case the review findings could be seriously biased. For these reasons it is important that systematic reviews search for and locate most relevant trials.

Locating all relevant trials is not an easy task. As we saw in Chapter 4, randomized trials in physiotherapy are indexed across a range of partially overlapping major medical literature databases such as Medline, Embase, CINAHL, AMED, and PsycINFO. The Cochrane Collaboration's Register of Clinical Trials and the Centre for Evidence-Based Physiotherapy's PEDro database attempt to provide more complete indexes of the clinical trial literature, but they rely on other databases to locate trials. Some trials are not indexed on any databases, or are so poorly indexed that they are unlikely ever to be found. So even the most thorough systematic reviews may sometimes miss relevant trials.

Health information scientists have developed optimal search strategies for the major medical literature databases. (See Box 5.3 for an example of an optimized search strategy for finding controlled trials in PubMed.) These search strategies are designed to assist reviewers to locate as many relevant clinical trials as possible.[33]

A substantial number of trials may not be indexed on major health literature databases; they may be published in obscure journals, or they may not have been published at all. Some high quality systematic reviews supplement optimized searches of health literature databases

---

[32] If a meta-analysis is conducted, it may provide less precise estimates of effects of intervention.

[33] The search strategies are designed for maximum sensitivity, so they are not appropriate for use by clinicians seeking answers to clinical questions. That is why, in Chapter 4, we used simpler search strategies to find evidence.

Box 5.4   Example of a comprehensive search strategy in a systematic review of ventilation with lower tidal volumes versus traditional tidal volumes in adults with acute lung injury and acute respiratory distress syndrome (Petrucci & Iacovelli 2003)

We searched the Cochrane Central Register of Controlled Trials (CENTRAL), *The Cochrane Library* issue 4, 2003, MEDLINE (January 1966 to October 2003), EMBASE and CINAHL (1982 to October 2003) using a combination of MeSH and text words. The standard methods of the Cochrane Anaesthesia Review Group were employed. No language restrictions were applied.

The MeSH headings and text words applied (MEDLINE) were:

Condition MeSH: 'respiratory distress syndrome, adult'. Text words: 'Adult Respiratory Distress Syndrome', 'Acute Lung Injury', 'Acute Respiratory Distress Syndrome', 'ARDS', 'ALI'
Intervention MeSH: 'respiration, artificial'. Text words: 'lower tidal volume', 'protective ventilation', 'LPVS', 'pressure-limited'

The search was adapted for each database (EMBASE, CINAHL).

The Cochrane MEDLINE filter for randomized controlled trials was used (Dickersin et al 1994), see additional Table 04. A randomized controlled trial filter was also used for EMBASE (Lefebvre 1996). All the searches were limited to patients 16 years and older.

An additional hand search was focused on:

- references lists
- abstracts and proceedings of scientific meetings held on the subject.

In particular, proceedings of the Annual Congress of the European Society of Intensive Care Medicine (ESICM) and of the American Thoracic Society (ATS) were searched over the last 10 years.

The following databases were also searched:

- Biological abstracts
- ISI web of science
- Current Contents.

Data from unpublished trials and 'grey' literature were sought by:

- The System for Information on Grey Literature in Europe (SIGLE)
- The Index to Scientific and Technical Proceedings (from the Institute for Scientific Information, accessing via BIDS)
- Dissertation abstracts (DA). This database includes: CDI – Comprehensive Dissertation Index, DAI – Dissertation Abstracts International, MAI – Master Abstract International, ADD – American Doctoral Dissertation
- Index to Theses of Great Britain and Ireland
- Current Research in Britain (CRIB). This database also includes Nederlanse Onderzoek Databank (NOD), the Dutch current research database
- Web Resources: the meta Register of Controlled Trials (mRCT) (www.controlled-trials.com).

An informal inquiry was made through equipment manufacturers (Siemens, Puritan-Bennet, Comesa) in order to obtain any clinical studies performed before the implementation and marketing of new ventilatory modes on ventilators.

The original author(s) were contacted for clarification about content, study design and missing data, if needed.

with other strategies designed to find trials that are not indexed. An example is shown in Box 5.4.

These heroic searches are enormously time consuming but they are thought to be justified because there is evidence that the trials which are most difficult to locate tend to have different conclusions to more easily located trials. It has been shown that unpublished studies and studies published in languages other than English tend to have more negative estimates of the effects of interventions than trials published in English (for example, Easterbrook et al 1991, Egger et al 1997, Stern & Simes 1997). Hence systematic reviews which search only for published trials are said to be exposed to 'publication bias', and systematic reviews which search only for trials reported in English are said to be exposed to 'language bias'. Reviewers perform exhaustive searches because they believe this will minimize publication bias and language bias.[34] But it is possible that exhaustive searches create a greater problem than they solve. The studies that are hardest to find may also be, on average, lower quality trials that are potentially more biased than trials that are easier to find (Egger et al 2003). Exhaustive searches may substitute one sort of bias for another.

What constitutes an adequate search? How much searching must reviewers do to satisfy us that they have reviewed a nearly complete and sufficiently representative selection of relevant trials? It is clearly insufficient to search only Medline: a review of studies of the sensitivity of Medline searches for randomized trials found that Medline searches, even those conducted by trained searchers, identified only a relatively small proportion of the trials known to exist (range 17–82%, mean 51%; Dickersin et al 1994). It is desirable that the reviewers perform sensitive searches of several medical literature databases (say, at least two of Medline, Embase, CINAHL, PsychINFO) and at least one of the specialist databases such as the Cochrane Collaboration's Central Register of Clinical Trials (CENTRAL) or PEDro.

A further consideration is the recency of the review. Systematic reviews tend to date rather quickly because, in most fields of physiotherapy, new trials are being published all the time (Moseley et al 2002). The recency of reviews is particularly critical in fields that are being very actively researched. In actively researched fields, a systematic review that involved a comprehensive search but which was published 5 years ago is unlikely to provide a comprehensive overview of the findings of all relevant trials. In fact, there is often a lag of several years between when a search is conducted and the review is eventually published, so the search may be considerably older than the year of publication of the review suggests. The year in which the search was conducted is usually given in the Methods section of the review. For example, the systematic review of spinal manipulation for chronic headache by Bronfort and colleagues, published in 2001, was based on literature searches conducted up to 1998. In general, if the search in a systematic review was published more than a few years ago it may be better to use a more recent systematic review or, if a more recent review is not available, to supplement the systematic review by locating individual randomized trials published since the review.

Was the quality of the reviewed studies taken into account?

Many randomized trials are poorly designed and provide potentially seriously biased estimates of the effects of intervention. Consequently, if a systematic review is to obtain an unbiased estimate of the effects of intervention, it must ignore low quality studies.

The simplest way to incorporate quality assessments into the findings of a systematic review is to list minimum quality criteria for trials that are

---

[34] As we shall see in Chapter 7, clinical guidelines may involve the production of multiple systematic reviews, so they can be multiply heroic. The time-consuming nature of literature searches in systematic reviews is one reason why clinical guidelines tend to be developed at a national level.

to be considered in a review. Most (but not all) reviews specify that trials must be randomized. The consequence is that non-randomized trials are effectively ignored.

Excluding non-randomized trials protects against the allocation bias that potentially distorts findings of non-randomized trials. However, as we have seen, randomization alone does not guarantee protection from bias. Even randomized trials are exposed to other sources of bias, so it is not sufficient to require only that trials be randomized; it is necessary to apply additional quality criteria. Some systematic reviewers stipulate that a trial must also be subject- and assessor-blinded if it is to be considered in the review. An example of this is the review of spinal manipulation by Ernst & Harkness (2001). This review only considered randomized 'double-blind' trials.[35]

An alternative way to take into account trial quality in a review is to assess the quality of the trial using a checklist or scale. Earlier in this chapter we mentioned that there are now many such checklists and scales of trial quality, derived both from expert opinion and empirical research about what best discriminates biased and unbiased studies. This diversity reflects the fact that we do not yet know the best way to assess trial quality. The most popular methods used to assess trial quality in systematic reviews of physiotherapy are the Maastricht scale (Verhagen et al 1998b), the Cochrane Back Review Group criteria (van Tulder et al 2003), the Jadad scale (1996) and the PEDro scale (Maher et al 2003). Two of these, the Maastricht scale and the PEDro scale, generate a quality score (that is, they are scales), and the other two do not (they are checklists). There is a high degree of consistency of the criteria used in these four scales: the scales with more extensive criteria include all of the criteria in the less extensive scales.

In well-conducted reviews, assessments of trial quality are considered when drawing conclusions: the findings of high quality trials are weighted more heavily than the findings of low quality trials, and the degree of confidence expressed in the review's conclusions is determined, at least in part, by consideration of the quality of the trials.

If a scale has been used to assess quality, the quality score can be used to set a quality threshold. Trials with quality scores below this threshold are not used to draw conclusions. For example, in their systematic review of the effects of stretching before sport on muscle soreness and injury risk, Herbert & Gabriel (2002) indicated that only those trials with scores of at least 3 on the PEDro scale were considered in the initial analysis. This is an extension of the approach of specifying minimum criteria for inclusion in the trial. Another common alternative is to use a less formal approach, and simply comment on the quality of trials when drawing conclusions from them.[36]

---

[35] See the comment in footnote 28 regarding problems with interpretation of the term 'double-blinding'.

[36] Detsky et al (1992) discuss four ways of incorporating quality in systematic reviews: using threshold score as an inclusion criterion; use of quality score as a weight in statistical pooling; plotting effect size against quality score; and sequential combination of trial results based on quality score.

Box 5.5   Assessing validity of systematic reviews

Was it clear which studies were to be reviewed?
Look for a list of inclusion and exclusion criteria (that defines, for example, the patients or population, intervention and outcomes of interest).

Were most relevant studies reviewed?
Look for evidence that several key databases were searched with sensitive search strategies, and that the search was conducted recently.

Was the quality of the reviewed studies taken into account?
Did the trials have to satisfy minimum quality criteria to be considered in the review? Alternatively, was trial quality assessed using a scale or checklist, and were quality assessments taken into account when conclusions were drawn?

We do not yet know which of these approaches is best. There is the risk that quality thresholds are too low (biased trials are still given too much weight) or too high (important trials are ignored), or that quality criteria do not really discriminate between biased and unbiased trials (so the conclusion becomes a lottery). However, it seems reasonable to insist that trial quality should be taken into account in some way. Some reviews do not consider trial quality at all, and others assess trial quality but do not use these assessments in any way when drawing conclusions. Such reviews potentially base their findings on biased studies. Readers of systematic reviews should check that trial quality was taken into account when formulating a review's conclusions.

In conclusion, when appraising the validity of a systematic review, readers should consider whether the review clearly defined the scope and type of studies to be reviewed, whether an adequate search was conducted, and whether the quality of trials was taken into account when formulating conclusions (see Box 5.5). When not all criteria are satisfied, the reader needs to weigh up the magnitude of the threats to validity.

CRITICAL APPRAISAL OF EVIDENCE ABOUT EXPERIENCES

So far in this chapter we have considered the appraisal of studies of effects of interventions. Such studies use quantitative methods. But we saw in Chapter 3 other studies use qualitative methods. Both kinds of studies make useful contributions to knowledge and should be regarded as complementary rather than conflicting.

The particular strength of qualitative research is that it 'offers empirically based insight about social and personal experiences, which necessarily have a more strongly subjective – but no less real – nature than biomedical phenomena' (Giacomini et al 2002).

In this section we consider appraisal of qualitative research of experiences. As pointed out in Chapter 3, we use the term 'experiences' as a shorthand way of referring to the phenomena that qualitative research might explore, which also include attitudes, meanings, beliefs, interactions and processes.

Before beginning the process of appraisal it is first necessary to ask if an appropriate method has been used to address the research question. If the aim of the study is to explore social or human phenomena, or to gain deep insight into experiences or processes, then a qualitative methodology is appropriate.

In all kinds of research, no matter which method is used, it is necessary to observe phenomena in a systematic way and to describe and reflect upon the research findings. This applies equally well to qualitative research: insight emerges from systematic observations and their competent interpretation. Just as with quantitative research of effects of therapy, qualitative research is not uniformly of high quality. Although the adequacy of checklists and guidelines has been vigorously debated, and although it has been claimed that qualitative research cannot be assessed by a 'cookbook approach', scientific standards and checklists do exist (Seers 1999, Greenhalgh 2001, Malterud 2001, Giacomini et al 2002). The framework we will use for critical appraisal of qualitative studies is drawn from those sources. All sources emphasize that there is no definitive set of criteria for appraisal, and that the criteria should be continually revised. Consequently we see these criteria as a guide that we expect to change with time.

Qualitative research uses methods that are substantively different from most quantitative research. The methods differ with regard to sampling techniques, data collection methods and data analysis. Consequently, the criteria used to appraise qualitative research must differ from those used to appraise quantitative research. When critically appraising the methodological quality of qualitative research, you need to ask questions that focus on other elements and issues than those that are relevant to research which includes numbers and graphs. Appraisal should focus on the trustworthiness, credibility and dependability of the study's findings – the qualitative parallels of validity and reliability (Gibson & Martin 2003). Since qualitative research often seeks to discern subjective realities, interpretation of the research is frequently greatly influenced by the researcher's perspective. Consequently, a clear account of the process of collecting and interpreting data is needed. This is sometimes referred to as a decision trail (Seers 1999). Subjectivity is thus accounted for, though not eliminated. Subjectivity becomes problematic only when the perspective of the researcher is ignored (Malterud 2001).

When readers look to reports of qualitative research to answer clinical questions about experiences, we suggest they routinely consider the following three issues.

Was the sampling strategy appropriate?

Why was this sample selected? How was the sample selected? Were the subjects' characteristics defined?

In qualitative research we are not interested in an 'on average' view of a population. We want to gain an in-depth understanding of the experience of particular individuals or groups. The characteristics of individual study participants are therefore of particular interest.

The sample in qualitative research is often made up of individual people, but it can also consist of situations, social settings, social interactions or documents. The sample is usually strategically selected to contain subjects with relevant roles, perspectives or experiences.

> The methods of sampling randomly from populations, or sampling consecutive patients satisfying explicit criteria, common in quantitative research, are replaced in qualitative research by a process of conscious selection of a small number of individuals meeting particular criteria – a process called purposive sampling (Giacomini et al 2002).

People may be selected because they are typical or atypical, because they have some important relationship, or just because they are the most available subjects. Sometimes sampling occurs in an opportunistic way: one person leads the researcher to another person, and that person to one more, and so on. This is called snowball sampling (Seers 1999). Often the goal of sampling is to obtain as many perspectives as possible. The author should explain and justify why the participants in the study were the most appropriate to provide access to the type of knowledge sought by the study. If there have been any problems with recruitment (for example, if there were many people that were invited to participate but chose not to take part), this should be reported. And, as the aim is to gain in-depth and rich insight, the number of observations is not predetermined. Instead, data collection continues until all phenomena have emerged. Nonetheless, readers should expect to see an explanation of the number of observations or people included in the study and why it is thought this number was sufficient (Seers 1999).

Was the data collection sufficient to cover the phenomena?

Was the method used to collect data relevant? Were the data detailed enough to interpret what was being researched?

A range of very different methods is used to collect data in qualitative research. These vary from, for example, participant observations, to in-depth interviews, to focus groups, to document analysis. The data collection method should be relevant and address the questions raised, and should be justified in the research report. A common method in physiotherapy research involves the use of observations or in-depth interviews to explore communication and interactions of physiotherapists and patients. In-depth interviews are also used to explore experiences, meanings, attitudes, views and beliefs, for example the experiences of being a patient, or of having a certain condition, as in a study that explored stroke patients' motivation for rehabilitation (Maclean 2000). Focus groups might be a relevant method of identifying barriers and facilitators to lifestyle changes or understanding attitudes and behaviours, as demonstrated by Steen & Haugli (2001), who conducted focus groups to explore the significance of group participation for people with chronic musculoskeletal pain.

Sometimes qualitative research uses more than one data collection method to obtain a broader or deeper understanding of what is being studied. The use of more than one method of data collection can help to confirm or extend the analysis of different facets of the experience being studied. For example, the data from observations of a mother playing with her child with cerebral palsy might be supplemented by interviewing the mother about her attitudes and experiences.

In observations or interviews, the researcher becomes the link between the participants and the data. Consequently, the information collected is likely to be influenced by what the interviewer or researcher believes or has experienced. A rigorous study clearly describes where the data collection took place, the context of data collection, and why this context was chosen. A declaration of the researcher's point of view and perspectives is important, as these might influence both data collection and analysis. A critical reflection on the potential implications of influence and role should follow.

Data collection should be comprehensive enough in both breadth (type of observations) and depth (extent of each type of observation) to generate and support the interpretations. That means that as much data as possible should be collected. Often a first round of data collection suggests whether it is necessary to continue sampling in order to confirm the preliminary findings. Enough participants should be interviewed or revisited until emerging theories are either confirmed or refuted and no new views are obtained. This is often called saturation (Seers 1999). The point of saturation is the point at which the sample size becomes sufficient. A description of saturation reassures the reader that sufficient data were collected.

Another important question to ask about data collection is whether ethical issues have been taken into consideration. The ethics of a study do not have a direct bearing on the study's validity but may, nonetheless, influence a reader's willingness to read and use the findings of the study. In qualitative research, peoples' feelings and deeper thoughts are revealed and it is therefore important that issues around informed consent and confidentiality are clarified. In such situations we would like to see the authors describe how they have handled the effects on the participants during and after the study. This issue was raised after the publication of a project that explored interactions between two physiotherapists and their patients. The authors were criticized because they had characterized one physiotherapist as competent and caring and the other as incompetent and non-empathic. This conclusion was criticized on ethical grounds, and raised the importance of careful explanation of the study aim to the participants, and also how the results are to be presented. One good way of handling this is to invite participants to read a draft of the research report.[37] Having participants verify that the researcher's interpretation is accurate and

---

[37] This is controversial. Very few researchers ask participants to read a draft of the research report.

representative is also a common method for checking trustworthiness of the analysis (Gibson & Martin 2003).

Were the data analysed in a rigorous way?

Was the analytical path described? Was it clear how the researchers derived categories or themes from the data, and how they arrived at the conclusion? Did the researchers reflect on their roles in analysing the data?

The process of analysis in qualitative research should be rigorous. This is a challenging, complex and time-consuming job. The aim of this process is often to make sense of an enormous amount of text, tape recordings or video materials by reducing, summarizing and interpreting the data. The researchers often extend their conceptual frameworks into themes, patterns, hypotheses or theories; but ultimately they must communicate what their data mean. An in-depth description of the decision trail gives the reader a chance to follow the interpretations that have been made and to assess these interpretations in the light of the data.

An indication of a rigorous analysis is that the data are presented in a way that is clearly separated from the interpretation of the data. There should be sufficient data (e.g. transcripts) to justify the interpretation. Sometimes the data and the interpretation of the data are mixed up, and then it can be difficult to know what is the author's view and what is a reflection of a participant. Separation of these elements makes it possible for the reader to draw his or her own interpretations from the data. The reader should be satisfied that sufficient data were presented to support the findings.

In the analysis phase, researchers should reflect upon their own roles and influences in data selection and analysis. The reader needs to consider that the researcher may have presented a selection of the data that primarily reflects the researcher's pre-existing personal views. It is helpful if, when analysing and reporting the study, the investigator distinguishes between the knowledge of the participants, the knowledge that the researcher originally brought to the project, and the insights the researcher has gained along the way. The data can be considered to be more trustworthy when the researcher considers contradictory data and findings that do not support a defined theory or pattern, and discusses the strengths and weaknesses of each finding.

There are several features that can strengthen a reader's trust in the findings of a study. One is the use by the researchers of more than one source for information when studying the phenomena, for example the use of both observation and interviews. This is often called triangulation. Triangulation might involve the use of more than one method, more than one researcher or analyst, or more than one theory. The use of more than one investigator to collect and analyse the raw data (multiple coders) also strengthens the study. This means that findings emerge through consensus between multiple investigators, and it ensures themes are not missed (Seers 1999).

Box 5.6 summarizes this section.

Box 5.6   Assessing validity of individual studies of experiences

Was the sampling/recruitment strategy appropriate?
Why was this sample selected? How was the sample selected? Were the subjects' characteristics defined?

Was the data collection sufficient to cover the phenomena?
Was the method used to collect data relevant? Were the data detailed enough to interpret what was being researched?

Were the data analysed in a rigorous way?
Was the analytical path described? Was it clear how the researcher derived categories or themes from the data, and how they arrived at the conclusion? Did the researcher reflect on his or her role in analysing the data?

CRITICAL APPRAISAL OF EVIDENCE ABOUT PROGNOSIS

In Chapter 2 we considered two sorts of questions about prognosis: questions about what a person's outcome will be, and questions about how much we should modify our estimates of prognosis on the basis of particular prognostic characteristics.

Subsequently, in Chapter 3, we considered the types of studies that are likely to provide us with the best information about prognosis and prognostic factors. The best information is likely to come from cohort studies or, occasionally, from systematic reviews of cohort studies, but sometimes we can also get useful information from clinical trials.

In this section we consider how we can assess whether studies of prognosis are likely to be valid. We begin by considering individual studies of prognosis and then consider, very briefly, systematic reviews of prognosis.

INDIVIDUAL STUDIES OF PROGNOSIS

Was there representative sampling from a well-defined population?

If we are to derive useful information about prognoses from clinical research, we must be able to use the findings of the research to make inferences about prognoses of some larger population. We can only do this if the subjects participating in the research (the 'sample') are representative of the population we are interested in.

When we read studies of prognosis we first need to know which population the study is seeking to provide a prognosis for (the 'target population'). The target population is defined by the criteria used to determine who was eligible to participate in the study. Most studies of prognosis describe a list of inclusion and exclusion criteria that clearly identify the target population. For example, Coste et al (1994) conducted an inception cohort study of the prognosis of people presenting for primary medical care for acute low back pain. They stated that 'all consecutive patients aged 18 and over, self-referring to participating doctors ($n = 39$) for a primary complaint of back pain between 1 June and 7 November 1991 were eligible. Only patients with pain lasting less than 72 hours and without radiation below the gluteal fold were included. Patients with malignancies, infections, spondylarthropathies, vertebral fractures, neurological signs, and low back pain during the previous 3 months were excluded, as were non-French speaking and illiterate patients.' The target population for this study is clear.

A closely related issue concerns how subjects entered the study. This is critical because it determines whether the sample is representative of the target population.[38] In the clinical populations that are of most interest to physiotherapists, representativeness is usually best achieved by selecting a recruitment site and then recruiting into the study, as far as is possible, all subjects presenting to that site who satisfy the inclusion criteria. Recruitment of *all* eligible subjects ensures that the sample is representative. Studies in which all (or nearly all) eligible subjects enter the study are sometimes said to have sampled 'consecutive cases'. Where not all people who satisfy the inclusion criteria enter the study, it is possible that those who do not enter the study will have systematically different prognoses from those subjects who do enter the study. In that case the study will provide a biased estimate of prognosis in the target population. When a study recruits 'all' subjects or 'consecutive cases' that satisfy inclusion criteria (as in the study by Coste, cited in the last paragraph) we can be relatively confident that the findings of the study apply to a defined population. The greater the proportion of eligible subjects that participates in the study, the more representative the sample is likely to be.

Researchers may find it difficult to gather data from consecutive cases, particularly when participation in the study requires extra measurements be made over and above those that would normally be made as part of routine clinical practice. An example of a study that did not sample in a representative way is a study of the 'outcomes' (prognosis) of children with developmental torticollis (Taylor & Norton 1997). The researchers sampled 'twenty-three children (14 male, nine female) … diagnosed with developmental torticollis by a physician. … Most of the children (74%) were referred to physical therapy by pediatricians … Data were collected retrospectively from the initial physical therapy evaluations of the 23 children whose parents agreed to a follow-up evaluation.' Such samples may not always be representative; they may comprise subjects with particularly good or particularly bad prognoses. Consequently, samples of convenience can provide biased prognoses for the target population.

---

[38] There are two ways to claim representativeness. The first approach is to clearly define the population of interest and then sample from that population in a representative way, or in as representative a way as possible. The alternative approach is to sample in a non-representative way and then use the characteristics of the sample to dictate about whom inferences can be made. With the former approach, inferences can be made about the sorts of people who satisfy the study's inclusion and exclusion criteria. With the latter approach, inferences are made about people with characteristics like the study sample's characteristics. Of the two approaches, the first is preferable because it provides samples that are representative of the real population from which they were drawn. The second approach provides samples that are representative of virtual populations from which the sample could be imagined to have been drawn.

Failures to sample in a representative way (i.e. to sample consecutive cases) or to sample from a population that is well defined (absence of clear inclusion and exclusion criteria) commonly threaten the validity of studies of prognosis.

> When you read studies looking for information about prognosis, start by looking to see whether the study recruited 'all' patients or 'consecutive cases'. If it did not, the study may provide biased estimates of the true prognosis.

Was there an inception cohort?

At any point in time, many people may have the condition of interest. Some will have just developed the condition, and others may have had the condition for very long periods of time.

A study of prognosis could sample from the whole population of people who currently have the condition of interest. But samples obtained from the whole population of people who currently have the condition (called 'survivor cohorts') will tend to consist largely of people who have had the condition for a long time, and that introduces a potential bias. The bias arises because the prognosis of people with chronic conditions is likely to be quite different from the prognosis of people who have just developed the condition. With many conditions, the people with long-standing disease are those who fared badly; they have not yet recovered. For this reason, survivor cohorts can tend to generate unrealistically bad prognoses. With life-threatening diseases the opposite may be true: the people who have long-standing disease are the survivors; they may have a better prognosis than those who died quickly, so survivor cohorts of life-threatening diseases might generate unrealistically good prognoses. Either way, survivor cohorts potentially provide biased estimates of prognosis.

The solution is to recruit subjects at a uniform (usually early) point in the course of the disease.[39] Studies which recruit subjects in this way are said to recruit 'inception cohorts' because subjects were identified as closely as possible to the inception of the condition. The advantage of inception cohorts is that they are not exposed to the biases inherent in studies of survivor cohorts.

We have already seen examples of prognostic studies that used survivor cohorts and inception cohorts. In the study of prognosis of developmental muscular torticollis (Taylor & Norton 1997), the age of children with torticollis at the time of initial evaluation ranged from 3 weeks to 10.5 months. Clearly those children attending for assessments at 10.5 months are survivors, and their prognoses are likely to be worse than average. In contrast, Coste et al (1994) obtained their estimates of the prognosis of low back pain from an inception cohort of subjects who developed their current episode of back pain within the preceding 72 hours. Consequently, the Coste study is able to provide a relatively unbiased estimate of the prognosis of people with acute low back pain, at

---

[39] Subjects recruited at the point of disease onset are sometimes called 'incident cases'.

least among those who visit a general medical practitioner with that condition.

Readers of studies of prognosis should routinely look for evidence of recruitment of an inception cohort.

> Studies that recruit inception cohorts may provide less biased estimates of prognosis than studies that recruit survivor cohorts.

While many studies provide good evidence of the prognosis of acute conditions, relatively few provide good evidence of the prognosis of chronic conditions. This is because the dual requirements of sampling *consecutive* cases from an *inception cohort* are frequently not satisfied in studies of chronic conditions. What would a good study of the prognosis of a chronic condition look like? If we wanted to know about the prognosis for people with chronic low back pain we would need to look for studies that identify consecutive cases presenting with a current episode of back pain that had lasted for a homogenous period, say, between 3 and 4 months. In practice, relatively few studies of the prognosis of chronic conditions sample consecutively from uniform points in the course of the condition, so we have relatively little good evidence of the prognosis of chronic conditions.

Was there complete or near-complete follow-up?

Like clinical trials of effects of therapy, prognostic studies can be biased by loss to follow-up. Bias occurs if those lost to follow-up have, on average, different outcomes to those who were followed up.

It is easy to imagine how this might happen. A study of the prognosis of low back pain might incompletely follow-up subjects whose pain has resolved, perhaps because these subjects feel well and are disinclined to return for follow-up assessment. Such a study would necessarily base estimates of prognosis on the subjects who could be followed up. These subjects would have, on average, worse outcomes, and so such a study would provide a biased (unduly pessimistic) estimate of prognosis. In contrast, a study of the prognosis of motor function following stroke might only follow up subjects discharged to home, perhaps because of difficulties following up subjects discharged to nursing homes. The subjects followed up are likely to have better prognoses, on average, than those who were not followed up, so this study would provide a biased (unduly optimistic) estimate of prognosis.

How much of a loss to follow-up can be tolerated? As with clinical trials, losses to follow-up of less than 10% are unlikely to seriously distort estimates of prognoses,[40] and losses to follow-up of greater than 20% are usually of concern, particularly if there is any possibility that outcomes influenced follow-up. It may be reasonable to apply the same 85% rule that we applied to clinical trials of the effects of therapy: as a rough rule of thumb, the study is unlikely to be seriously biased by loss to follow-up if follow-up is at least 85%.

---

[40] Unless the probability of loss to follow-up is highly correlated with outcome.

An example of a study with a high degree of follow-up is the study of the prognosis of pregnancy-related pelvic pain by Albert et al (2001). These researchers followed 405 women who reported pelvic pain when presenting to an obstetric clinic during pregnancy. It was possible to verify the presence or absence of post-partum pain in all but 18 women, giving a post-partum loss to follow-up of just 4%. Such a low rate of loss to follow-up is unlikely to be associated with significant bias. On the other hand, Jette et al (1987) conducted a randomized trial to compare the effects of intensive rehabilitation and standard care on functional recovery over the 12 months following hip fracture. This study incidentally provides information about prognosis following hip fracture. However, loss to follow-up in the standard care group at 3, 6 and 12 months was 35%, 53% and 57%, respectively. The prognosis provided by this study is potentially seriously biased by a large loss to follow-up.

In large studies with long follow-up periods, or studies of serious disease, or studies of elderly subjects, it is likely that a substantial proportion of subjects will die during the follow-up period. (For example, in Allerbring & Heagerstam's (2004) study of orofacial pain, 13/74 patients had died at the 9–19 year follow-up, and in Jette et al's (1987) study of hip fracture, 29% of subjects died within 12 months). Should these subjects be counted as lost to follow-up? For all practical purposes the answer is 'no'. If we know a subject has died, we know that subject's outcome: this particular form of loss to follow-up is informative, and does not bias estimates of prognosis. We can consider death an outcome, which means that risk of death is considered as part of the prognosis, or we could focus on prognosis in survivors.

It is relatively easy to identify losses to follow-up in clinical trials and prospective cohort studies. In retrospective studies of prognosis it can be more difficult to ascertain the proportion lost to follow-up because it is not always clear who was entered into the study. In retrospective studies, loss to follow-up should be calculated as the proportion of all *eligible* subjects for whom follow-up data were available.

See Box 5.7 for a summary of this section.

Box 5.7   Assessing validity of individual studies of prognosis

Was there representative sampling from a well-defined population?
Did the study sample consecutive cases that satisfied clear inclusion criteria?

Was there an inception cohort?
Were subjects entered into the study at an early and uniform point in the course of the condition?

Was there complete or near complete follow-up?
Look for information about the proportion of subjects for whom follow-up data were available at key time points. Alternatively, calculate loss to follow-up from numbers of subjects entered into the study and the numbers followed up.

SYSTEMATIC REVIEWS OF PROGNOSIS

In Chapter 3 we pointed out that the preferred source of information about prognosis is systematic reviews. Systematic reviews of prognosis differ from systematic reviews of therapy in several ways. They need to employ different search strategies to find different sorts of studies, and they need to employ different criteria to assess the quality of the studies included in the review. Nonetheless, the methods of systematic reviews of prognosis are fundamentally similar to the methods of systematic reviews of the effects of therapy, so the process of assessing the validity of systematic reviews of prognosis is essentially the same as evaluating the validity of systematic reviews of therapy. That is, it is useful to ask if it was clear which trials were to be reviewed, if most relevant studies were reviewed, and if the quality of the reviewed studies was taken into account. As these characteristics of systematic reviews have already been considered in detail, we shall not elaborate on them further here.

CRITICAL APPRAISAL OF EVIDENCE ABOUT DIAGNOSTIC TESTS

Chapter 3 argued that questions about diagnostic accuracy are best answered by cross-sectional studies that compare the findings of the test in question with the findings of a reference standard. What features of such studies confer validity?

INDIVIDUAL STUDIES OF DIAGNOSTIC TESTS

Was there comparison with an adequate reference standard?

Interpretation of studies of diagnostic accuracy is most straightforward if the reference standard is perfectly accurate, or close to it. But it is difficult to know if the reference standard is accurate. Assessment of the accuracy of the reference standard would require comparing its findings with another reference standard, and we would then need to know *its* accuracy. So, realistically, we have to live with imperfect knowledge of the reference standard. Claims of the adequacy of a reference standard cannot be based on data. Instead they must rely on face validity. That is, ultimately our assessments of the adequacy of the reference standard must rely on our assessment of whether the reference standard appears to be the sort of measurement that would be more-or-less perfectly accurate.

An example of a reference standard that has apparent face validity is open surgical or arthroscopic confirmation of a complete tear of the anterior cruciate ligament. It is reasonable to believe that the diagnosis of a complete tear could be made unambiguously at surgery. On the other hand, the diagnosis of partial tears is more difficult, and the surgical presentation may be ambiguous. Thus open surgical exploration and arthroscopic examination are excellent reference standards for diagnosis of complete tears, but less satisfactory reference standards for partial tears.

When the reference standard is imperfect, the accuracy of the diagnostic test of interest will tend to be underestimated. This is because when the reference standard is imperfect we are asking the clinical test to do something that is impossible: if the test is to perform well, its findings must correspond with the incorrect findings of the reference standard as well as the correct ones.[41] Readers of studies of the accuracy of diagnostic tests that use imperfect reference standards should recognize that the true accuracy of the test may be higher than the observed accuracy.[42]

Was the comparison blind?

Studies of the accuracy of diagnostic tests can be biased in just the same way as randomized trials by the expectations of the person taking the measurements. If the person administering the diagnostic test (the 'assessor') is aware of the findings of the reference standard then, when the test's findings are difficult to interpret, he or she may be more inclined to interpret the test in a way that is consistent with the reference standard. In theory this could also happen in the other direction. When the reference standard is difficult to interpret, the assessor of the reference standard might be more inclined to interpret the findings in a way that is consistent with the diagnostic test. Either way, the consequence is the same: the effect will be to bias (inflate) estimates of diagnostic test accuracy.

It is relatively straightforward for the researcher to reduce the possibility of this bias. The simple solution is to ensure that the assessor is unaware, at the time he or she administers the diagnostic test, of the

---

[41] Some statistical techniques have been developed to correct estimates of the accuracy of diagnostic tests when there is error in the reference standard, but these techniques require knowledge of the degree of error in the reference standard or necessitate tenuous assumptions. They are not widely used in studies of diagnostic test accuracy.

[42] Two special problems arise in the studies of the accuracy of diagnostic tests used by physiotherapists. The first is that, while it is sometimes quite straightforward to determine if a test can accurately detect the presence or absence of a particular pathology, it may be difficult to determine if the test can accurately detect if that pathology is the cause of the person's symptoms. Consider the clinical question about whether, in people with stiff painful shoulders, O'Brien's test accurately discriminates between those people with and without complete tears of rotator cuff muscles. An answer to this question could be provided by a study that compared the findings of O'Brien's test and arthroscopic investigation. If, however, the question was whether O'Brien's test accurately discriminates between those people *whose symptoms are or are not due to* complete tears of rotator cuff muscles, it would be necessary for the reference standard to ascertain whether a patient's symptoms were due to the rotator cuff tear. Many older people have rotator cuff tears that are asymptomatic, so the arthroscopic finding of the presence of a rotator cuff tear cannot necessarily be interpreted as indicating that the person's symptoms are due to the tear. There is no reference standard for determining if symptoms are due to a rotator cuff tear, so we cannot ascertain if O'Brien's test can accurately determine if a rotator cuff tear is a cause of a person's symptoms.

A second problem arises in the diagnosis of conditions that are defined by a simple clinical presentation. For example, sciatica is defined by the presence of pain radiating down the leg. As the condition is defined in terms of pain radiating down the leg, there can be no reference standard beyond asking the patient where he or she experiences the pain. So it is generally not useful to ask questions about the diagnostic accuracy of tests for sciatica. There is no need to know the accuracy of tests for sciatica because it is obvious whether someone has sciatica from the clinical presentation. More generally, there is no point in testing the accuracy of a test for a diagnosis that is obvious without testing.

findings of the reference standard. If the assessor is unaware of the findings of the reference standard then the estimate of diagnostic accuracy cannot be inflated by assessor bias.

> Readers of studies of the accuracy of diagnostic tests should determine whether the clinical test and reference standard were conducted independently. That is, readers should ascertain if each test was conducted blind to the results of the other test.

Confirmation of the independence of the tests implies that estimates of diagnostic test accuracy from these trials were probably not distorted by assessor bias. The findings of studies which provide no evidence of the independence of tests should be considered potentially suspect.

A reasonably frequent scenario is that the diagnostic test is administered prior to the administration of the reference standard. When this is the case, the assessment of the diagnostic test is blind to the reference standard. This is more important than blinding the reference standard to the diagnostic test because the tester will usually feel less inclined to modify interpretation of the reference standard on the basis of a finding from the diagnostic test than he or she might feel inclined to modify interpretation of the diagnostic test on the basis of a finding on the reference standard. Consequently, studies in which the diagnostic test is consistently recorded prior to administration of the reference standard need not be a cause for serious concern.

Did the study sample consist of subjects in whom there was diagnostic uncertainty?

The last criterion we will consider is the least obvious, and yet there is some evidence that it is the criterion that best discriminates between biased and unbiased studies of diagnostic test accuracy.

In Chapter 3 we saw that there were two sorts of designs used in studies of the accuracy of diagnostic tests. The first type, sometimes called a cohort study, samples subjects who are suspected of having, but are not known to have, the condition that is being tested for. That is, cohort studies sample from the population that we would usually test in clinical practice. In clinical practice we only test people who we suspect of having the condition; we don't test if the diagnosis is not suspected, nor do we test if the diagnosis has been confirmed.

> Cohort studies provide the best way to evaluate diagnostic accuracy because they involve testing the discriminative accuracy of the diagnostic test in the same spectrum of patients that the test would be applied to in the course of clinical practice.

Such studies provide us with the best estimates of diagnostic test accuracy.

The alternative to the cohort design is the case–control design. Case–control studies recruit samples of subjects who clearly do and clearly do not have the diagnosis of interest. In Chapter 3 we saw the example of a study of the accuracy of Phalen's test for diagnosis of carpal tunnel syndrome which recruited one group of subjects (cases) with

> **Box 5.8   Assessing validity of individual studies of diagnostic tests**
>
> *Was there comparison with an adequate reference standard?*
> Were the findings of the test compared with the findings of a reference standard that is considered to have near-perfect accuracy?
>
> *Was the comparison blind?*
> Were the clinicians who applied the clinical tests unaware of the findings of the reference standard?
>
> *Did the study sample consist of subjects in whom there was diagnostic uncertainty?*
> Was there sampling of consecutive cases satisfying clear inclusion and exclusion criteria?

clinically and electromyographically confirmed carpal tunnel syndrome and another group (controls) who did not complain of any hand symptoms. The advantage of the case–control design is that it makes it relatively easy to obtain an adequate number of subjects with and without the diagnosis of interest. But there is a methodological cost: in case–control studies the test is subject to relatively gentle scrutiny. Case–control studies only require the test to discriminate between people who obviously do and obviously do not have the condition of interest. That is an easier task than the real clinical challenge of making accurate diagnoses on people who are suspected of having the diagnosis. Only cohort studies can tell us about the ability of a test to do that.

Analyses by Lijmer et al (1999) suggest that the strongest determinant of bias in studies of diagnostic test accuracy is the use of case–control designs.

> Readers should probably be suspicious of the findings of case–control studies of diagnostic test accuracy.

See Box 5.8 for a summary of this section.

SYSTEMATIC REVIEWS OF DIAGNOSTIC TESTS

The same criteria can be used to assess systematic reviews of diagnostic tests as were used to assess systematic reviews of the effects of interventions or systematic reviews of prognosis. Consequently, we shall not elaborate further on appraisal of systematic reviews of studies of diagnostic test accuracy.

References

Albert H, Godskesen M, Westergaard J 2001 Prognosis in four syndromes of pregnancy-related pelvic pain. Acta Obstetrica et Gynecologica Scandinavica 80:505–510

Allerbring M, Haegerstam G 2004 Chronic idiopathic orofacial pain. A long term follow-up study. Acta Odontologica Scandinavica 62:66–69

Anyanwu AC, Treasure T 2004 Surgical research revisited: clinical trials in the cardiothoracic surgical literature. European Journal of Cardiothoracic Surgery 25:299–303

Beecher HK 1955 The powerful placebo. JAMA 159: 1602–1606

Brody H 2000 The placebo response: recent research and implications for family medicine. Journal of Family Practice 49:649–654

Bronfort G, Assendelft WJ, Evans R et al 2001 Efficacy of spinal manipulation for chronic headache: a systematic review. Journal of Manipulative and Physiological Therapeutics 24:457–466

Campbell D, Stanley J 1963 Experimental and quasi-experimental designs for research. Rand-McNally, Chicago

Chalmers TC, Celano P, Sacks HS et al 1983 Bias in treatment assignment in controlled clinical trials. New England Journal of Medicine 309:1358–1361

Colditz GA, Miller JN, Mosteller F 1989 How study design affects outcomes in comparisons of therapy. I: Medical. Statistics in Medicine 8:441–454

Cook TD, Campbell DT 1979 Quasi-experimentation: design and analysis issues for field settings. Houghton Mifflin, Boston

Coste J, Delecoeuillerie G, Cohen de Lara A et al 1994 Clinical course and prognostic factors in acute low back pain: an inception cohort study in primary care practice. BMJ 308:577–580

Dean CM, Shepherd RB 1997 Task-related training improves performance of seated reaching tasks after stroke. A randomized controlled trial. Stroke 28:722–728

de Bie RA, de Vet HC, Lenssen TF et al 1998 Low-level laser therapy in ankle sprains: a randomized clinical trial. Archives of Physical Medicine and Rehabilitation 79:1415–1420

Department of Clinical Epidemiology and Biostatistics 1981 How to read clinical journals: I. why to read them and how to start reading them critically. Canadian Medical Association Journal 124:555–558

Detsky AS, Naylor CD, O'Rourke K et al 1992 Incorporating variations in the quality of individual randomized trials into meta-analysis. Journal of Clinical Epidemiology 45:255–265

Dickersin K, Scherer R, Lefebvre C 1994 Systematic reviews: identifying relevant studies for systematic reviews. BMJ 309:1286–1291

Dickinson K, Bunn F, Wentz R et al 2000 Size and quality of randomised controlled trials in head injury: review of published studies. BMJ 320:1308–1311

Easterbrook PJ, Berlin JA, Gopalan R et al 1991 Publication bias in clinical research. Lancet 337:867–872

Ebenbichler GR, Erdogmus CB, Resch KL et al 1999 Ultrasound therapy for calcific tendinitis of the shoulder. New England Journal of Medicine 340:1533–1538

Egger M, Zellweger-Zahner T, Schneider M et al 1997 Language bias in randomised controlled trials in English and German. Lancet 347:326–329

Egger M, Bartlett C, Holenstein F et al 2003 How important are comprehensive literature searches and the assessment of trial quality in systematic reviews? Empirical study. Health Technology Assessment 7:1–76

Ernst E, Harkness E 2001 Spinal manipulation: a systematic review of sham-controlled, double-blind, randomized clinical trials. Journal of Pain and Symptom Management 22:879–889

Fung KP, Chow OK, So SY 1986 Attenuation of exercise-induced asthma by acupuncture. Lancet 2(8521–22): 1419–1422

Giacomini M, Cook D, Guyatt G 2002 Qualitative research. In: Guyatt G, Rennie D and the Evidence-Based Medicine Working Group (eds) Users' guide to the medical literature. A manual for evidence-based physiotherapy practice. [Book with CD-ROM.] American Medical Association, Chicago

Gibson B, Martin D 2003 Qualitative research and evidence-based physiotherapy practice. Physiotherapy 89:350–358

Gould SJ 1997 The mismeasure of man. Penguin, London

Green J, Forster A, Bogle S 2002 Physiotherapy for patients with mobility problems more than 1 year after stroke: a randomised controlled trial. Lancet 359:199–203

Green S, Buchbinder R, Glazier R et al 1998 Systematic review of randomised controlled trials of interventions for painful shoulder: selection criteria, outcome assessment, and efficacy. BMJ 316:354–360

Greenhalgh T 2001 How to read a paper. BMJ Books, London

Gruber W, Eber E, Malle-Scheid D 2002 Laser acupuncture in children and adolescents with exercise induced asthma. Thorax 57:222–225

Guyatt GH, Rennie D 1993 Users' guides to the medical literature. JAMA 270:2096–2097

Herbert RD, Gabriel M 2002 Effects of pre- and post-exercise stretching on muscle soreness, risk of injury and athletic performance: a systematic review. BMJ 325:468–472

Hinman RS, Crossley KM, McConnell J et al 2003 Efficacy of knee tape in the management of osteoarthritis of the knee: blinded randomised controlled trial. BMJ 327:125

Hrobjartsson A, Götsche PC 2001 Is the placebo powerless? An analysis of clinical trials comparing placebo with no treatment. New England Journal of Medicine 344:1594–1602

Jadad AR, Moore RA, Carroll D et al 1996 Assessing the quality of reports of randomized clinical trials: is blinding necessary? Controlled Clinical Trials 17:1–12

Jette AM, Harris BA, Cleary PD et al 1987 Functional recovery after hip fracture. Archives of Physical Medicine and Rehabilitation 68:735–740

Kienle GS, Kiene H 1997 The powerful placebo effect: fact or fiction? Journal of Clinical Epidemiology 50:1311–1318

Kjaergard LL, Frederiksen SL, Gluud C 2002 Validity of randomized clinical trials in gastroenterology from 1964–2000. Gastroenterology 122:1157–1160

Kleinhenz J, Streitberger K, Windeler J et al 1999 Randomised clinical trial comparing the effects of acupuncture and a newly designed placebo needle in rotator cuff tendinitis. Pain 83:235–241

Kunz R, Oxman AD 1998 The unpredictability paradox: review of empirical comparisons of randomised and non-randomised clinical trials. BMJ 317:1185–1190

Lavori PW, Louis TA, Bailar JC et al 1983 Designs for experiments: parallel comparisons of treatment. New England Journal of Medicine 309:1291–1299

Lijmer JG, Mol BW, Heisterkamp S et al 1999 Empirical evidence of design-related bias in studies of diagnostic tests. JAMA 282:1061–1066

McLachlan Z, Milne EJ, Lumley J et al 1991 Ultrasound treatment for breast engorgement: a randomised double blind trial. Australian Journal of Physiotherapy 37:23–28

Maclean N, Pound P, Wolfe C et al 2000 Qualitative analysis of stroke patients' motivation for rehabilitation. BMJ 321:1051–1054

McMahon AD 2002 Study control, violators, inclusion criteria and defining explanatory and pragmatic trials. Statistics in Medicine 21:1365–1376

Maher CG, Sherrington C, Herbert RD et al 2003 Reliability of the PEDro scale for rating quality of randomized controlled trials. Physical Therapy 83:713–721

Malterud K 2001 Qualitative research: standards, challenges and guidelines. Lancet 358:483–489

Moher D, Pham B, Cook D et al 1998 Does quality of reports of randomised trials affect estimates of intervention efficacy reported in meta-analyses? Lancet 352:609–613

Moher D, Schulz KF, Altman DG 2001 The CONSORT statement: revised recommendations for improving the quality of reports of parallel group randomized trials. BMC Medical Research Methodology 1:2

Moher D, Sampson M, Campbell K et al 2002 Assessing the quality of reports of randomized trials in pediatric complementary and alternative medicine. BMC Pediatrics 2:2

Moseley AM, Herbert RD, Sherrington C et al 2002 Evidence for physiotherapy practice: a survey of the Physiotherapy Evidence Database (PEDro). Australian Journal of Physiotherapy 48:43–49

Nathan PE, Stuart SP, Dolan SL 2000 Research on psychotherapy efficacy and effectiveness: between Scylla and Charybdis? Psychological Bulletin 126:964–981

Pengel HL 2004 Outcome of recent onset low back pain. PhD thesis, School of Physiotherapy, University of Sydney

Petrucci N, Iacovelli W 2003 Ventilation with lower tidal volumes versus traditional tidal volumes in adults for acute lung injury and acute respiratory distress syndrome (Cochrane review). The Cochrane Library, Issue 3. Wiley, Chichester

Powell J, Heslin J, Greenwood R 2002 Community based rehabilitation after severe traumatic brain injury: a randomised controlled trial. Journal of Neurology, Neurosurgery and Psychiatry 72:193–202

Quinones D, Llorca J, Dierssen T et al 2003 Quality of published clinical trials on asthma. Journal of Asthma 40:709–719

Raghunathan TE 2004 What do we do with missing data? Some options for analysis of incomplete data. Annual Review of Public Health 25:99–117

Robinson KA, Dickersin K 2002 Development of a highly sensitive search strategy for the retrieval of reports of controlled trials using PubMed. International Journal of Epidemiology 31:150–153

Sackett DL, Straus SE, Richardson WS et al 2000 Evidence-based medicine. How to practice and teach EBM, 2nd edn. Churchill Livingstone, Edinburgh

Schiller L 2001 Effectiveness of spinal manipulative therapy in the treatment of mechanical thoracic spine pain: a pilot randomized clinical trial. Journal of Manipulative and Physiological Therapeutics 24:394–401

Schulz KF, Grimes DA 2002 Allocation concealment in randomised trials: defending against deciphering. Lancet 359:614–618

Schulz K, Chalmers I, Hayes R et al 1995 Empirical evidence of bias: dimensions of methodological quality associated with estimates of treatment effects in controlled trials. JAMA 273:408–412

Schwartz D, Lellouch J 1967 Explanatory and pragmatic attitudes in therapeutical trials. Journal of Chronic Diseases 20:637–648

Seers K 1999 Qualitative research. In: Dawes M, Davies P, Gray A et al (eds) Evidence-based practice. A primer for health care professionals. Churchill Livingstone, London

Soares HP, Daniels S, Kumar A et al 2004 Bad reporting does not mean bad methods for randomised trials: observational study of randomised controlled trials performed by the Radiation Therapy Oncology Group. BMJ 328:22–24

Steen E, Haugli L 2001 From pain to self-awareness: a qualitative analysis of the significance of group participation for persons with chronic musculoskeletal pain. Patient Education and Counselling 42:35–46

Stern JM, Simes RJ 1997 Publication bias: evidence of delayed publication in a cohort study of clinical research projects. BMJ 315:640–645

Taylor JL, Norton ES 1997 Developmental muscular torticollis: outcomes in young children treated by physical therapy. Pediatric Physical Therapy 9:173–178

van der Heijden GJ, Leffers P, Wolters PJ et al 1999 No effect of bipolar interferential electrotherapy and pulsed ultrasound for soft tissue shoulder disorders: a randomised controlled trial. Annals of the Rheumatic Diseases 58:530–540

van Tulder M, Furlan A, Bombardier C et al 2003 Updated method guidelines for systematic reviews in the Cochrane Collaboration back review group. Spine 28:1290–1299

Verhagen AP, de Vet HC, de Bie RA et al 1998a The Delphi list: a criteria list for quality assessment of randomized clinical trials for conducting systematic reviews developed by Delphi consensus. Journal of Clinical Epidemiology 51:1235–1241

Verhagen AP, de Vet HC, de Bie RA et al 1998b Balneotherapy and quality assessment: interobserver reliability of the Maastricht criteria list and the need for blinded quality assessment. Journal of Clinical Epidemiology 51:335–341

Vickers AJ, de Craen AJM 2000 Why use placebos in clinical trials? A narrative review of the methodological literature. Journal of Clinical Epidemiology 53:157–161

Zar HJ, Brown G, Donson H et al 1999 Home-made spacers for bronchodilator therapy in children with acute asthma: a randomised trial. Lancet 354(9183):979–982

Chapter 6

What does this evidence mean for my practice?

CHAPTER CONTENTS

OVERVIEW

Interpretation of clinical research involves assessing, firstly, the relevance of the research. This may involve consideration of the type of subjects and outcomes in the study, as well as the way in which the intervention was applied (for studies of the effectiveness of an intervention), or the context of the phenomena being studied (for studies of experience), or the way in which the test was administered (for studies of the accuracy of a diagnostic test). Relevant studies can provide answers to clinical questions. Estimates of the average effects of interventions can be obtained from the difference in outcomes of treated and control groups. Answers to questions about experiences might be in the form of descriptions or theoretical insights or theories. Prognoses may be quantitative estimates of the expected magnitude of an outcome or the probability of an event. The accuracy of diagnostic tests is best expressed in terms of likelihood ratios.

WHAT DOES THIS RANDOMIZED TRIAL MEAN FOR MY PRACTICE?

IS THE EVIDENCE RELEVANT TO ME AND MY PATIENT/S?

If, having asked the questions about validity in Chapter 5, we are satisfied that the evidence is likely to be valid, we can proceed to the second step of critical appraisal. This involves assessing the relevance (or 'generalizability', or 'applicability' or 'external validity') of the evidence. This is an important step. Indeed, one of the major criticisms of randomized trials and systematic reviews of effects of therapies has been that they often do not address the questions asked by physiotherapists and patients.

Readers should ask the following three questions about relevance.

Are the subjects in the study similar to the patients to whom I wish to apply the study's findings?

We read clinical trials and systematic reviews because we want to use their findings to assist clinical decision-making. This can only be done if we are prepared to make inferences about what will happen to *our* patients on the basis of outcomes in *other* patients (the subjects in clinical trials). How reasonable is it to use clinical trials to make inferences about effects of therapy on our patients?

The process of using trials to make inferences about our patients is convoluted. First, we use the sample to make inferences about a hypothetical population: the universe of all people from which the sample could be considered to have been randomly selected (Efron & Tibshirani 1993). This is the role of inferential statistics; we will consider this step in detail in the next section. Then we 'particularize' (Lilford & Royston 1998) from the hypothetical population to individual patients or particular sets of patients. That is, we make inferences about individual patients from our understanding of how hypothetical populations behave. We will consider this second step a little further.

We can most confidently use clinical trials to make inferences about the effects of therapy on our own patients when the patients and interventions in those trials are similar to the patients and interventions we wish to make inferences about. Obviously, the more similar the patients in a trial are to our patients, and the more similar the interventions in a trial are to the interventions we are interested in, the more confidently we can use those trials to inform our clinical decisions. In this section we consider the issue of making inferences about particular patients: how similar must patients in a trial be to the particular patients we are interested in? How can we decide if patients are similar enough to reasonably make such inferences?

Immediately we run into a problem. On what dimensions do we measure similarity? What characteristics of subjects are we most concerned about? Is it critical that the patients have the same diagnosis, or the same disease severity, or the same access to social support, or the same attitudes to therapy? Or do they need to be similar in all these dimensions? To answer these questions we need to know, or at least have some feeling for, the major 'effect modifiers'. That is, we need to know what factors most influence how patients respond to a particular therapy. We would like major effect modifiers of subjects in a clinical trial to be similar to the patients we want to make inferences about. But, as we shall see below, it is very difficult to obtain objective evidence about effect modifiers. Consequently, when we make decisions about whether subjects in a trial are sufficiently similar to the patients we wish to make inferences about, we must base our decisions on our personal impressions of the importance of particular factors.

One factor that sometimes generates particular controversy is the diagnosis. First, diagnostic labels are often applied inconsistently. One physiotherapist's reflex sympathetic dystrophy is another physiotherapist's shoulder–hand syndrome, and one physiotherapist's posterior tibial compartment syndrome is another physiotherapist's tibial stress syndrome. The precise clinical presentation of patients in a clinical trial may not be clear from descriptions of their diagnoses. When this is the case it may be difficult to know precisely to whom the trial findings can be applied. A greater problem arises when several diagnostic taxonomies co-exist or overlap, because readers may want the diagnosis to be based on a taxonomy that is not reported. Thus, a trial of manipulation for low back pain might report that subjects have acute non-specific low back pain (a taxonomy based on duration of symptoms), but some readers will ask if these patients had disc lesions or facet lesions (they are interested in a pathological taxonomy); others will ask if the patients had stiff joints (their taxonomy is based on palpation findings); and others will ask if the patients had a derangement syndrome (they use a taxonomy based on McKenzie's theory of low back pain). There are many taxonomies for classifying low back pain, and patients cannot be (or never are) classified according to all taxonomies. The reason we have many taxonomies is that we do not know which taxonomies best differentiate prognosis or responses to therapy. That is, we do not know which taxonomy is the strongest effect modifier. A consequence of the diversity of taxonomies is that readers of clinical trials are frequently not satisfied that the patients in a trial are 'similar enough' to the patients about whom they wish to make inferences.

But there is a paradox here. Readers of clinical trials may be least prepared to use the findings of clinical trials when they most need them. For some interventions there is an enormous diversity in the indications for therapy applied by different therapists. A case in point is manipulation for neck pain (Jull 2002). A small number of physiotherapists, and many chiropractors, would routinely manipulate people with neck pain. Others may restrict manipulation to only those patients with non-irritable symptoms who do not respond to gentler mobilization techniques. Yet other physiotherapists never manipulate necks, under any circumstances. Conscientious and informed physiotherapists sit at either end of the spectrum. This diversity of practice suggests that at least some therapists, possibly all, are not applying therapy to an optimal spectrum of cases. We just do not have precise information on who is best treated with manipulation. That is, we do not know with any certainty what the important effect modifiers are for treatment of neck pain with manipulation. Under these circumstances, when there is a diversity of practice with regards to indications for therapy, the readers of a clinical trial may not be prepared to accept the trial's findings because the subjects in the trial did not necessarily satisfy the reader's impressions of appropriate indications for therapy. When we least know who best to apply therapy to, physiotherapists are most reluctant to accept the findings of clinical trials. The paradox is that, when readers most need information from clinical trials, they may be most prepared to ignore them.

A simplistic solution to the problem of identifying subgroups of patients who would most benefit from therapy might involve more detailed analysis of trial data. Readers could look for analyses designed to see if subgroups of patients, patients with certain characteristics, respond particularly well or particularly badly to therapy. This information could inform decisions about whether appropriate inclusion and exclusion criteria were used in subsequent clinical trials. Unfortunately, it is usually very difficult to identify subgroups of responders and non-responders with subgroup analyses. This is because subgroup analyses are typically exposed to a high risk of statistical errors: they will typically fail to detect true differences between subgroups when they exist *and* they may be prone to identify spurious differences between subgroups as well.[1] One of the consequences is that subgroup analyses must usually be considered to be exploratory rather than definitive. Usually the best estimate of the effect of an intervention is the estimate of the average effect of the intervention in the whole population (Yusuf et al 1991).

> The best that a clinical trial can tell us about the effects of an intervention on patients with particular characteristics is the average effect of the intervention on the heterogenous population from which that patient was drawn.

That said, common sense must prevail. Some characteristics of subjects in trials could well be important. For example, trials of motor training for patients with acute stroke may well not be relevant to patients with chronic stroke because the mechanisms of recovery in these two groups could be quite different. Occasionally, trials sample from populations for whom the intervention is patently not indicated. Such trials should not be used to assess the effectiveness of the therapy. The reader must assess whether subjects in a trial *could* be those for whom therapy is indicated, or *could be* similar enough to those patients they want to make inferences about, given the current understanding of the mechanisms of therapy.

There is a simple conclusion from this rather philosophical discussion. It is difficult to know with any certainty which patients an intervention is

---

[1] These issues have been studied intensively. Accessible treatments of this subject are those by Yusuf et al (1991), Moyé (2000) and Brookes et al (2001). Alternatively, readers might prefer to consult the light-hearted and equally illuminating reports of the effects of DICE therapy (Counsell et al 1994) and the analysis of effects of astrological star sign in the ISIS II trial (Second International Study of Infarct Survival Collaborative Group 1988).

likely to benefit most. Consequently, readers of clinical trials should not be too fussy about the characteristics of subjects in a clinical trial.

> If patients in a trial are broadly representative of the patients we want to make inferences about, then we should be prepared to use the findings of the trial for clinical decision-making. It is only when there are strong grounds to believe that the patients in a trial are clearly different to those for whom therapy is indicated that we should be dismissive of a trial's findings on the basis of the subjects in the trial.

To some, this approach seems to ignore everything that theory and clinical experience can tell us about who will respond most to therapy. The reader appears to be faced with a choice between accepting the findings of clinical trials without considering the characteristics of patients in the trial, or ignoring clinical trials altogether. That is, there appears to be a choice between the unbiased but possibly irrelevant conclusions of high quality clinical trials and relevant but possibly biased clinical intuition. This suggests a compromise: a sensible way to proceed is to use estimates of the effects of therapy as a starting point, but to modify these estimates on the basis of clinical intuition. We will return to this idea in more detail later in the chapter.

Were interventions applied appropriately?

We have just considered how the selection of patients in a clinical trial may affect our decision about the trial's relevance to our patients. Exactly the same considerations apply to the way in which interventions were applied. Just as some readers will choose to ignore clinical trials whose subjects differ in some way from the patients about whom the reader wishes to make inferences, we could choose to ignore clinical trials that apply the intervention in a way that differs from the way that we might apply it.

A specific example concerns electrotherapy. There have now been a large number of clinical trials in electrotherapy (at the time of writing, around 700 randomized trials). For the most part they are not very flattering. Most of the relevant high quality trials suggest that electrotherapies have little clinically worthwhile effect. Nonetheless, Laakso and colleagues (2002) have argued that it would not be appropriate to dismiss electrotherapies as ineffective because all possible permutations of doses and methods of administration have not yet been subjected to clinical trials. They argue that trials may not yet have investigated the optimal modes for administering interventions and that future clinical trials may identify optimally effective modes of administration that produce clinically worthwhile effects.

The counterargument mirrors that in the preceding section. It is very difficult to identify precise characteristics of optimally administered therapy. Indeed, it would seem impossible to expect that we could know with any certainty about how *best* to apply a therapy before we have first established with some certainty that the therapy is generally effective. As there are usually many ways an intervention could be applied, it will usually be impossibly inefficient to examine all possible ways of administering the therapy in randomized trials. The same paradox applies: when we don't know how best to apply a therapy there is likely to be diversity of practice, and when there is diversity of practice readers are least inclined to accept the findings of clinical trials because, they argue, therapy was not applied in the way they consider to be optimal. But this is not a workable approach: when we don't know the best way to apply therapy we cannot be too fussy about how therapy is applied in a clinical trial.

On the other hand, where theory provides clear guidelines about how a therapy ought to be administered, there is no point in basing clinical decisions on trials that have clearly applied therapy in an inappropriate way. Several clinical trials have investigated the effects of inspiratory muscle training on dyspnoea in people with chronic airways disease (reviewed by Lotters et al 2002). But many of these trials (30 of 57 identified by Lotters et al) utilized training intensities of less than 30% of maximal inspiratory pressure. Laboratory research suggests that much higher training intensities (perhaps >60% of maximal force) are required to increase strength, at least in appendicular muscles (McDonagh & Davies 1984). So it would be inappropriate to base conclusions about the effects of inspiratory muscle training on studies which use low training intensities.

What practical recommendations can be made?

> A sensible approach to critical appraisal of clinical trials might be to consider whether the intervention was administered in a theoretically reasonable way. We should choose to disregard clinical trials that apply therapy in a way that is clearly and unambiguously inappropriate. However, where there is uncertainty about how best to apply a therapy we should be prepared to accept the findings of the trial, even if the therapy was administered in a way that differs to the way we may have chosen to provide the therapy, at least until better evidence becomes available.

We conclude this section by considering how trial design influences what can be inferred about intervention. In Chapter 3 we indicated that there are three broad types of contrasts in controlled clinical trials: trials can either compare an intervention with no intervention, standard intervention plus a new intervention with standard intervention alone, or two interventions. The nature of the contrast between groups determines what inferences can be drawn from the trial. Thus, a trial which randomizes subjects to receive either an exercise programme or no intervention can be used to make inferences about how much more effective exercise is than no intervention, whereas a trial which randomizes subjects to receive either advice to remain active and an exercise programme or advice alone can be used to make inferences about how much more effective exercise and advice are than advice alone. In one sense, both trials tell us about the effects of an exercise programme, but they tell us something slightly different: the former tells us about the effects of exercise in isolation, whereas the latter tells us about the supplementary effects of exercise, over and above the effects of advice. The two may differ if there is an interaction between the co-interventions. (In this example, we might expect that the effects of exercise would be smaller if all subjects received advice to remain active.)

Are the outcomes useful?

Good therapeutic interventions are those that make people's lives better. When we ask questions about the effects of an intervention, we most need to know if the therapy improves the quality of people's lives.

What is a 'better' life? Is it a life free from suffering, or a happy life, a life filled with satisfaction, or something else? If clinical trials are to tell us about the effects of an intervention, what are they to measure? Clinical trials may provide indirect measures of people's suffering, but they rarely report the effects of therapy on happiness or satisfaction. The closest clinical trials get to telling us about outcomes that are really worth knowing about is probably 'health-related quality of life'. Health-related quality of life is usually assessed with patient-administered questionnaires.

In principle there are two sorts of measures of health-related quality of life: generic measures, designed to allow comparison across disease types, and disease-specific measures (Guyatt et al 1993). Two examples of generic measures of quality of life are the SF-36 and the EuroQol. Examples of specific measures of quality of life are those designed for people suffering from respiratory disease (the Chronic Respiratory Disease Questionnaire; Guyatt et al 1987) and rheumatoid arthritis (the RAQol; e.g. Tijhuis et al 2001). Disease-specific measures of quality of life focus on the dimensions of quality of life that most affect people with that disease, so they tend to be more sensitive, and they usually provide more useful information for clinical decision-making.

But many clinical trials, probably a majority, do not attempt to directly measure quality of life. Instead they measure variables that are thought to directly relate to, or are a component of, quality of life. Examples include measures of pain, disability or function, dyspnoea and exercise capacity. In so far as these measures are related to quality of life, they can help us make decisions about intervention.

Sometimes the variables that relate most closely to quality of life cannot easily be measured. A work-around used in many trials is to measure more easily measured outcomes that are known to be related to the construct of interest. The measured outcome (sometimes referred to as a 'surrogate' measure) acts as a proxy for the construct of real interest. An example arises in trials of the effects of an exercise programme for post-menopausal women with osteoporosis. Exercise programmes are offered to post-menopausal women with or at risk of osteoporosis, with the aim of reducing fracture risk. But it is very difficult to conduct trials which assess the effects of exercise on fracture risk. Such trials must monitor very large numbers of people for long periods of time in order to observe enough fractures.[2] The easier alternative is to assess the effects of exercise on bone density. Many trials have measured the effects of exercise programmes on bone density because the effects of exercise on bone density can be assessed in much smaller trials. Other examples of surrogate measures in clinical trials in physiotherapy are measures of postural sway (sometimes used as a surrogate for falls risk in trials of falls prevention programmes; Sherrington et al 2004) and measurement of performance on lung function tests (used as a surrogate for respiratory morbidity in trials of interventions for cystic fibrosis; McIlwaine et al 2001).

---

[2] For example, according to the usual conventions, if the 1-year fracture risk in control subjects was 5% and we wanted to be able to reliably detect reductions in risk of 2% or more, we would need to see 3000 subjects in the trial.

Trials that measure surrogate measures potentially provide us with answers to our clinical questions. However, there are two reasons why such trials may appear to be more useful than they really are. First, our primary interest in clinical trials stems from their potential to provide us with clinically useful estimates of the effects of intervention (more on this in the next section), yet it may be very difficult to get a sense for the effect of an intervention by looking at surrogate measures. It is easier to interpret a trial that tells us exercise reduces 1-year fracture risk from 5% to 3% than a trial that tells us exercise increases bone density by $6\,mg/cm^3$ at 1 year.[3] A more serious concern is that the surrogate and the construct of interest may become uncoupled as a result of intervention. That is, it may be that the surrogate measure and the outcome of interest respond differently to intervention. There have been notorious examples from medicine in which drugs that had been shown to have beneficial effects on surrogate outcomes were subsequently shown to produce harmful effects on clinically important outcomes. For example, encainide and flecainide were known to reduce ventricular ectopy (a surrogate outcome) following myocardial infarction, but a randomized trial (Echt et al 1991) showed that these drugs substantially increased mortality[4] (a clinically important outcome). We can rarely be sure that surrogate measures provide us with valid indications of the effect of therapy on the constructs we are truly interested in (de Gruttola et al 2001).

One of the reasons that not all clinical trials measure quality of life is the concern that such measures may not be sensitive to effects of intervention. Indeed, some trialists believe that generic quality of life measures such as the SF-36 are generally not useful in clinical trials because they may change little, even when there are apparent changes in a patient's condition. It is true that outcome measures in clinical trials are only useful if they are sensitive to clinically important change. However, there may be circumstances in which interventions produce effects that are clinically evident but not clinically important. An example might be an intervention that produces more muscle activity in the hemiparetic hand after stroke, but which does not produce appreciable improvements in hand function. Outcomes measures in clinical trials must be capable of detecting changes that are important to patients,[5] but they need not always be sensitive to clinically evident change.

---

[3] The best way to make sense of this result would be to look at well-designed epidemiological studies which try to quantify the effects of bone density on fracture risk.

[4] Over the mean 10-month follow-up in this trial, 23 of 743 subjects receiving placebo therapy, and 64 of 746 patients receiving encainide or flecainide died. As we shall see later in this chapter, this implies that encainide and flecainide killed one in every 18 patients to whom it was administered.

[5] This does not mean that the outcome measure must be sensitive to change in *individual* patients. One factor that limits sensitivity to change of measures on individual patients is random measurement error. Random measurement error can be quantified with a range of indices, including the minimal change detectable with 90% certainty, or MDC90. But random measurement errors are of much less concern in clinical trials because they average out across subjects. Trials with equal sample sizes in each group can detect effects of the order of $MDC90 \times (2/n)^{-2}$, where n is the number of subjects in each group. Thus a trial with 100 subjects in each group may be able to detect effects of the order of one-fifth of the change that is detectable on a single patient.

Some clinical trials do not measure outcomes that matter to patients. This may be because the trialists are interested in questions about the mechanisms by which interventions have their effects, rather than in whether the intervention is worth applying in clinical practice. For example, Meyer et al (2003) randomized subjects with reduced ventricular function to either a 2-month high intensity residential exercise training programme or to a control group. They measured indices of ventilatory gas exchange, blood lactate and arterial blood gas levels, cardiac output and pulmonary artery and wedge pressures. The effect of exercise on these outcomes may be of considerable interest because it is important to know the physiological effects of exercise in the presence of ventricular failure. However, the outcomes have no intrinsic importance to patients, so the trial cannot tell us if the intervention has effects that will make it worth implementing. Trials such as this tell us about mechanisms of therapy, but they give us little information that can help us decide if the therapy is worth applying. These trials are of use to theoreticians interested in developing ways of providing therapy, but they do not help clinicians decide whether they should use the therapy in clinical practice.

> In summary, when critically appraising a clinical trial it is sensible to consider if the trial measures outcomes that matter to patients. If not, the trial is unlikely to be able to guide clinical decision-making.

WHAT DOES THE EVIDENCE SAY?[6]

The third and last part of the process of critical appraisal of studies of the effects of interventions involves assessing whether the therapy does more good than harm.

Does the intervention do more good than harm?

In controlled clinical trials, attention is often focused on the 'p value' of the difference between groups. The p value is used to determine if the difference between groups is likely to represent a real effect of intervention or could have occurred simply by chance: 'p' is the probability of the observed difference in groups occurring by chance alone. A small probability (conventionally, $p < 5\%$) means that it is unlikely that the difference would have occurred by chance alone, so it is said to constitute evidence of an effect of intervention.[7] Higher probabilities (conventionally, probabilities $\geqslant 5\%$)

---

[6] This section is reproduced, with only minor changes, from Herbert RD (2000a, 2000b): We are grateful to the publishers of the Australian Journal of Physiotherapy for granting permission to reproduce this material.

[7] This is a conventional interpretation of p values. However, critics argue that this interpretation is incorrect. The contemporary view is not consistent with either the Fisherian or Neyman–Pearson approaches to statistical inference (Gigerenzer 1989). Moreover, there are some powerful arguments supporting the view that p should not provide a measure of the strength of evidence or belief for or against a hypothesis. In the internally consistent Neyman–Pearson view of statistical inference, p serves no other function than to act as a criterion for optimally accepting or rejecting hypotheses. The strength of the evidence supporting one hypothesis over another is given by the ratio of their likelihoods, not by p values. And the strength of belief for or against a hypothesis requires consideration of prior probabilities. Readers interested in exploring these ideas further could consult the marvellous expositions of these ideas by Barnett (1982) and Royall (1997).

indicate that the effect could have occurred by chance alone. High p values are usually interpreted as a lack of evidence of an effect of intervention.

A consequence of this tortuous logic is to distract readers from the most important piece of information that a trial can provide, that is, information about the magnitude of the intervention's effects. If clinical trials are to influence clinical practice they must determine more than simply whether the intervention has an effect. They must, in addition, ascertain how big the effect of intervention is. Good clinical trials provide unbiased estimates of the size of the effect of an intervention. Such estimates can be used to determine if the intervention has a big enough effect to be clinically worthwhile.

What is a clinically worthwhile effect? That depends on the costs and risks of the intervention. Costs most obviously include monetary costs (to the patient, health provider or funder), but they also include the inconvenience, discomfort and side-effects of the intervention. When costs are conceived of in this way it is apparent that all interventions come at some cost. If an intervention is to be clinically worthwhile its positive effects must exceed its costs; it must do more good than harm. Clinical trials often provide information about the size of effects of interventions, but they rarely provide information about all of the costs of intervention.

> Thus the evaluation of whether an intervention provides a clinically worthwhile effect usually requires weighing evidence about beneficial effects of the intervention (provided by clinical trials) against subjective impressions of the costs and risks of the intervention.

Continuous and dichotomous outcomes

In subsequent sections we will consider how we can use clinical trials to tell us about what the effects of a particular intervention are likely to be. We will go about this in a slightly different way, depending on whether outcomes are measured on continuous or dichotomous scales.[8] Outcomes can be considered to be measured on continuous scales when it is the *amount* of the outcome that has been measured on each patient. Examples of outcomes measured on continuous scales are pain intensity measured on a visual analogue scale, disability measured on an Oswestry scale, exercise capacity measured as 12 minute walking distance, or shoulder subluxation measured in millimetres. These contrast with dichotomous outcomes, which can only have one of two values. Dichotomous variables

---

[8] Purists will object to classification of outcomes as either continuous or dichotomous. Their first objection might be that we should add further classes of outcomes. Some outcomes are 'polytomous': they can have more than two values (like continuous variables) but can only take on discrete values (like dichotomous variables). An example is the walking item of the Motor Assessment Scale, which can have integer values of 1–6. For our purposes we can treat most polytomous outcomes (all with more than a few levels on their scale) as if they were continuous outcomes. Another class of outcomes are 'time-to-event' outcomes. As the name suggests, measurement of time-to-event outcomes involves measuring the time taken until an event (such as injury) occurs. Yet another form of outcomes are counts of events. Clinical trials that report time-to-event data or count data often provide the data in a form that enables the reader to extract dichotomous data. We will not consider polytomous, time-to-event or count data any further here.

are usually *events* that either happen or do not happen to each subject. Examples of dichotomous variables are death, respiratory complications, ability to walk independently, ankle sprains, and so on.

We shall first consider how to obtain estimates of the size of the effects of intervention from clinical trials with continuous outcomes. Then we shall consider how to obtain estimates of the effect of intervention on dichotomous outcomes.

Continuous outcomes

All interventions have variable effects. With all interventions, some patients benefit from the intervention but others experience no effect, or even harmful effects. Thus, strictly speaking, we cannot talk of 'the effect' of an intervention. What useful information can a clinical trial provide if it cannot tell us about how all patients (or any individual patient) will respond to intervention? Clinical trials can provide an estimate of the average effects of intervention.

> Fortunately, the *average* effect of intervention is usually the *most likely* or *expected* effect of intervention.[9]

Thus, while clinical trials cannot tell us about what the effect of an intervention will be for a particular patient, they can give us an unbiased 'best guess'.[10]

A sensible way to use estimates, from clinical trials, of the effects of intervention is to consider them as a starting point for predicting the effect on any particular patient. This can then be modified up or down depending on the characteristics of the particular patients to whom the intervention is to be applied.[11] For example, Cambach et al (1997) found that a 3-month community-based pulmonary rehabilitation programme produced modest effects on 6-minute walking distance (39 metres) and quality of life (17 points on the 100-point Chronic Respiratory Disease Questionnaire). We could reasonably anticipate bigger effects than this among people who have very supportive home environments and access to good exercise facilities, and we might expect relatively poor effects among people who have co-morbidities, such as rheumatoid arthritis, that make exercise more difficult.

The advantage of this approach is that it combines the objectivity of clinical trials (which provide unbiased estimates of average effects of intervention) with the richness of clinical acumen (which may be able to distinguish

---

[9] This bold statement is true in one sense but not in another. The mean effect in the population is the *expectation* of the effect (Armitage & Berry 1994). The difficulty arises because we can only estimate, and cannot know, the population mean. The mean effect of the intervention observed in the study sample is a 'maximum likelihood estimator' of the mean effect in the hypothetical population from which the sample could be considered to have been randomly drawn (Barnett 1982). This implies that the estimated mean effect would have been most likely to have been observed if the mean effect in the population was equal to the estimated mean effect. It is *not* equivalent to saying that the mean effect observed in the sample is the most likely value of the mean effect in the population.

[10] The same limitation applies to all sources of information about effects of intervention – this is not a unique limitation of clinical trials.

[11] Later in this chapter we will see that there are complementary statistical techniques for modifying estimates of treatment effects on the basis of baseline severity or risk.

between probable good and poor responders to intervention).[12] Of course, care must be taken when using clinical reasoning to modify estimates of effects provided by clinical trials. A conservative approach would be to ensure that the estimate of the effect of intervention is modified downwards as often as it is modified upwards, although it may be reasonable to depart from this approach if the patients in the trial differ markedly, on average, from the clinical population being treated. Particular caution ought to be applied when a clinical trial provides evidence of no effect of intervention.

Weighing benefit and harm: is the effect clinically worthwhile?

The easiest way to make decisions about whether an intervention has a clinically worthwhile effect is to first nominate the smallest effect that is clinically worthwhile. This is a subjective decision that involves consideration of patients' perceptions of both the benefits and costs of intervention.[13,14] Then we can use estimates of the effects of intervention to decide if intervention will do more good than harm.

The process of weighing benefit and harm can be done in two ways. Individual therapists can develop personal 'policies' about particular interventions. Such policies might stipulate that particular interventions will, or will not, be routinely offered to patients with certain conditions.

---

[12] Some of our colleagues object to this approach on the grounds that clinical acumen is not all it is cracked up to be. It would be very interesting to see some empirical tests of the accuracy of clinical judgements of who will respond most and least to intervention.

[13] Some researchers have conducted surveys in an attempt to discern what patients consider to be the smallest clinically worthwhile effects. (For a discussion of methods used to estimate the smallest worthwhile effects, see Jaeschke et al 1989 and Hajiro & Nishimura 2002). Such studies potentially provide very useful information for physiotherapists making 'policies' about management. To be meaningful, estimates of smallest clinically worthwhile effects must be intervention-specific because they involve consideration of the costs of the intervention. However, few studies have provided intervention-specific estimates of the smallest worthwhile effect. Occasionally researchers have stipulated what they consider to be minimally clinically worthwhile effects of intervention (e.g. Schonstein et al 2003). These recommendations carry relatively little authority because they are based on the opinions of the researchers, rather than the opinions of patients, but at least they make statements about what is clinically worthwhile more transparent. Blanket statements about what constitutes a worthwhile effect of interventions for a particular condition (such as 'we considered a 10-mm difference on the VAS and a 2-point or greater difference on the RDQ as clinically relevant', Assendelft et al 2003) are less useful because 'clinically relevant' effects must be intervention-specific.

[14] The process of deciding what is a clinically worthwhile effect is most straightforward when we conceive of treatment effects in terms of the difference between outcomes of a group receiving intervention and a group not receiving intervention. Then the smallest worthwhile effect is that which makes the intervention worth its costs. Alternatively, if we are interested in how much benefit is obtained by *adding* an intervention to a standard therapy, then we must think of the smallest worthwhile effect in terms of how much of a difference in outcomes would make the costs of adding the new therapy worthwhile. A trickier scenario arises when we wish to compare the effectiveness of two interventions. Then we must decide if the better outcomes produced by one intervention is worth its *extra* costs over and above the costs of the other intervention. Sometimes the two interventions will be very similar in terms of their costs, in which case *any* difference in the outcome of the two interventions could be considered to indicate that the intervention with the better outcome is worthwhile. And sometimes the better therapy will be associated with less cost, in which case it will *always* be worthwhile.

For example, some therapists have a personal policy not to offer ultrasound therapy to people with ankle sprains. This policy can be defended on the grounds that, on average, ultrasound does not appear to produce benefits that most patients would consider minimally worthwhile (van der Windt et al 2004). To make this decision, the physiotherapist has to anticipate patient preferences and make decisions that he or she believes are in the patients' best interests.

Alternatively, decisions about therapy can be negotiated individually with patients. This involves discerning what individual patients want from therapy, and what their values and preferences are (see p. 161). Some patients are intervention-averse, and will only be interested in intervention if it makes a big difference to quality of life. Others are intervention-tolerant (or even intervention-hungry!) and are prepared to try interventions that are expected to have little effect. As an example, there is quite strong evidence that electrical stimulation of rotator cuff muscles can prevent glenohumeral subluxation after hemiparetic stroke (Ada & Foongchomcheay 2002), but this does not mean that all patients with hemiparetic stroke should be given electrical stimulation. Instead, the benefits (a mean reduction of subluxation by 6.5 mm) should be weighed against 'costs' (application of a moderately uncomfortable modality for several hours each day for several weeks). Some patients will consider the expected benefit of therapy worthwhile and others will not. This provides a legitimate basis for variations in practice. Quite different decisions about interventions might be made for patients with similar clinical presentations but different values and preferences. The physiotherapist's role is to elicit patient preferences and assist in the process of making decisions about intervention, as discussed in Chapter 1.

To illustrate this process we will consider if the application of a pneumatic compression pump produces clinically worthwhile reductions in post-mastectomy lymphoedema. We might begin by nominating the smallest reduction in lymphoedema that would make the costs of the compression therapy worthwhile. Most therapists, and perhaps even most patients, would agree that a short course of daily compression therapy would be clinically worthwhile if it produced a sustained 75% reduction in oedema. Most would also agree that a 15% decrease was not clinically worthwhile. Somewhere in between these values lies the smallest clinically worthwhile effect. This value is best arrived at by discussion with the particular patients for whom the intervention is intended. Let us assume for the moment that a particular patient (or typical patients) considers that the smallest reduction in oedema that would make therapy worthwhile is around 40%.

Does compression therapy produce reductions in lymphoedema of this magnitude? Perhaps the best answer to this question comes from a randomized trial by Dini et al (1998) that compared 2 weeks (10 days) of daily intermittent pneumatic compression with a control (no treatment) condition. We will use the findings of this trial to estimate what the effect of compression therapy is likely to be.

Estimating the size of an intervention's effects

For continuous outcomes, the best estimate of the effect of an intervention is simply the difference in the means (or, in some trials, the medians) of the intervention and control groups. In the trial by Dini et al (1998), oedema was measured by measuring arm circumference at seven locations, summing the measures, and then taking the difference of the summed circumference of affected and unaffected arms (positive numbers indicate that the affected arm had a larger circumference than the unaffected arm). After the 2-week experimental period the oedema was 14 cm (SD 6) in both the control group and in the intervention group. Thus the best estimate of the effect of intervention (compared to no intervention) is that it has no effect on oedema. Clearly the effect is smaller than the smallest clinically worthwhile effect, which we had decided might be about 40%. Our expectation should be that when pressure therapy is applied to this population in the manner described by Dini et al, there will be little effect. Our best guess is that the effect of the intervention will be, on average, not clinically worthwhile.

Another example comes from a trial by O'Sullivan and colleagues (1997). These authors examined the effects of specific segmental exercise for people with painful spondylolysis or spondylolysthesis. Subjects were randomly allocated to groups that received either a 10-week programme of training of the deep spinal stabilizing muscles (10–15 minutes of exercise daily) or routine care from a medical practitioner. Pain intensity was measured after the intervention period on a 100-mm visual analogue scale (maximum score of 100). To interpret the findings of this study we could begin by nominating the smallest clinically worthwhile effect. Patients with spondylolysthesis often experience chronic pain or recurrent episodes of pain, so they may be satisfied with the intervention even if it had relatively modest effects: a 20% reduction in pain intensity, if sustained, may be perceived as worthwhile. The trial found that, after intervention, mean pain in the intervention group was 19 mm and mean pain in the control group was 48 mm, indicating that the effect of specific muscle training was, on average, 29 mm (or $29/48 = 60\%$ of the pain level in the control group). Effects of this magnitude are considerably greater than the threshold of 20% and are likely to be perceived as worthwhile by most patients. Of course, some patients may perceive that therapy would only be worthwhile if it gave them complete relief of symptoms; these patients would consider the treatment effect too small to be worthwhile.

In the two examples just used, outcomes were measured in terms of the amount of oedema and the degree of pain intensity *at the end of the experimental period*. Some trials, instead, report the *change* in outcome variables over the intervention period. In such trials the measure of the effect of intervention is still the difference of the means (this time of the difference of the mean *change*) in intervention and control groups.[15]

---

[15]Some readers will wonder why we do not always use change scores rather than end scores to estimate the effects of intervention. At first glance, change scores seem to take account of differences between groups at baseline, whereas end scores do not. It is true that change scores may be preferred over end scores, but not because they take better account of baseline differences. When the correlation between baseline scores and end scores is greater than 0.5 (as is usually the case), change scores will have less variability than end scores, so that (as we shall see shortly) when these conditions are satisfied we can get more precise estimates of the effect of intervention from change scores than end scores (Cohen 1988). (In fact, even change scores are not optimally efficient.

Estimating uncertainty   Even when clinical trials are well designed and conducted, their findings are associated with uncertainty. This is because the difference between group means observed in the study is only an estimate of the true effect of intervention derived from the sample of subjects in the clinical trial. (Our estimate of the effects of compression therapy has uncertainty associated with it because the estimate was obtained from the 80 subjects employed in the study by Dini et al (1998), not from all patients in the population we want to make inferences about.) The outcomes in this sample, as in any sample, approximate but do not exactly equal the average outcomes in the populations which the sample represents. Thus the average effect of intervention reported in the study approximates but does not equal the true average effect of intervention. Rational interpretation of the clinical trial requires consideration of how good an approximation the study provides.

> That is, to properly interpret a study's findings it is necessary to know how much uncertainty is associated with its results.

The degree of uncertainty associated with the effect of an intervention can be described with a confidence interval (Gardner & Altman 1989). Most often the 95% confidence interval is used. Roughly speaking, the 95% confidence interval is the range within which we can be 95% certain that the true average effect of intervention actually lies.[16] (Note that the confidence interval describes the degree of uncertainty about the average effect on the population, not the degree of uncertainty of the effect on individuals.) The 95% confidence interval for the difference between means in the trial by Dini et al extends from approximately −3 to +3 cm (methods used to calculate confidence intervals are presented in Box 6.1 on pages 141–142. This suggests that we can suppose that the true average effect of pressure therapy lies somewhere between a reduction in oedema of 3 cm and an increase in oedema of 3 cm. All of the values encompassed by the 95% confidence interval are smaller than what we nominated as the smallest clinically worthwhile effect. (We had nominated a smallest worthwhile effect of 40%; as the initial oedema was 14 cm, this corresponds to a reduction in

Covariate-adjusted scores will always be more efficient again, so covariate-adjusted scores are preferred wherever they are available.) But change scores do not better account for baseline differences, at least not in the sense of removing bias due to baseline differences. In randomized trials, baseline differences are due to chance alone. Averaged across many trials, baseline differences will be zero. So, averaged across many trials, analyses of change scores and analyses of end scores will give the same result. Both give unbiased estimates of the average effect of intervention.

[16] This interpretation is easy to grasp and easy to use but, strictly speaking, incorrect (see footnote 9). One justification for perpetuating the incorrect interpretation is that it may be a reasonable approximation; 95% confidence intervals for differences between means correspond closely to 1/32 likelihood intervals (Royall 1997), which means that they correspond to the interval most strongly supported by the trial data. Also, in the presence of 'vague priors' (that is, in the presence of considerable uncertainty about the true effect prior to the conduct of the trial), 95% confidence intervals usually correspond quite closely to Bayesian 95% credible intervals that can more legitimately be interpreted as 'the interval within which the true value probably lies' (Barnett 1982).

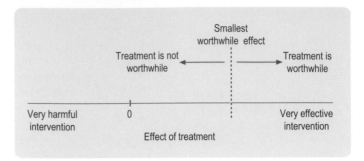

Figure 6.1   'Tree plot' of effect size. The tree plot consists of a horizontal line representing the effect of intervention. At the extremes are very harmful and very effective interventions. The smallest worthwhile effect is represented as a vertical dotted line. This divides the tree plot into two regions: the region to the left of this line represents effects of intervention that are too small to be worthwhile, whereas the region to the right of this line represents interventions whose effects are worthwhile.

oedema of $40\% \times 14$ cm or about 6 cm.) Thus we can conclude that not only is the best estimate of the magnitude of the effect less than the smallest clinically worthwhile effect (0 cm < 6 cm), but also that no value of the effect that is plausibly consistent with the findings of this study exceeds the smallest clinically worthwhile effect. These data strongly suggest that pressure therapy does not produce clinically worthwhile reductions in lymphoedema.

Some readers will find confidence intervals easier to interpret if they sketch the confidence intervals on a 'tree' plot,[17] as in Figure 6.1. The tree plot consists of a line along which effects of intervention could lie. The middle of the line represents no effect (difference between group means of 0). The usual convention is that the right end of the line represents a very good effect (intervention group mean minus control group mean is a large positive number) and the left end represents a very harmful intervention (intervention group mean minus control group mean is a large negative number). For any trial we can draw three variables on this graph (Figure 6.2A): the smallest clinically worthwhile effect (in our example this is 6 cm), the best estimate of the effect of intervention (the difference between group means from Dini et al's randomized controlled trial, or 0 cm), and the 95% confidence interval about that estimate (-3 cm to $+3$ cm). The region to the right of the smallest clinically worthwhile effect is the domain of clinically worthwhile effects of intervention. The graph for the Dini trial (Figure 6.2A) clearly shows that there is not a clinically worthwhile effect, because neither the best estimate of the effect of intervention nor any point encompassed by the 95% confidence interval lie in the region of a clinically worthwhile effect.

Living with uncertainty   In the example that was just used, the effect of intervention was clearly not large enough to be clinically worthwhile. This is a helpful result because

[17] We call these tree plots because they resemble one element of a forest plot. (For an example of a forest plot, see Figure 6.6.)

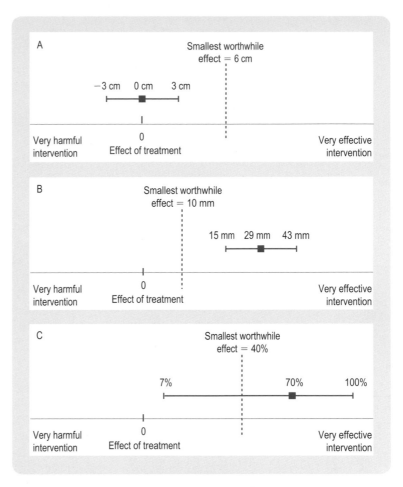

Figure 6.2   **A** Data from Dini et al (1998) on effects of pressure therapy on post-mastectomy oedema. The smallest clinically worthwhile effect has been nominated as a reduction of oedema by 40% of initial oedema levels (or about 6 cm). The best estimate of the size of the treatment effect (no effect at all) has been illustrated as a small square, and the 95% confidence interval about this estimate (−3 to +3 cm) is shown as a horizontal line. The effect of intervention is clearly smaller than the smallest clinically worthwhile effect. **B** Data from O'Sullivan et al (1997) on effects of specific exercise on pain intensity in people with spondylolisthesis and spondylolysis. The mean effect is a reduction in pain of 29 mm on a 100 mm visual analogue scale (VAS) (95% CI 15 to 43 mm). This is clearly more than the smallest worthwhile effect, which we nominated as a 10 mm reduction (or approximately 20% of the initial pain levels of 48 mm). **C** Data from Sand et al (1995) on effects of a programme of electrical stimulation on urine leakage in women with stress urinary incontinence. The smallest clinically worthwhile effect has been nominated as 40%. The best estimate of the size of the treatment effect (a 70% reduction in leakage) is very worthwhile (much more than a 40% reduction in leakage). However, the 95% confidence interval for this estimate is very wide (7 to 100%). (In this particular case the confidence intervals are not symmetrical because it is not possible to reduce leakage by more than 100%.) The confidence intervals include effects of intervention that are both smaller than the smallest worthwhile effect and greater than the worthwhile effect. Thus, while the best estimate of the treatment effect is that it is clinically worthwhile, this conclusion is subject to a high degree of uncertainty.

it gives us some certainty about the effect (in this case, the lack of any worthwhile effect) of the intervention. In other examples, such as with the trial by O'Sullivan et al (1997) on specific muscle training for people with spondylolysis and spondylolysthesis, we may find clear answers in the other direction (Figure 6.2B). We have already seen that the mean effect of treatment reported in the O'Sullivan trial was 29 mm, substantially more than the smallest worthwhile effect (20% of 48 mm or about 10 mm). The 95% confidence interval for this effect is approximately 15 to 43 mm.[18] Consequently, the entire confidence interval falls in the region that is greater than the smallest worthwhile effect. Again this is helpful because it tells us with some certainty that the intervention produces clinically worthwhile effects.

Unfortunately, the results will often be less clear. Ambiguity arises when the confidence interval spans the smallest clinically worthwhile effect, because then it is plausible both that the intervention does and does not have a clinically worthwhile effect. Part of the confidence interval is less than the smallest clinically worthwhile effect and part of the confidence interval is greater than the smallest clinically worthwhile effect; either result could be the true one. For example, Sand et al (1995) showed that 15 weeks of pelvic floor electrical stimulation for women with genuine stress incontinence produced large reductions in urine leakage (average of 32 ml or 70% reduction) compared to sham stimulation. This result is shown on a tree plot in Figure 6.2C. The mean difference suggests a large and worthwhile effect of intervention, but the 95% confidence interval spanned from a 7% to a 100% reduction. There is, therefore, a high degree of uncertainty about how big the effect actually is, and because the lower end of the confidence interval includes trivially small reductions in urine loss it is not certain, on the basis of this trial alone, that the intervention is worthwhile.

This situation, when the confidence interval spans the smallest worthwhile effect, arises commonly for two reasons. First, the designers of clinical trials conventionally use sample sizes that are sufficient only to rule out no effect of intervention if there truly is a clinically worthwhile effect, but such samples may be too small to prevent their confidence intervals spanning the smallest clinically worthwhile effect. Second, many interventions have modest effects (their true effects are close to the smallest clinically worthwhile effect), so their confidence intervals must be very narrow if they are not to span the smallest clinically worthwhile effect. Consequently few studies provide unambiguous evidence of an effect, or lack of effect, of intervention.

There are two ways to respond to the uncertainty that is often provided by single trials. First, we can accept uncertainty and proceed on the

---

[18] Try and do the calculations yourself using the formula in Box 6.1. The key data are that (a) mean pain intensity was 48 mm in the control group and 19 mm in the exercise group, (b) the standard deviations were 23 in the control group and 21 in the exercise group, and (c) both groups contained 21 subjects.

basis of the best available evidence. In this approach, clinical decisions are based on the difference between group means. When the difference exceeds the smallest clinically worthwhile effect the intervention is thought to be worthwhile, and when the difference between group means is less than the smallest clinically worthwhile effect the intervention is thought to be insufficiently effective. With this approach the role of confidence

---

Box 6.1   A method for calculating confidence intervals for differences between means

When confidence intervals about differences between group means are not explicitly supplied in reports of clinical trials, it is usually an easy matter to calculate these from the data reported in trials.

The confidence intervals for the difference between the means for two groups can be calculated from the difference between the two means (*difference*), their standard deviations and the group sizes. An approximate 95% confidence interval is given by first obtaining the average of the two standard deviations (SD_{av}) and the average of the group sizes (n_{av}). Then the 95% confidence interval (95% CI) for the difference between the two means is calculated from:

$$95\% \text{ CI} \approx difference \pm (3 \times SD_{av})/\sqrt{n_{av}}$$

(Herbert 2002a).[19] (The '$\approx$' symbol means 'is approximately equal to'.) In other words, the confidence interval spans an interval from $(3 \times SD)/\sqrt{n_{av}}$ below the difference in group means to $(3 \times SD)/\sqrt{n_{av}}$ above the difference in group means.

This equation is an approximation to the more complex equation that should be used when trialists analyse their data, but it is an adequate approximation for readers of clinical trials to use for clinical decision-making.[20] It has the advantage that it is simple enough to be routinely calculated whenever a clinical trial does not report the confidence interval for the difference between group means.[21]

In the trial by Dini et al (1998) on 80 subjects (average group size of 40), the authors reported mean measures of oedema for both intervention and control groups (14 cm for both groups), and the standard deviations about those means (6.0 cm for both groups), but they did not report the 95% confidence interval for the difference between means. The 95% confidence interval can be calculated from this data and is:

$$95\% \text{ CI} \approx (14 - 14) \pm (3 \times 6)/\sqrt{40}$$
$$95\% \text{ CI} \approx 0 \pm 3$$
$$95\% \text{ CI} \approx -3 \text{ to } +3 \text{ cm}$$

---

[19] The derivation is as follows. If we assume equal group sizes (n) and equal standard deviations (SD) in the two groups, the standard error of the difference in means (SE_{diff}) is $SD\sqrt{(2/n)}$. For reasonably large samples, the 95% CI is $\approx$ *difference* $\pm 1.96\ SE_{diff}$, or *difference* $\pm 1.96\ SD\sqrt{(2/n)}$, which is $\approx$ *difference* $\pm 3\ SD/\sqrt{n}$. A simple estimate of the SD is given by SD_{av}, and we can substitute n_{av} for n. Hence the 95% CI is approximated by the *difference* $\pm 3\ SD_{av}/\sqrt{n_{av}}$.

[20] The procedures described above for calculating the confidence interval of the difference between two means will tend to produce overly conservative confidence intervals (confidence intervals that are too broad) in some circumstances. In particular, this procedure will tend to produce confidence intervals that are too broad when the study is a cross-over study, a study in which subjects are matched prior to randomization, or a study in which

statistical procedures (such as ANCOVA) are used to partition out explainable sources of variance. Less often, if the sample size is small and the group sizes are very unequal, the confidence interval may be too narrow. In such studies it is highly desirable that the authors report confidence intervals for the differences between groups.

[21] In fact, if you are prepared to do the calculations roughly, they are easy enough to do without a calculator. Rough calculations can be justified because small differences in the width of confidence intervals are unlikely to make any difference to the clinical decision. The hard part of the equation is in taking the square root of the sample size. But you can take advantage of the fact that square roots are insensitive to approximation. You will probably make the same clinical decision if you calculate that the square root of 40 is 6.3246, or if you just say it is 'about 6'.

Box 6.1   (Contd)

Often papers will report standard errors of the means (*SEs*), rather than standard deviations. In that case the calculation is even simpler:[22,23]

$$95\% \text{ CI} \approx \textit{difference} \pm 3 \times SE_{av}$$

Many trials have more than two groups (as there may be more than one intervention group, or more than one control). The reader must then decide which between-group comparison is (or are) of most interest, and then the 95% confidence intervals for differences between these groups can be calculated in the same way as above. Similarly, most trials report several, and sometimes many, outcomes. It is tedious to calculate 95% confidence intervals for all outcomes, and the best approach is usually to decide which few outcomes are of greatest interest, and then calculate 95% confidence interval for those outcomes only.

Sometimes a degree of detective work is required to find the standard deviations or standard errors. If the standard deviations or standard errors are not explicitly given, they may sometimes be obtained from the error bars in figures. In other trial reports there may be inadequate reporting of trial outcomes and it will not be possible to calculate 95% confidence intervals. Such trials are difficult to interpret. Some trials report medians and interquartile ranges, or sometimes ranges, instead of means and standard deviations, which makes it more difficult to estimate confidence intervals for these trials.[24]

[22] Some readers will wonder why the 95% CI is $\pm 3\, SE_{av}$, and not $\pm 2\, SE_{av}$ (or $\pm 1.96\, SE_{av}$). The explanation is that the 95% CI for the difference between two means is equal to the difference $\pm 1.96\, SE_{diff}$, not the difference $\pm 1.96\, SE_{av}$. When sample sizes and SDs of both groups are equal, $SE_{diff} = \sqrt{2}\, SE_{av}$.
[23] Occasionally papers will report the 95% CI for *each* group's mean. This is unhelpful, because we really want to know the 95% CI for the *difference* between the two means. It is possible, albeit tedious, to convert the 95% CIs for the two group means into a CI for the difference between the two means. To do so we take advantage of the fact that the 95% CI for a group mean is $\approx 4\, SE$ wide.

Here's what to do:
Take the 95% CI for the control group's mean and determine its width by subtracting the lower limit of the confidence interval from the upper limit. Then divide the width of the confidence interval by 4 to get the standard error for the control group mean. Repeat the procedure to calculate the standard error for the intervention group. Then take the average of the two SEs to get the SE_{av}. Then you can calculate the 95% CI for the difference between groups as the *difference* $\pm 3\, SE_{av}$.
[24] As a rough approximation you can use the equation presented above by treating medians like means and approximating the SD as three-quarters of the inter-quartile range or one-quarter of the range.

intervals is to provide an indicator of the degree of self-doubt that should be applied, but they do not otherwise affect clinical decisions. An alternative is to seek more certainty by determining if the findings of individual studies are replicated in other, similar studies. This is one of the reasons why systematic reviews of randomized controlled trials are potentially a very useful source of information about the effects of intervention. As we saw earlier in this chapter, systematic reviews can combine the results of individual trials in a meta-analysis, effectively providing a single result from many studies. The combined result is derived from a relatively large sample size, so it usually provides a more precise estimate of effects of intervention (its confidence intervals are relatively narrow), and it is more likely it will provide unambiguous information about the effect of intervention (narrow confidence intervals are less likely to span the smallest clinically worthwhile effect). We shall consider the role of meta-analysis further later in this chapter.

Dichotomous outcomes

The examples in the preceding section were of clinical trials in which outcomes were measured as continuous variables. Other outcomes are measured as 'dichotomous' variables. This section considers how we might estimate the size of effects of intervention on dichotomous variables.

Dichotomous outcomes are discrete events – things that either do or do not happen – such as dead/alive, injured/not injured, or satisfied with treatment/not satisfied with treatment. These variables can take on one of two values, so we don't conventionally talk about their mean values.[25] Instead we quantify outcomes of intervention in terms of the proportion of subjects that experienced the event of interest, usually within some specified period of time. This tells us about the 'risk' of the event for individuals from that population.[26,27] A good example is provided by a trial of the effects of prophylactic chest physiotherapy on respiratory complications following major abdominal surgery (Olsen et al 1997). In this study the event of interest was the development of a respiratory complication. Of subjects in the control group, 52/192 experienced respiratory complications within 6 days of surgery, so the risk of respiratory complications for these subjects was ($100 \times 59/192 =$) 27%.

In clinical trials with dichotomous outcomes we are interested in whether intervention reduces the risk of the event of interest. Thus we need to determine if the risk differs between intervention and control groups. The magnitude of the risk reduction, which tells us about the degree of effectiveness of the intervention, can be expressed in a number of different ways (Guyatt et al 1994, Sackett et al 2000). Three common measures are the *absolute risk reduction* (ARR), *number needed to treat* (NNT) and *relative risk reduction* (RRR).

Absolute risk reduction

The absolute risk reduction is simply the difference in risk between intervention and control groups. In the trial by Olsen et al (1997), a relatively small proportion of subjects in the intervention group (10/172 = 6%) experienced respiratory complications, so the risk of respiratory complications for subjects in the group was relatively small compared to the 27% risk in the control group. The absolute reduction in risk is 27% − 6% = 21%. This means that treated subjects were at a 21% lower risk than control group subjects of experiencing respiratory complications in the 6 days following surgery. Big absolute risk reductions indicate intervention is

---

[25] It would be unconventional, but not necessarily inappropriate, to talk about the mean value of a dichotomous outcome. If the alternative events are assigned values of 0 and 1, then their mean is the risk of the alternative assigned a value of 1.

[26] We refer to the risk of an event when the event is undesirable, but we don't usually talk of the risk of a desirable event. (For example, it seems natural to talk of the risk of getting injured, but not of the risk of not getting injured). There are two ways to deal with this. Given the 'risk' of a desirable event, we can always estimate the risk of the undesirable alternative. The risk (in %) of undesirable event = 100 − the risk (in %) of desirable event. Thus if the risk of not getting injured is 80%, the risk of getting injured is 20%. Alternatively, we could replace the word 'risk' with 'probability' and talk instead about the probability of not getting injured.

[27] Rothman & Greenland (1998: 37) point out that the word 'risk' has several meanings. They call the proportion of subjects experiencing the event of interest the 'average risk' or, less ambiguously, the 'incidence proportion'.

very effective. Negative absolute risk reductions indicate that risk is greater in the intervention group than in the control group and that the intervention is harmful. (An exception to this rule is when the event is a positive event, such as return to work, rather than a negative event.)

It is possible to put confidence intervals about the absolute risk reduction (as it is about any measure of the effect of intervention), just as we did for estimate of the effects of intervention on continuous outcomes. Box 6.2 on page 148 explains how to calculate and interpret the 95% CI for the absolute risk reduction.

Number needed to treat   Understandably, many people have difficulty appreciating the magnitude of absolute risk reductions. A consequence is that it is often difficult to specify the smallest clinically worthwhile effect in terms of absolute risk reduction, especially when the risk in control subjects is low. How big is a 21% reduction in absolute risk? Is a 21% absolute risk reduction clinically worthwhile? A second measure of risk reduction, the number needed to treat, makes the magnitude of an absolute risk reduction more explicit. The number needed to treat is obtained by taking the inverse of the absolute risk reduction. In our example, the absolute risk reduction is 21%, so the number needed to treat is 1/21%, or ~5.[28,29] This is the number of people that would need to be treated, on average, to prevent the event of interest happening to one person. In our example, one respiratory complication is prevented for every 5 people given the intervention. For the other 4 out of every 5 patients the intervention made no difference: some would not have developed a respiratory complication anyhow, and the others developed a respiratory complication despite intervention. A small number needed to treat (such as 5) is better than a large number needed to treat (such as 100) because it indicates that a relatively small number of patients need to be treated before the intervention makes a difference to one of them.

Figure 6.3 illustrates why it is that a reduction in risk from 27% to 6% corresponds to a number needed to treat of 5 (Cates 2003). This figure illustrates the outcomes of 100 typical patients who did not receive the intervention and another 100 typical patients who did receive the intervention. Twenty-seven of the 100 control group patients experienced a respiratory complication, whereas only 6 of the 100 treated patients experienced a respiratory complication (6% of 20 is about 1). That is, for every 100 people who received the intervention, 21 fewer experienced a respiratory complication. Twenty-one out of 100 people (or 1 in 5) benefit from this intervention. That is why we say the number needed to treat is 5. Conversely, 79 of the 100 people who received the intervention did not benefit from intervention (73 were not going to get a respiratory complication even if they did not have the intervention, and 6 experienced a respiratory complication despite intervention). In other words, 4 of every 5 patients do not benefit from this intervention.

The number needed to treat is very useful because it makes it relatively easy to nominate what the smallest clinically worthwhile effect might be. With the number needed to treat, we can more easily weigh up

---

[28] Remember that a percentage is a fraction, so 1/21% is the same as 1/0.21, not 1/21.
[29] Usual practice is to round NNTs to the nearest whole number.

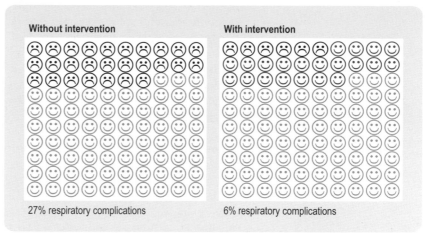

Figure 6.3   Diagram illustrating the relationship between the absolute risk reduction and the number needed to treat. The diagram is based on a diagram by Cates (2003) and it uses an example data from the trial by Olsen et al (1997). Each face represents 1% of the population. Sad faces represent people who experienced respiratory complications. Smiley faces represent people who did not experience respiratory complications. The left panel shows outcomes in a population that did not receive the intervention and the right panel shows outcomes in a population that did receive the intervention. The first 6 people (6% of the population) experienced a complication with or without intervention (i.e., in the left and right panels), so intervention made no difference to these subjects. The next 21 people, highlighted grey in the diagram, experienced respiratory complications without intervention but not with intervention. These subjects benefited from intervention. The remaining 73 people did not experience respiratory complications with or without intervention, so intervention made no difference to these people. Thus, overall, 21 of 100 people benefited from intervention; we say the absolute risk reduction was 21%. Another way of saying this is that about 1 in every 5 treated patients (21/100 people) benefited from treatment, so the number to treat was 5.

the benefits of preventing the event in one subject against the costs and risks of giving the intervention. (Note that the benefit is received by a few, but costs are shared by all). In our example, most would agree that a number needed to treat of 10 would be worthwhile, because preventing one respiratory complication is a very desirable thing, and the risks and costs of this simple intervention are minimal, so little is lost from ineffectively treating 9 out of every 10 patients. Most would agree, however, that a number needed to treat of 100 would be too small to make the intervention worthwhile. There may be little risk associated with this intervention, but it probably incurs too great a cost (too much discomfort caused to patients, for example) to ineffectively treat 99 people to make the prevention of one respiratory complication worthwhile. What, then, is the largest number needed to treat for prophylactic chest physiotherapy we would accept as being clinically worthwhile (what is the smallest clinically worthwhile effect)? When we polled some experienced cardiopulmonary therapists they indicated that they would not be prepared to instigate this therapy if they had to treat more than about 20 patients to prevent one respiratory complication. That is, they nominated a number needed to treat of 20 as the smallest clinically worthwhile effect. This corresponds to an absolute risk reduction of 5%. It would be interesting to survey patients facing major abdominal surgery to determine what they considered to be the smallest clinically worthwhile effect. The effect of intervention demonstrated in the trial by Olsen et al (number needed to treat = 5) is greater than most therapists would consider to be minimally clinically worthwhile (number needed to treat ~20; remember that a small number needed to treat indicates a large effect of intervention).

Clearly, there is no one value for the number needed to treat that can be deemed to be the smallest clinically worthwhile effect. The size of the smallest clinically worthwhile effect will depend on the seriousness of the event and the costs and risks of intervention. Thus the smallest clinically worthwhile effect for a 3 month exercise programme may be as little as 2 or 3 if the event being prevented is infrequent giving way of the knee, whereas the smallest clinically worthwhile effect for the use of incentive spirometry in the immediate post-operative period after chest surgery may be a number needed to treat of many hundreds if the event being prevented is death from respiratory complications.[30] When intervention is ongoing, the number needed to treat, like the absolute risk reduction, should be related to the period of intervention. A number needed to treat of 10 for a 3 month course of therapy aimed at reducing respiratory complications in children with cystic fibrosis is similar in the size of its effect to another therapy which has a number needed to treat of 5 for a 6 month course of therapy.

Relative risk reduction

A more commonly reported but less immediately helpful way of expressing the reduction in risk is as a proportion of the risk of untreated patients. This is termed the relative risk reduction. The relative risk reduction is obtained by dividing the absolute risk reduction by the risk in the control group. Thus the relative risk reduction produced by prophylactic chest physiotherapy is 21%/27%, which is 78%. In other words, prophylactic chest physiotherapy reduced the risk of respiratory complications by 78% *of the risk in untreated patients*. You can see that the relative risk reduction (78%) looks much larger than the absolute risk reduction (21%), even though they are describing exactly the same effect.[31] Which, then, is the best measure of the magnitude of an intervention's effects? Should we use the absolute risk reduction, its inverse (the number needed to treat), or the relative risk reduction?

---

[30] A simple way of weighing up benefit and harm is to assign (very subjectively) a number to describe the benefit of intervention. The benefit of intervention is described in terms of how much worse the event being prevented is than the harm of the intervention. In the example of prevention of respiratory complications with prophylactic chest physiotherapy, we might judge that respiratory complications are 10 times as bad (unpleasant, expensive, etc.) as the intervention of prophylactic physiotherapy. If the benefit is greater than the number needed to treat, the benefit of therapy outweighs its harm. In our example, respiratory complications are 10 times as bad as prophylactic physiotherapy, and the NNT is 5, so the therapy produces more benefit than harm.
[31] In fact the relative risk reduction always looks larger than the absolute risk reduction because it is obtained by dividing the absolute risk reduction by a probability, and probabilities must be less than 1.

The relative risk reduction has some properties that make it useful for comparing the findings of different studies, but it can be deceptive when used for clinical decision-making. This might best be illustrated with an example. Lauritzen et al (1993) showed that the provision of hip protector pads to residents of nursing homes produced large relative reductions in risk of hip fracture (relative risk reduction of 56%). This might sound as if the intervention has a big effect, and it may be tempting to conclude on the basis of this statistic that the hip protectors are clinically worthwhile. However, the incidence of hip fractures in the study sample was about 5% per year (Lauritzen et al 1993), so the absolute reduction of hip fracture risk with hip protectors in this population is 56% *of 5%*, or just less than 3%. By converting this to a number needed to treat we can see that 36 people would need to wear hip protectors for 1 year to prevent one fracture.[32] When the risk reduction is expressed as an absolute risk reduction or, better still as a number needed to treat, the effects appear much smaller than when presented as a relative risk reduction. (Nonetheless, because hip fractures are serious events, a 1-year number needed to treat of 36 may still be worthwhile.) This example illustrates that it is probably better to make decisions about the effects of interventions in terms of absolute risk reductions or numbers needed to treat than relative risk reductions.

The importance of baseline risk

In general, even the best interventions (those with large relative risk reductions) will only produce small absolute risk reductions when the risk of the event in untreated subjects (the 'baseline risk') is low. Perhaps this is intuitively obvious – if few people are likely to experience the event, it is not possible to prevent it very often. There are two very practical implications. First, even the best interventions are unlikely to produce clinically worthwhile effects if the event that is to be prevented is unlikely. The converse of this is that an intervention is more likely to be clinically worthwhile when it reduces risk of a high risk event. (For a particularly clear discussion of this issue see Glasziou & Irwig 1995.) Second, as the magnitude of the effect of intervention is likely to depend very much on the risk to which untreated subjects are exposed, care is needed when applying the results of a clinical trial to a particular patient if the risk to patients in the trial differs markedly from the risk in the patient for whom the intervention is being considered. If the risk in control subjects in the trial is much higher than in the patient in question, the effect of intervention will tend to be overestimated (that is, the absolute risk reduction calculated from trial data will be too high, and the number needed to treat will be too low).[33]

---

[32]Some people find NNTs per year hard to conceptualize. If a 1-year NNT for wearing hip protectors of 36 means nothing to you, try looking at it in another way. If 36 people need to wear hip protectors for 1 year to prevent one fracture, that is a bit like (though not exactly the same as) having to wear a hip protector for 36 years to prevent a hip fracture. Then the decision becomes easier still: would you wear a hip protector for 36 years if you thought it would prevent a hip fracture?

[33]The underlying assumption here is that measures of relative effects of treatment are constant regardless of baseline risk. This has been investigated by a number of authors, notably Furukawa et al (2000), Deeks & Altman (2001) and Schmid et al (1998). McAlister (2000) provides an excellent commentary on this literature.

There is a simple work-around that makes it possible to apply the results of a clinical trial to patients with higher or lower levels of risk. The approach described here is based on the method used by Straus & Sackett (1999; see also McAlister et al 2000). The absolute risk reduction or number needed to treat is calculated as described above, directly from the results of the trial, but is then adjusted by a factor, let's call it f, which describes how much more risk subjects are at than the untreated (control) subjects in the trial. An f of greater than 1 is used when the patients to whom the result is to be applied are at a greater risk than control subjects in the trial, and an f of less than 1 is used when patients to whom the result is to be applied are at a lower risk than untreated subjects in the trial. The absolute risk reduction is adjusted by multiplying by f, and the number needed to treat is adjusted by dividing by f.

The following example illustrates how this approach might be used. A physiotherapist treating a morbidly obese patient undergoing major abdominal surgery might estimate that the patient was at twice the risk of respiratory complications as subjects in the trial by Olsen et al (1997). To obtain a reasonable estimate of the effects of intervention (that is, to take into account the greater baseline risk in this subject than in subjects in the trial), the number needed to treat (which we previously calculated as 5) could be divided by 2. This gives a number needed to treat of 2.5 (which rounds to 3) for morbidly obese subjects. Thus we can anticipate an even larger effect of prophylactic physiotherapy among high-risk patients.[34] This approach can be used to adjust estimates of the likely effects of intervention for any individual patient up or down on the basis of therapists' perceptions of their patients' risks.

See Box 6.3 for a summary of this section.

Box 6.2   Estimating uncertainty of effects on dichotomous outcome

As with trials that measure continuous outcomes, many trials with dichotomous outcomes do not report confidence intervals about the absolute risk reduction, number needed to treat or relative risk reduction. Almost all, however, supply sufficient data to calculate the confidence interval. A very rough 95% confidence interval for the absolute risk reduction can be obtained simply from the average sample size (n_{av}) of the experimental and control groups:

$$95\% \text{ CI} \approx \textit{difference in risk} \pm 1/\sqrt{n_{av}}$$

(Herbert 2000b).[35] This approximation works well enough (it gives an answer that is close enough to that provided by more complex equations) when the average risk of the events of interest in treated and control groups is greater than ~10% and less than ~90%.

To illustrate the calculation of confidence intervals for dichotomous data, recall that in the study by Olsen et al (1997) the risk to control subjects was 27%, the risk to experimental subjects was 6%, and the average size of each group was 182, so:

$$95\% \text{ CI} \approx (27\% - 6\%) \pm 1/\sqrt{182}$$

[35]The 'proof' is as follows. If we assume that the sample sizes of the two groups are equal, the normal approximation for the 95% CI for the ARR reduces to the $ARR \pm 1.96 \times \sqrt{[(R_c(1 - R_c) + R_t(1 - R_t)]}/\sqrt{n}$, where R_c and R_t are the risks in the control and treated groups and n is the number of subjects in each group. To a very rough approximation, the term $1.96 \times \sqrt{[(R_c(1 - R_c) + R_t(1 - R_t)]} = 1$, provided $0.1 < R < 0.9$. Thus, to a very rough approximation, the 95% CI for the ARR $\approx ARR \pm 1/\sqrt{n}$. We can substitute n_{av} for n, so the 95% CI for the ARR $\approx ARR \pm 1/\sqrt{n_{av}}$.

---

[34]To see if you've got the hang of this, try using the data from our earlier example to calculate the number needed to treat with hip protectors to prevent a hip fracture in a high risk population with a 1-year risk of hip fracture of 20%.

95% CI ≈ 21% ± 0.07

95% CI ≈ 21% ± 7%

Thus the best estimate of the absolute risk reduction is 21% and its 95% confidence interval extends from 14% to 28%.

This result has been illustrated on a tree plot of the absolute risk reduction in Figure 6.4. The logic of this tree plot is exactly the same as that used for the tree plot of a continuous variable which was presented earlier.[36] Again, we plot the smallest clinically worthwhile effect (absolute risk reduction of 5%, corresponding to a number needed to treat of 20), the effect of intervention (absolute risk reduction of 21%) and its confidence interval (14% to 28%) on the graph. In this example the estimated absolute risk reduction and its confidence interval are clearly greater than the smallest clinically worthwhile effect, so we can confidently conclude that this intervention is clinically worthwhile. For morbidly obese patients (for whom we could multiply the absolute risk reduction by an f of 2 to take into account their greater untreated risk), the intervention is even more worthwhile.

In the example we just used we calculated absolute risk reduction and the 95% confidence intervals for the absolute risk reduction. We could, if we wished, have calculated the number needed to treat and the 95% confidence interval for the number needed to treat. As we have already seen, it is a simple matter to calculate the number needed to treat (NNT) from the absolute risk reduction (ARR) – we just invert the absolute risk reduction to obtain the number needed to treat.[37] The same applies to the ends of the confidence intervals (the 'confidence limits'). Once we have calculated the confidence limits for the absolute risk reduction we can obtain the 95% confidence interval for the number needed to treat by inverting the confidence limits of the absolute risk reduction. There is, however, a complication with the interpretation of confidence intervals for the number needed to treat (Altman 1998). When the confidence interval for the absolute risk reduction includes zero, confidence intervals for the number needed to treat don't appear to make sense. The problem and explanation are best illustrated with an example.

Pope et al (2000) investigated the effects of stretching before sport on all-injury risk in army recruits undergoing a 12-week training programme. Subjects were randomly allocated to groups that stretched or did not stretch prior to activity. Of the 803 subjects in the control group, 175 were injured

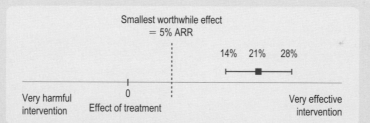

Figure 6.4   A 'tree plot' of the size of the treatment effect reported by Olsen et al (1997). The tree plot consists of a horizontal line representing treatment effect. At the extremes are very harmful and very effective treatments. The smallest clinically worthwhile effect is represented as a vertical dotted line. This example shows the effect (expressed as an absolute risk reduction, ARR) of chest physiotherapy on risk of respiratory complications following upper abdominal surgery. The smallest clinically worthwhile effect has been nominated as an absolute reduction in risk of 5%. The best estimate of the size of the treatment effect (21%) and all of the 95% confidence interval about this estimate (14 to 28%) fall to the right of the line of the smallest worthwhile effect. Thus the treatment effect is clearly greater than the smallest worthwhile effect.

[36] You will often see forest plots of the effects of intervention on dichotomous outcomes arranged so that beneficial treatment effects are to the left and harmful effects to the right. One of the reasons for this is that most forest plots are of the relative risk or odds ratio, and, by convention, smaller relative risks or odds ratios correspond to more beneficial effects of intervention.

Here we have decsribed the effect of intervention in terms of the absolute risk reduction. Larger absolute risk reductions correspond to more beneficial effects, so the natural convention is to plot beneficial effects of intervention to the right.
[37] The same operation is used to convert an NNT into an ARR: the ARR = 1/NNT.

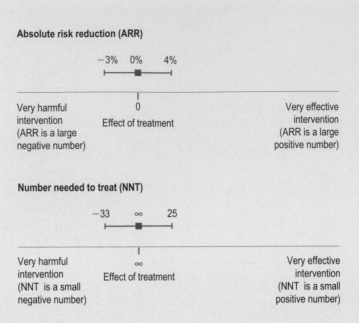

Figure 6.5 Explanation of confidence intervals for NNTs. The data of Pope et al (2000) suggest stretching before exercise reduces injury risk (ARR) by 0% (95% CI −3 to 4%) in army recruits undergoing a 12-week training programme (tree plot shown in top panel). When, as in this example, the confidence interval for the ARR includes zero, the confidence interval for the NNT looks a little strange. In this example the estimated NNT is infinity and the 95% CI extends from −33 to 25; bizarrely, the estimated effect (infinity) does not seem to lie within its confidence intervals (−33 to 25). The explanation is that the tree plot for the NNT has a strange number line. A tree plot for the NNT is drawn in the lower panel, and it has been scaled and aligned so that it corresponds exactly to the tree plot for the ARR shown in the upper panel. The NNT of infinity lies in the middle of the tree plot (no effect of intervention). Smaller numbers lie at the tails of the number line. On this bizarre number line the estimated NNT always lies within its confidence interval.

(risk of 21.8%) and 158 of the 735 subjects in the stretch group were injured (risk of 21.5%). Thus the effect of stretching was an absolute risk reduction of 0.3%, with an approximate 95% confidence interval from −3% to +4%. If we re-cast these estimates in terms of numbers needed to treat, we get a number needed to treat of 333 and an approximate 95% confidence interval for the number needed to treat of −33 to 25. The interpretation of the number needed to treat of 333 is quite straightforward. It means that 333 people would need to stretch before activity for 12 weeks to prevent one injury.[38,39] But the confidence limits are, at first, a little perplexing, because the estimate of 333 does not appear to lie within the confidence interval (−33 to 25).

The explanation is that numbers need to treat lie on an unusual number scale (Figure 6.5; Altman 1998). In fact it is easiest to visualize the number scale as the inverse of the normal number scale that we use for the absolute risk reduction. Instead of being centred on zero, like the number scale for the absolute risk reduction, the number scale for the number needed to treat is centred on 1/0, or infinity. This number scale is big in the middle and little at the edges! If we refer back to our example, you can see that, on this strange number scale, the best estimate of the number needed to treat (333) really does lie within the 95% confidence interval of −33 to 25!

---

[38] Following the same approach as in footnote 35, this is a bit like saying we would need to stretch before activity for 333 × 12 weeks, or 77 years, to prevent an injury.

[39] This analysis differs slightly from the analysis reported in the trial by Pope et al (2000) because the authors of the original trial report used more sophisticated methods to analyse the data than are used here.

Box 6.3   Is the evidence relevant to me and my patient/s?

Are the subjects in the study similar to the patients I wish to apply the study's findings to?
Look at the inclusion and exclusion criteria used to determine eligibility for participation in the trial or systematic review.

Were interventions applied appropriately?
Look at how the intervention was applied.

Are the outcomes useful?
Determine if the outcomes matter to patients.

Does the therapy do more good than harm?
Obtain an estimate of the size of the effect of treatment. Assess whether the effect of therapy is likely to be large enough to make it worth applying.

WHAT DOES THIS SYSTEMATIC REVIEW OF EFFECTS OF INTERVENTION MEAN FOR MY PRACTICE?

In the preceding section we considered how to assess whether a particular clinical trial provides us with relevant evidence, and what that evidence means for clinical practice. Now we turn our attention to interpreting systematic reviews of the effects of intervention.

IS THE EVIDENCE RELEVANT TO ME AND MY PATIENT/S?

Making decisions about the relevance of a systematic review is very much like making decisions about the relevance of a clinical trial. (See 'Is the evidence relevant to me and my patient/s?' at the beginning of this chapter.) All of the same considerations apply. Just as with individual trials, we need to decide whether the review is able to provide information about the subjects, interventions and outcomes we are interested in.

With systematic reviews, decisions about relevance of subjects, interventions and outcomes can be made at either of two levels. The simpler approach is to look at the question addressed by the review and the criteria used to include and exclude studies in the review. In most systematic reviews there are explicit statements about the review question and the criteria used to determine what trials were eligible for the review. For example, a Cochrane systematic review by the Outpatient Service Trialists (2004) stipulated that the objective of the review was to 'assess the effects of therapy-based rehabilitation services targeted towards stroke patients resident in the community within 1 year of stroke onset/discharge from hospital following stroke'. The review was explicitly concerned with the effects of therapist-based rehabilitation services (defined at considerable length in the review) on death, dependency or performance in activities of daily living of patients who had experienced a stroke, were resident in a community setting, and had been randomized to treatment within

1 year of the index stroke. This clear statement of the scope of the review is typical of Cochrane systematic reviews.

To some readers, particularly those with a specific interest in the field of the review, this level of detail may be insufficient. These readers may be interested in the precise characteristics of subjects included in each trial, or the precise nature of the intervention, or the precise method used to measure outcomes. It may be possible to obtain this level of information if the review separately reports details of each trial considered in the review. This information is often presented in the form of a table. Typically the table describes the subjects, interventions and outcomes measured in each trial. When systematic reviewers provide this degree of detail the reader can decide for himself or herself which trials study relevant subjects, interventions and outcomes. It may be that a particular trial has investigated the precise combinations of subjects, interventions and outcomes that are of greatest interest.

By way of example, if you were interested in the potential effects of weight-supported walking training for a particular patient who recently had a stroke, you might consult the recent Cochrane review by Moseley et al (2004). This review assessed the effects of treadmill training or body weight support in the training of walking after stroke, so it included all trials with subjects who had suffered a stroke and exhibit an abnormal gait pattern. The authors describe, in the text of their review, that five of the 11 trials in the review were clearly of ambulatory patients, and they provided detailed information about the subjects, interventions and outcomes of these trials. When systematic reviews provide the details of each of the reviewed studies, readers can base their conclusions on the particular trials that are most relevant to their own clinical questions.

WHAT DOES THE EVIDENCE SAY?

Good systematic reviews provide us with a wealth of information about the effects of interventions. They usually provide a detailed description of each of the individual trials included in the review and may, in addition, provide summary statements or conclusions that indicate the reviewers' interpretation of what the trials collectively say. Either or both may be helpful to the reader. In the following section we consider how to interpret the data presented in systematic reviews.

We begin by considering how systematic reviews can draw together the evidence from individual clinical trials into summary statements about the effects of intervention. As readers of systematic reviews, we want these summary statements to tell us both about the strength of the evidence and, if the evidence is strong enough to draw some conclusions, about the size of the effect of the intervention.

There are several distinctly different approaches that reviewers use to generate summary statements. Unfortunately, not all generate summary statements that are entirely satisfactory. As we shall see, a common problem is that the effect of the intervention is given in simplistic terms: the intervention is said to be either 'effective' or 'ineffective'. Statements about the effects of intervention that are not accompanied by estimates of the magnitudes of those effects are of little use for clinical decision-making. Readers should be wary of systematic reviews with simplistic summary statements.

The simplest method used to generate summary statements about the effects of intervention is called *vote counting*. Vote counting is used in many narrative reviews and some systematic reviews. In the vote counting approach, the reviewer assigns one 'vote' to each trial, and then counts up the number of studies that do and do not find evidence for an effect of intervention. Some reviewers apply a simple rule: the conclusion with the most votes wins! Other reviewers are more conservative: they stipulate that a certain (high) percentage of trials must conclude there is a significant effect of intervention before there is collective evidence of an effect. Sometimes the vote counting threshold is not made explicit. In that case the reviewer informally assesses the proportion of significant trials and decides if 'most' trials are significant or not, without explicitly stating the threshold that defines 'most'. But regardless of what threshold is used, vote counting generates one of two conclusions: either there is evidence of an effect, or there is not.

An example of the use of vote counting comes from a systematic review of preventive interventions for back and neck problems (Linton & van Tulder 2001). This review reports that 'Six of the nine randomised controlled trials did not find any significant differences on any of the outcome variables compared between the back school intervention and usual care or no intervention or between different types of back or neck schools … Thus, there is consistent evidence from randomized controlled trials that back and neck schools are not effective interventions in preventing back pain' (pp 789–783). In this review, there were more non-significant than significant trials of back and neck schools so the authors concluded back and neck schools are not an effective intervention.

The shortcomings of vote counting have been understood since the very early days of systematic reviews. Hedges & Olkin (1980, 1985) showed that vote counting is toothless; it lacks statistical power. That is, even when an intervention is effective the vote counting approach is likely to conclude that there is no evidence of 'an effect of' intervention. The power of the vote counting procedure is determined by the threshold required to satisfy the reviewer that there is an effect (for example, 50% of trials or 66% of trials), the number of trials, and the statistical power of the individual trials. (The statistical power of an individual trial refers to the probability that the trial will detect a clinically meaningful effect if such an effect truly exists. Many trials have low statistical power because they are too small; that is, many trials have too few subjects to enable them to detect clinically meaningful effects of intervention if such effects exist.) Typically, the power of the vote counting approach is low. A remarkably bad property of the vote counting approach is that the power of vote counting may actually decrease with an increasing number of trials (Hedges & Olkin 1985). Consequently, the probability of detecting an effect of intervention may decrease as evidence accrues. For this reason, systematic reviews that use vote counting and conclude there is no evidence of an effect of intervention should be treated with suspicion.

There is a second serious problem with vote counting. Vote counting provides a dichotomous answer: it concludes that there *is* or *is not* evidence that the intervention is effective. Earlier in this chapter it was argued that there is little value in learning if the intervention is effective. What we need to know, instead, is how effective the intervention is. The 'answer' provided by vote counting methods is not clinically useful.

An alternative to vote counting is the *levels of evidence approach*. This approach differs from vote counting in that it attempts to combine information about both the quality of the evidence and the effects of the intervention. In some versions of this approach, the reviewer defines 'strong evidence', 'moderate evidence', 'weak evidence' (or 'limited evidence') and 'little or no evidence'. Usually the definitions are based on the quantity, quality and consistency of evidence. A typical example is given in Box 6.4.

As an example, the same systematic review that used vote counting to examine effects of back and neck schools also used levels of evidence criteria to examine the effects of exercise for preventing neck and back pain (Linton & van Tulder 2001). Strong ('Level A') evidence was defined as 'generally consistent findings from multiple randomized controlled trials'. It was concluded that 'there is consistent evidence that exercise may be effective in preventing neck and back pain (Level A)'.

One of the problems with the levels of evidence approach is that different authors use slightly different criteria to define levels of evidence. Indeed, some authors use different criteria in different reviews. For example, van Poppel et al (1997) define limited evidence as 'only one high quality randomized controlled trial or multiple low quality randomized controlled trials and non-randomized controlled clinical trials (high or low quality). Consistent outcome of the studies', whereas Berghmans et al (1998) define limited evidence as 'one relevant RCT of sufficient methodologic quality or multiple low quality RCTs.' These small differences in wording are not just untidy; they can profoundly affect the conclusions

---

Box 6.4   Levels of evidence criteria of van Poppel et al (1997)

Level 1 (strong evidence): multiple relevant, high quality randomized clinical trials (RCTs) with consistent results.

Level 2 (moderate evidence): one relevant, high quality RCT and one or more relevant low quality RCTs or non-randomized controlled clinical trials (CCTs) (high or low quality). Consistent outcomes of the studies.

Level 3 (limited evidence): only one high-quality RCT or multiple low-quality RCTs and non-randomized CCTs (high or low quality). Consistent outcomes of the studies.

Level 4 (no evidence): only one low-quality RCT or one non-randomized CCT (high or low quality), no relevant studies or contradictory outcomes of the studies.

Results were considered contradictory if less than 75% of studies reported the same results, otherwise outcomes were considered to be consistent.

that are drawn. Even apparently small differences in definitions of levels of evidence can lead to surprisingly different conclusions. Ferreira and colleagues (2003) applied four different sets of levels of evidence criteria to six Cochrane systematic reviews and found only 'fair' agreement (kappa = 0.33) between the conclusions reached with the different criteria. Application of the different criteria to one particular review, of the effects of back school for low back pain, lead to the conclusion that there was 'strong evidence that back school was effective' or 'weak evidence' or 'limited evidence' or 'no evidence', depending on which criteria were used. As the conclusions of systematic reviews can be very sensitive to the criteria used to define levels of evidence, readers of systematic reviews should be reluctant to accept the conclusions of systematic reviews which use the levels of evidence approach.

Another significant problem with the levels of evidence approach is that it, too, is likely to lack statistical power. This is because most levels of evidence criteria are based on vote counting. For example the definition of 'strong evidence' used by van Poppel et al (1997) ('multiple relevant, high quality randomized clinical trials with consistent results') is based on vote counting because it requires that there be 'consistent' findings of the trials. In fact the levels of evidence approach is likely to be even less powerful than vote counting because it usually invokes additional criteria relating to trial quality. That is, to meet the definition of strong evidence there must be at least a certain proportion of significant trials (vote counting) *and* the trials must be of a certain quality. Thus, in general, the levels of evidence approach will have even less power than vote counting.

A quick inspection of the systematic reviews in physiotherapy that use vote counting or levels of evidence approaches shows that only a small proportion conclude there is strong evidence of an effect of intervention. This low percentage may indicate that there is not yet strong evidence of the effects of many interventions, but an equally plausible explanation is that true effects of intervention have been missed because the levels of evidence approach lacks the statistical power required to detect such effects.

Recent efforts have focused on developing qualitative methods of summarizing evidence that do not have the shortcomings of vote counting and levels of evidence approaches. One promising initiative is the GRADE project, which seeks to summarize several dimensions of the quality of evidence and the strength of recommendations (GRADE Working Group 2004). The GRADE scale assesses dimensions of study design, study quality, consistency (the similarity of estimates of effect across studies) and directness (the extent to which people, interventions and outcome measures are similar to those of interest). It uses the following definitions of the quality of evidence:

- *High quality evidence.* Further research is very unlikely to change our confidence in the estimate of effect.
- *Moderate quality evidence.* Further research is likely to have an important impact on our confidence in the estimate of effect and may change the estimate.

- *Low quality evidence.* Further research is very likely to have an important impact on our confidence in the estimate of effect and may change the estimate.
- *Very low quality evidence.* Any estimate of effect is very uncertain.

The breadth of this scale and its emphasis on the magnitude of the effect makes it attractive. It will probably be subject to empirical investigation in the next few years.

An alternative to vote counting and the levels of evidence approach is *meta-analysis*. As with vote counting, meta-analysis provides a tool for summarizing effects of interventions but it does not usually incorporate information about the quality of evidence. It involves extracting estimates of the size of the effect of intervention from each trial and then statistically combining ('pooling') the data to obtain a single estimate based on all the trials.

An example of meta-analysis is provided in the systematic review, of effects of pre- and post-exercise stretching on muscle soreness, risk of injury and athletic performance, by Herbert & Gabriel (2002). This systematic review identified five studies that reported useful data on the effects of stretching on muscle soreness. The results of the five studies were pooled in a meta-analysis to produce a single pooled estimate of the effects of stretching on subsequent muscle soreness.

To conduct a meta-analysis the researcher must first describe the magnitude of the effect of intervention reported in each trial. This can be done with any of a number of statistics. In trials which report continuous outcomes, the statistic most used to describe the size of effects of intervention is the mean difference between groups. This is the same statistic we used to describe the size of effects of interventions when appraising individual trials earlier in this chapter, and it has the same interpretation. Alternatively, some reviews will report the standardized mean difference between groups (usually calculated as the difference between group means divided by a pooled estimate of the within-group standard deviation).[40] The advantage of dividing the difference between means by the standard deviation is that it makes it possible to pool the findings of studies which report findings on different scales. However, when the size of the effect of intervention is reported on a standardized scale it can be very difficult to interpret, because it is difficult to know how big a particular standardized effect size must be to be clinically worthwhile.

When outcomes are reported on a dichotomous scale, different statistics are used to describe the effects of intervention. Unfortunately, the statistics we preferred to use earlier in this chapter to describe the effects of intervention on dichotomous outcomes in individual trials (the absolute risk reduction and number needed to treat) are not well suited to meta-analysis. Instead, in meta-analysis the effect of intervention on dichotomous outcomes is most often reported as a relative risk or an odds ratio.[41]

---

[40] There are several minor variations of this statistic.
[41] A number of other measures, notably the hazard ratio, are also used, though rarely.

The relative risk is simply the ratio of risks in intervention and control groups. Thus, if the risk in the intervention group is 6% and the risk in the control group is 27% (as in the trial by Olsen et al (1997) that we examined earlier in this chapter), the relative risk is 6/27 or 0.22. Relative risks of less than 1.0 indicate that risk in the intervention group was lower than in the control group, and risks of greater than 1 indicate that the risk in the intervention groups was higher than in the control group. A relative risk of 1.0 indicates that both groups had the same risk, and implies there was no effect of the intervention. The further the relative risk departs from 1, the bigger the effect of the intervention.

The odds ratio is similar to relative risk except that it is a ratio of odds, instead of a ratio of risks (or probabilities). Odds are just another way of describing probabilities,[42] so the odds ratio behaves in some ways very like the relative risk. In fact when the risk in the control group is low, the odds ratio is nearly the same as the relative risk. When the risk in the control groups is high (say >15%), the odds ratio diverges from the relative risk. This divergence happens in a simple way: the odds ratio always departs from 1.0 more than the relative risk.

Usually the summary statistic for each trial is presented either in a table, or in a forest plot such as the one reproduced in Figure 6.6. This is a particularly useful feature of systematic reviews. They provide, at a glance, a summary of the effects of intervention from each trial.

Regardless of what summary statistic is used to describe the effect of intervention observed in each trial, meta-analysis proceeds in the same way. The summary statistics from each trial are combined to produce a pooled estimate of the effect of intervention. The pooled estimate is really just an average of the summary statistics provided by each trial. But the average is not a simple average because some trials are given more 'weight' than others. The weight is determined by the standard error of the summary statistic, which is nearly the same as saying that the weight is determined by sample size: bigger studies (those with lots of subjects) provide more precise estimates of the effects of intervention, so they are given more influence on the final pooled (weighted average) estimate of the effect of intervention.

The allure of meta-analysis is that it can provide more precise estimates of the effects of intervention than individual trials. This is illustrated in the meta-analysis of effects of stretching before or after exercise on muscle soreness, mentioned earlier (Herbert & Gabriel 2002). None of the five studies included in the meta-analysis found a statistically significant effect of stretching on muscle soreness, and all found the effects of stretching on muscle soreness was near zero. However, most of the individual studies were small and had quite wide confidence intervals, meaning that individually they could not rule out small but marginally

---

[42] The odds is the ratio of the risk of the event happening to the 'risk' of the event not happening. So if the risk is 33%, the ratio of risks is 33/67 or 0.5. If the risk is 80%, the odds are 80/20, or 4, and so on. You can convert risks (probabilities, R) to odds (O) with the equation $O = R/(1 - R)$. And you can convert back from odds to risks with $R = O/(1 + O)$.

WHAT DOES THIS EVIDENCE MEAN FOR MY PRACTICE?

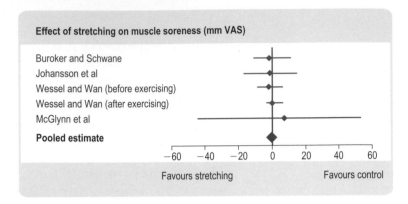

Figure 6.6   An example of a forest plot. Forest plots summarize the findings of several randomized trials of intervention, in this case the effects of stretching on post-exercise muscle soreness. Each row corresponds to one randomized trial; the names of the trial authors are given at the left. For each trial, the estimate of effect of intervention is shown as a diamond. (In this case the effect of intervention is expressed as the average reduction in muscle soreness, given in mm on a 100 mm soreness VAS.) The horizontal lines indicate the extent of the 95% confidence intervals, which can be loosely interpreted as the range within which the true average effect of stretching lies. The big symbol at the bottom is the pooled estimate of the effect of intervention, obtained by statistically combining the findings of all of the individual studies. Note that the confidence intervals of the pooled estimate are narrower than the confidence intervals of individual studies. (Data from Herbert and Gabriel (2002).)

worthwhile effects. Pooling estimates of the effects of stretching from all five trials in a meta-analysis provided a more precise estimate of the effects of stretching (Figure 6.6). The authors concluded that 'the pooled estimate of reduction in muscle soreness 24 hours after exercising was only 0.9 mm on a 100 mm scale (95% confidence interval −2.6 mm to 4.4 mm) … most athletes will consider effects of this magnitude too small to make stretching to prevent later muscle soreness worthwhile.' The meta-analysis was able to provide a very precise estimate of the average effect of stretching (between −2.6 and 4.4 mm on a 100 mm scale), which permitted a clear conclusion to be drawn about the ineffectiveness of stretching in preventing muscle soreness.

> The important difference between meta-analysis and both the vote counting and the levels of evidence approaches is that meta-analysis focuses on estimates of the *size* of the effect of the intervention, rather than on whether the effect of intervention was statistically significant or not.

This is important for two reasons. First, as we have already seen, information about the size of the effects of intervention is critically important for clinical decision-making. Rational clinical decision-making requires information about how much benefit intervention gives, not just information about whether intervention is 'effective' or not. Second, by using estimates of effects of interventions, meta-analysis accrues more information about the effects of intervention than vote counting or the levels of evidence approach. Consequently meta-analysis is much more powerful than either vote counting or the levels of evidence approach. Under some conditions, meta-analysis is statistically optimal. That is, meta-analysis can provide the maximum possible information about the effects of an intervention, so it is less likely than vote counting or the levels of evidence approach to conclude that there is 'not enough evidence' of the effects of intervention if there really is a worthwhile effect of the intervention. For this reason meta-analysis is the strongly preferred method of synthesizing findings of trials in a systematic review.

Why is meta-analysis not used in all systematic reviews? One reason is that some trials do not provide enough information about the effects of intervention for meta-analysis. For example, the review by Ferreira et al (2003) on the effects of manipulation for acute low back pain identified 34 relevant trials, of which four trials did not report enough data to permit inclusion in a meta-analysis. Another reason why meta-analysis is not used in all reviews is that the pooled estimates of effects of intervention provided by meta-analysis are only interpretable if each of the trials is trying to estimate something similar. Meta-analysis is only interpretable if the estimates to be pooled are from trials that measure similar outcomes and apply similar sorts of intervention to similar types of patients. (That is, the trials need to be 'homogeneous' with respect to outcomes, interventions and patients.) The trials need not be identical – they just need to be sufficiently similar for the pooled estimate to be interpretable. However, the practical reality is that when several trials investigate the effects of an intervention they typically recruit subjects from quite different sorts of populations, apply interventions in quite different sorts of ways, and use quite different outcome measures. (That is, they are typically 'heterogeneous'.) Ferreira et al (2003) reported that only 11 of 34 trials could be included in meta-analyses 'due primarily to heterogeneity of outcome measures and comparison groups'. In these circumstances it is often difficult for the reader to decide if it was appropriate or inappropriate statistically to pool the findings of the trials in a meta-analysis. In fact this issue, of when it is and is not appropriate to pool estimates of effects of intervention in a meta-analysis, is one of the most difficult methodological issues in systematic reviews. Readers of meta-analyses must carefully examine the details of the individual trials to decide whether the pooled estimate is interpretable. The reader needs to ask: 'Is it reasonable to combine estimates of the effect of interventions from these studies?'

These impediments to meta-analysis (insufficient data for meta-analysis, and heterogeneity of subjects, interventions or outcomes) may be thought to provide a justification for using vote counting or the levels of evidence approach. But, as we have seen, vote counting and the levels of evidence approach lack statistical power and, at any rate, do not provide useful summaries of the effects of intervention because they do not estimate the size of effects of intervention. And the levels of evidence approach has the additional problem that it is sensitive to the precise definitions of each of the levels of evidence, which are somewhat arbitrary. That is not to say that reviews which employ vote counting or the levels of evidence approach are not useful. Such reviews may still provide the reader with results of a comprehensive literature search and an assessment of quality, and perhaps a detailed description of the trials and their findings. But their conclusions should be regarded with some caution.

When meta-analysis is not possible, vote counting and levels of evidence are not a good alternative. So what is? The best information we can get from a systematic review, if meta-analysis is not appropriate or not possible, is a detailed description of each of the trials included in the review. Fortunately, as we have seen, estimates of effects of intervention provided by each trial are usually given in a table or a forest plot, and this information is often complemented by information about the methodological quality of each trial and the details of the patients, interventions and outcomes in each trial.

> So even if meta-analysis has not been conducted, or if it has been conducted inappropriately, we can still get useful information from systematic reviews. The reviews fulfil the very useful role of locating and summarizing relevant trials.

Readers may find the prospect of examining the estimates of individual trials less attractive than being presented with a summary meta-analysis. In effect, the reader is provided with many answers ('the effect on a particular outcome of applying intervention in a particular way to a particular population was X, and the effect on another outcome of applying intervention in another way to another population was Y') , rather than a simple summary ('the intervention has effect Z'). Also, because the findings of individual studies are not pooled, conclusions must be based on the (usually imprecise, and possibly less credible) estimates of the effects of intervention provided by individual trials. Nonetheless, this is the only truly satisfactory alternative to meta-analysis when meta-analysis is not appropriate or not possible because, unlike vote counting and the levels of evidence approach, the description of estimates of effects of intervention provided by individual trials provides clinically interpretable information.

To summarize this section, systematic reviews which use vote counting or the levels of evidence approach do not generate useful conclusions about effects of intervention, and may conclude there is insufficient evidence of effects of intervention even when the data say otherwise. Systematic reviews that employ meta-analysis potentially provide better evidence of effects of intervention because meta-analysis involves explicit quantification of effects of interventions, and is statistically optimal. However, meta-analysis is not always possible, and even when meta-analysis is possible, it may not be appropriate. When a meta-analysis has been conducted, readers must examine whether the trials pooled in the meta-analysis were sampled from sufficiently similar populations, used sufficiently similar interventions, and measured outcomes in sufficiently similar ways. Where meta-analysis is not appropriate or possible, or has not been done, the best approach is to inspect details of individual trials.

WHAT DOES THIS STUDY OF EXPERIENCES MEAN FOR MY PRACTICE?

It is said that the strength of the quantitative approach lies in its *reliability* (repeatability), by which is meant that replication of quantitative studies should yield the same results time after time, whereas the strength of qualitative research lies in *validity* (closeness to the truth). That is, good qualitative research can touch what is really going on rather than just skimming the surface (Greenhalgh 2001). Specifically, high quality interpretive research offers an understanding of roles and relationships. This implies that qualitative research can help physiotherapists better understand the context of their practice and their relationships with patients and their families. But this requires that the research findings be presented clearly, and that the findings are transferable to other settings.

WAS THERE A CLEAR STATEMENT OF FINDINGS?

Are the findings explicit? Is it clear how the researchers arrived at their conclusion?

What do findings from qualitative research look like? The product of a qualitative study is a narrative that tries to represent faithfully and accurately the social world or phenomena being studied (Giacomini et al 2002). The findings may be presented as descriptions or theoretical insights or theories.

The interpretation of findings is closely related to the analytical path. This was discussed in Chapter 5, but we revisit these ideas here. The findings should be presented explicitly and clearly and it should be clear how the researchers arrived at their conclusion. Interpretation is an integral part of qualitative inquiry, and there is an emerging nature of qualitative research in the way that the research alters as the data are collected. In qualitative research the results are an interpretation of the data, so it is not reasonable to expect separation of what the researchers found from what they think it means (as in quantitative research) (Greenhalgh 2001). Consequently, in qualitative research, the results and the discussion are sometimes presented together. If so, it is still important that the data and the interpretation are linked in a logical way. As described in Chapter 5, the analytical path should be clearly described so that readers can follow the way to the conclusion. Triangulation can improve the credibility of the study and strengthen the findings.

The findings are often grouped into themes, patterns or categories, and by developing hypothesis and theories. The theoretical framework can be likened to reading glasses worn by the researcher when she or he asks questions about the materials (Malterud 2001). A frequent shortcoming in report-writing in qualitative research is to omit information about whether the presented categories represent empirical findings or whether they were identified in advance. It is not sufficient for a researcher simply to say that the materials were coded for typical patterns, resulting in some categories. The reader needs to know the principles and choices underlying pattern recognition and category foundation (Malterud 2001). Hjort and colleagues (1999) describe their arrival at categories with a two-step approach in a study carried out among patients with rheumatoid arthritis. The aim of the study was to describe and analyse patients' ideas and perceptions about home exercise and physical activity. Five categories emerged from the first step of open coding and categorization, ending up with three idealized types of people: the action-oriented, the compliant and the resigned. By integrating results such as these into practice, physiotherapists are more likely to be able to identify and understand individual needs and may be better equipped to collaborate with patients.

Findings are often supplied with quotations. Quotations and stories can be used to illustrate insights gained from the data analysis. One important function of quotations in the results section is to demonstrate that the findings are based on data (Greenhalgh 2001). Statements such as 'The participants became aware of their breathing' would be more credible if one or two verbatim quotes from the interviews were reproduced to illustrate them. For example:

> Breathing – it always comes back to breathing. I stop, become aware of how I breathe, and discover again and again that when I start to breathe deeply, my body relaxes. I do this several times a day, especially at work.
> (Steen & Haugli 2001)

Quotes and examples should be indexed so that they can be traced back to an identifiable subject or setting (Greenhalgh 2001).

It is a challenge to present complex material from qualitative research in a clear, transparent and meaningful way without overloading the reader with details and theories that do not relate directly to the phenomenon that is studied. Still, readers should look for whether the results of a qualitative research report address the way the findings relate to other theories in the field. An empirically developed theory need not agree with existing beliefs (Giacomini et al 2002). But, regardless of whether it agrees or not, authors should describe its relationship to prevailing theories and beliefs in a critical manner (Giacomini et al 2002).

HOW VALUABLE IS THE RESEARCH?

Does the study contribute to existing knowledge or understanding? Have avenues for further research been identified? Can the findings be transferred to other populations or settings?

The aim of most research, and almost all useful research, is to produce information that can be shared and applied beyond the study setting. No study, irrespective of the method used, can provide findings that are universally transferable. Nonetheless, studies whose findings cannot be generalized to other contexts in some way can have little direct influence on clinical decision-making. Thus, readers should ask if a study's findings are generalizable. One criterion for the generalizability of a qualitative study is whether it provides a useful 'road map' for the reader to navigate similar social settings.

A common criticism of qualitative research is that the findings of qualitative studies pertain only to the limited setting in which they were obtained. Indeed, it has been argued that issues of generalizability in qualitative research have been paid little attention, at least until quite recently (Schofield 2002). A major factor contributing to disregard of issues of generalizability (or 'external validity'[43]) appears to be a widely shared view that external validity is unimportant, unachievable or both (Schofield 2002). However, several trends, including the growing use of qualitative studies in evaluation and policy-oriented research, have led to an increased awareness of the importance of structuring qualitative research in a way that enhances understanding of other situations. Generalizability can be enhanced by studying the typical, the common and the ordinary, by conducting multisite studies, and by designing studies to fit with future trends (Schofield 2002).

Still, the generalizability of qualitative research is likely to be conceptual rather than numerical. Interpretive research offers clinicians an understanding of roles and relationships, not effect sizes or rates or other quantifiable phenomena. Many studies of interest to clinicians focus on communication among patients, therapists, families and caregivers. Other studies describe behaviours of these groups, either in isolation or during interactions with others (Giacomini et al 2002). A study that explored views held by health professionals and patients about the role of guided self-management plans in asthma care suggested that attempts to introduce such plans in primary care were unlikely to be successful because neither patients nor professionals were enthusiastic about guided self-management plans (Jones et al 2000). Neither health professionals nor patients felt positive towards guided self-management plans, and most patients felt that the plans were largely irrelevant to them. A fundamental mismatch was apparent between the views of professionals and patients on the characteristics of a 'responsible' asthma patient, and on what patients should be doing to control their symptoms. Studies like this provide findings that could, for example, help clinicians to understand why patients with asthma might not 'comply' with treatment plans. This might suggest (but would not prove the effectiveness of) modifications to care processes, and it suggests ways that practice could be made more patient-centred.

WHAT DOES THIS STUDY OF PROGNOSIS MEAN FOR MY PRACTICE?

This section considers how we can interpret good quality evidence of the prognosis of particular conditions. That evidence may be in the form of a cohort study, or a clinical trial, or even a systematic review of prognosis.

IS THE STUDY RELEVANT TO ME AND MY PATIENT/S?

The first step in interpreting evidence of prognosis is very much the same as for studies of the effects of therapy. We need to consider whether the patients in the study are similar to the patients that we wish to make inferences about, and whether the outcomes are those that are of interest to patients. These issues are very similar to those discussed at length with

---

[43] 'External validity' is another term for 'generalizability' or 'applicability' (Campbell & Stanley 1966).

randomized trials or systematic reviews of the effects of therapy, so we will not elaborate further on them here. Instead we focus on some issues that pertain particularly to interpretation of evidence of prognosis.

When we ask questions about prognosis we could be interested in the natural course of the condition (what happens to people who are untreated) or, instead, we might be interested in the clinical course of the condition (what happens to people treated in the usual way). We can learn about the natural course of the condition from studies that follow untreated cohorts, and we learn about the clinical course of the condition from studies that followed treated cohorts.[44] What clinical value can this information have? How is this information relevant to clinical practice?

Perhaps the most important role of prognostic information is that it can be used to inform patients of what the likely outcome of having a particular condition is likely to be. For some conditions, particularly relatively minor ailments, one of the main reasons that patients seek out professionals is to obtain a clear prognosis. People are naturally curious about what their futures are likely to be, and they often ask about their prognoses. They may seek reassurance that their conditions are not serious, or that the conditions will resolve without intervention. In responding, physiotherapists are required to be fortune tellers, and it is best, where possible, that they be evidence-based fortune tellers! We need to be provisioned with good quality evidence about prognosis for the conditions we often see. Of course, we should not divulge prognoses just because we know what they are. Some patients do not want to know their prognoses, particularly if the prognosis is bleak. It may take a great deal of wisdom to know if, when and how to inform patients of poor prognoses.

Information about the natural history of a condition also tells us if we should be alarmed about prognosis, and if we should look for some way to manage the condition. For example, the parents of a young child with talipes valgus (also called pes calcaneovalgus or pes abductus or pes valgus) might be interested in the natural history of the condition because they want to know if it is likely to become a persistent problem, or if it is something that will resolve with time. If the natural course was one of ongoing disability we might consider investigating interventions that might improve outcomes. But if, as is the case for talipes valgus in very young children, the long-term prognosis is favourable (Widhe et al 1988), then we will probably not consider intervention, and we would probably choose simply to monitor development of the child's foot.

We can extend this idea further. Information about the natural course of a condition sets an upper limit for the benefit that can be provided by intervention. For example, we may learn that the prognosis for a 42-year-old male with primary shoulder dislocation is good: the risk of subsequent re-dislocation is around 6% within 4 years (te Slaa et al 2004). Theoretically, then, the best possible intervention is one which reduces the risk of dislocation by around 6% over 4 years. The implication is that

---

[44]Some controlled trials may be able to tell us about both the natural course of the condition (using data from an untreated control group) and the clinical course of the condition (using data from the intervention group).

there is little point in considering interventions (such as a long-term exercise programme) to prevent re-subluxation, because, even if the intervention prevented all dislocations (an unrealistically optimistic scenario), the number needed to treat for 10 years would be 11. That is, even in this unrealistically optimistic scenario, the intervention would prevent only one subluxation for every 11 patients who exercised for 10 years. Most patients would consider this benefit (an average of 110 years of exercise to prevent one subluxation) insufficient to make the intervention worthwhile. This example illustrates how information about a good prognosis might discourage consideration of intervention.

In a similar vein, prognostic information can be used to supplement decisions about therapy. Early in this chapter we considered whether the effects of particular interventions were big enough to be clinically worthwhile and we used the example of a clinical trial that showed that, in the general population of patients undergoing upper abdominal surgery, prophylactic chest physiotherapy produced substantial reductions in risk of respiratory complications (number needed to treat = 5). Then we noted that the effects would be twice as big (number needed to treat of 2 or 3) in a morbidly obese population at twice the risk of respiratory complications. The information required for these calculations, about the prognosis (risk of respiratory complications) in morbidly obese patients, can be obtained from studies of prognosis. That is, prognostic studies can be used to scale estimates of the effects of therapy to particular populations.

A particular consideration in studies of prognosis concerns whether the follow-up was sufficiently prolonged to be useful. For some conditions (such as acute respiratory complications of surgery) most of the interest focuses on a short follow-up period (days or weeks), whereas for other conditions (such as cystic fibrosis or Parkinson's disease) the long-term prognosis (prognosis over years or even decades) is of more interest. Readers should ascertain whether follow-up was sufficiently prolonged to capture important prognoses.

WHAT DOES THE EVIDENCE SAY?

What does prognosis look like? Essentially prognoses come in two styles. Prognoses about events (dichotomous outcomes) are expressed in terms of the risk of the event. And prognoses about continuous outcomes are expressed in terms of the expected value of the outcome (usually the mean outcome, but sometimes the median outcome). Usually prognoses have to be associated with a time frame to be useful. Thus we say 'in patients who have undergone ACL [anterior cruciate ligament] reconstruction, the 5 year risk of injury of the contralateral ACL is approximately 11%' (Deehan 2000; this is a prognosis about a dichotomous variable) or 'In the 3 months following hemiparetic stroke, hand function recovers, on average, by approximately 2 points on the 6 point Hand Movement Scale' (Katrak et al 1998; this is a prognosis about a continuous variable).

This means that calculating prognosis is straightforward. For dichotomous outcomes we need only determine the proportion of people (that is, the risk of) experiencing the event of interest. And for continuous outcomes

Figure 6.7 An example of survival curves from a randomized trial of the effects of pre-exercise stretching on risk of injury. The survival curves show the cumulative probability of army recruits in stretch (S) and control groups (C) remaining injury free over the course of a 12 week training programme. Redrawn from Pope et al 2000.

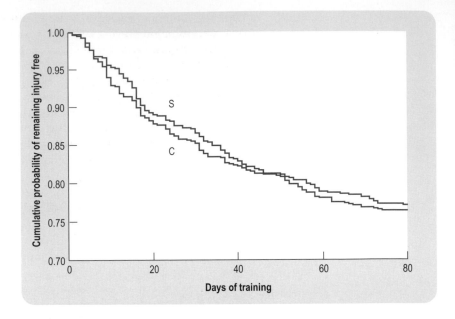

we need only determine the mean (or median) outcome. But while the calculations are straightforward, finding the data can be difficult. Often the prognostic information is contained in studies that were not explicitly designed to measure prognosis. It can require a degree of detective work to snoop out key data that appear incidentally, perhaps in among statistical summaries or in the headings to tables.

Sometimes outcome data are presented in the form of survival curves such as the one illustrated in Figure 6.7. Survival curves are particularly informative because they indicate how the risk of experiencing an event changes with time.[45] The risk for any particular prognostic time frame can be obtained from this curve. Figure 6.7 gives an example of a survival curve that shows the risk of lower limb musculoskeletal injury in army recruits undergoing military training. As the study was a randomized trial, there are two survival curves: one for each group. However the curves are very similar, so either curve could be used to generate information about risk of injury in army recruits undergoing training. The curves show that risk of injury in the first fortnight is 6 or 8%, and risk of injury in the first 10 weeks is 22 or 23%.

Estimates of prognosis, like estimates of the effects of intervention, are at best only approximations, because they are obtained from finite samples of patients. Earlier in this chapter we considered how to quantify the uncertainty associated with estimates of effects of intervention using

---

[45] The survival curve is not just the proportion of survivors at any one point in time, because if the probability of surviving was calculated in this way it would be biased by loss to follow-up. Instead, the survival curve is calculated by estimating survival over each successive increment of time, and then obtaining the product of the successive probabilities of surviving each successive time interval.

confidence intervals. We saw that large studies were associated with relatively narrow confidence intervals. The same applies for estimates of prognosis: large studies provide more certainty about the prognosis.

It may be useful to determine the degree of uncertainty to attach to an estimate of prognosis. This is best done by inspecting the confidence intervals associated with the prognosis. If we are lucky, the paper will report confidence intervals for estimates of prognosis, but if not it is a relatively easy matter to calculate the confidence ourselves, at least approximately. Again, there are some simple equations that we can use to obtain approximate confidence intervals for estimates of prognosis. These are given in Box 6.5.

Box 6.5   Confidence intervals for prognosis

These equations are similar to those we used to generate confidence intervals for estimates of effects of intervention.[46] When outcomes are measured on continuous scales we can calculate the approximate 95% confidence interval for the mean outcome at some point in time:

$$95\% \text{ CI} \approx mean \pm 3 \times SD/\sqrt{2N}$$

where N is the number of subjects in the group of interest.

When the outcome is measured on a dichotomous scale we can calculate an approximate 95% confidence interval for the risk of an event within some time period:

$$95\% \text{ CI} \approx risk \pm 1/\sqrt{2N}$$

To illustrate the use of these formulae, consider the study of long-term prognosis of whiplash-associated disorder conducted by Bunketorp et al (2004). These authors followed-up patients who had presented to hospital emergency departments with a whiplash injury 17 years earlier.

At 17 years, the mean total score on the 100-point Neck Disability Index was 22 (*SD* 22 *N* = 99). This is the expected level of disability in a patient in this population 17 years after injury. The mean score of 22 indicates that on average patients had quite mild disability. We can calculate an approximate 95% confidence interval for this prognosis:

$$95\% \text{ CI} \approx mean \pm 3 \times SD/\sqrt{2N}$$
$$95\% \text{ CI} \approx 22 \pm (3 \times 22)/\sqrt{2 \times 99}$$
$$95\% \text{ CI} \approx 22 \pm 5$$
$$95\% \text{ CI} \approx 17 \text{ to } 27$$

Thus we expect an average level of disability in this population of between 18 and 28 points on the Neck Disability Index 17 years after whiplash injury.

Fifty-five of 108 subjects reported persistent pain related to the initial injury. That is, in this cohort the risk of persistent pain after 17 years was 55/108 or 51%. The 95% confidence interval for this prognosis is:

$$95\% \text{ CI} \approx risk \pm 1/\sqrt{2N}$$
$$95\% \text{ CI} \approx 51\% \pm 1/\sqrt{2 \times 108}$$
$$95\% \text{ CI} \approx 51\% \pm 7\%$$
$$95\% \text{ CI} \approx 44 \text{ to } 58\%$$

We could say that we anticipate a risk of persistent pain of between 44 and 58% at 17 years.

---

[46] The only difference is that, for prognosis of continuous variables, we now need to estimate a confidence interval for the mean of a single group (rather than for the difference in the means of control and experimental groups, as we did for effects of therapy). Likewise for prognosis of dichotomous variables, we now need to estimate a confidence interval for the risk of a single group (rather than for the absolute risk reduction, which is the difference in the risks of control and experimental groups, as we did for effects of therapy). The width of the confidence intervals for estimates of prognosis differ from those used to estimate the size of effects of intervention only in that we use 2N (twice the number of subjects in the group of interest) rather than n_{av} (the average number of subjects in each group) in the denominator.

Up to now we have considered how to obtain global prognoses for broadly defined groups. But prognosis often varies hugely from person to person. Some people have characteristics that are likely to make their prognosis much better or much worse than average. For example, the prognosis of return to work in young head-injured adults probably varies enormously with degree of physical and psychological impairment, age, level of education and social support. Ideally, we would use information about prognostic variables such as these to refine the prognosis for any individual.

Many studies aim to identify prognostic variables, and to quantify how prognosis differs across people with and without (or with varying degrees of) the prognostic variables. The simplest approach involves separately reporting prognosis for subjects with and without a prognostic factor (or, for continuous variables, for people with low and high levels of the prognostic factor). An example comes from the prospective cohort study by Albert et al (2001) of prognosis of pregnant women with pelvic pain that we examined in Chapter 5. These authors separately reported prognoses for women with each of four syndromes of pelvic pain.

More recent studies tend to use a different and more complex approach. These studies develop multivariate predictive models to ascertain the degree to which prognosis is independently associated with each of a number of prognostic factors. The results are often reported in a table describing the importance and strength of the independent associations with each prognostic factor. Interpretation of the independent associations of prognostic factors is beyond the scope of this book. Suffice it to say that information about the independent associations of prognostic factors with prognosis is potentially important for two reasons. First, this can tell us how much the presence of a particular prognostic factor modifies prognosis. Second, we can potentially generate more precise estimates of prognosis if we take into account the prognostic factor when making the prognosis.

WHAT DOES THIS STUDY OF THE ACCURACY OF A DIAGNOSTIC TEST MEAN FOR MY PRACTICE?

In the final section of this chapter we consider the interpretation of high quality studies of the accuracy of diagnostic tests.

IS THE EVIDENCE RELEVANT TO ME AND MY PATIENT/S?

The interpretation of the relevance of evidence about the accuracy of diagnostic tests is very similar to the interpretation of studies of the effects of therapy and prognosis. Most importantly, we need to consider whether the patients in the study are similar to the patients about which we wish to make inferences.

An additional consideration is the skill of the tester. Many of the diagnostic tests used by physiotherapists require manual skill to implement and clinical experience to interpret. When reading studies of diagnostic tests that require skill and experience it is good practice to look for an indication that the test was conducted by people with appropriate levels of training and expertise. This is particularly critical when the test performs poorly. Then you want to be satisfied that it was the test, rather than the tester, that was incapable of generating an accurate diagnosis.

Another issue concerns the setting in which the tests were conducted. Tests may perform well in one setting (say, a private practice that sees a broad spectrum of cases) and poorly in other settings (say, in a specialist clinic). We will revisit this issue towards the end of this chapter. For now we simply allude to the idea that readers will obtain the best estimates of the accuracy of diagnostic tests from studies conducted in clinical settings similar to their own.

WHAT DOES THE EVIDENCE SAY?[47]

We say that a test is positive when its findings are indicative of the presence of the condition, and we say the test is negative when its findings are indicative of the absence of the condition. However, most tests are imperfect. Thus, even good clinical tests will sometimes be negative when the condition being tested for is present (false negative), or positive when the condition being tested for is absent (false positive). Thus the process of applying and interpreting diagnostic tests is probabilistic – the findings of a test often increase or decrease suspicion of a particular diagnosis but, because most tests are imperfect, it is rare that a single test clearly rules in or rules out a diagnosis. Good diagnostic tests have sufficient accuracy for positive findings greatly to increase suspicion of the diagnosis and negative tests greatly to reduce suspicion of the diagnosis.

The most common way of describing the accuracy of diagnostic tests (the concordance of the findings of the test and the reference standard) is in terms of sensitivity and specificity. Sensitivity is the probability that people who truly have the condition, as determined by testing with the reference standard, will test positive. It is estimated from the proportion (or percentage) of people who truly have the condition that test positive. Specificity is the probability that people who do not have the condition (again, as determined by testing with the reference standard) will test negative. It is estimated from the proportion (or percentage) of people who truly have the condition that test positive. Clearly, it is desirable that sensitivity and specificity are as high as possible – that is, it is desirable that sensitivity and specificity are close to 100%.

Though widely used, there is a major limitation to the use of sensitivity and specificity as indexes of the accuracy of diagnostic tests (Anonymous 1981). Fundamentally, sensitivity and specificity are quantities that we do not need to know about. Sensitivity tells us the probability that a person who has the condition will test positive. Yet when we test patients in the course of clinical practice we *know* if the test was positive or negative so

---

[47] This next section has been reproduced with only minor changes from Herbert (2005). We are grateful to the publisher for permission to reproduce this material.

we don't need to know the probability of a positive test occurring. More-over, we *don't know*, when we apply the test in clinical practice, if the person actually has the condition. If we did, there would be no point in carrying out the test. There is no practical value in knowing the probability that the test is positive when the condition is present. Instead, we need to know the probability of the person having the condition if the test is posi-tive. There is a similar problem with specificities – we don't need to know the probability of a person testing negative when he or she does not have the condition, but we do need to know the probability of the person hav-ing the condition when he or she tests negative.

Likelihood ratios

Likelihood ratios provide an alternative way of describing the accuracy of diagnostic tests (Sackett et al 1985). Importantly, likelihood ratios can be used to determine what we really need to know about. With a little numerical jiggery-pokery,

> likelihood ratios can be used to determine the probability that a person with a particular test finding has the diagnosis that is being tested for.

The likelihood ratio tells us how much more likely a particular test result is in people who have the condition than it is in people who don't have the condition. As most tests have two outcomes (positive or negative), this means we can talk about two likelihood ratios – one for positive test outcomes (we call this the positive likelihood ratio) and one for negative test outcomes (we call this the negative likelihood ratio).

The positive likelihood ratio tells us how much more likely a positive test finding is in people who have the condition than it is in those who don't. Obviously it is desirable for tests to be positive more often in people who have the condition than in those who don't, so consequently it is desirable to have positive likelihood ratios with values greater than 1. In practice, positive likelihood ratios with values greater than about 3 are useful, and positive likelihood ratios with values greater than 10 are very useful.

The negative likelihood ratio tells us how much more likely a negative test finding is in people who have the condition than those who don't. This means that it is desirable for tests to have negative likelihood ratios of less than 1. The smallest value negative likelihood ratios can have is zero. In practice, tests with negative likelihood ratios with values less than about a third (0.33) are useful, and tests with negative likelihood ratios of less than about one-tenth (0.10) are very useful.

Many studies of diagnostic tests only report the sensitivity or the specificity of the tests, but not likelihood ratios. Fortunately it is an easy matter to calculate likelihood ratios from sensitivity and specificity:

$$LR+ = sensitivity/(100 - specificity)$$
$$LR- = (100 - sensitivity)/specificity$$

where $LR+$ is the positive likelihood ratio and $LR-$ is the negative likelihood ratio, and sensitivity and specificity are given as percentages.[48,49]

Therefore, if sensitivity is 90% and specificity is 80%, the positive likelihood ratio is $90/(100 - 80) = 4.5$ and the negative likelihood ratio is $(100 - 90)/80 = 0.125$. In this example, the positive likelihood ratio is big enough to be quite useful and the negative likelihood ratio is small enough to be very useful.

Likelihood ratios provide more relevant information than sensitivities and specificities. So it is a worthwhile practice, when reading papers of the accuracy of diagnostic tests, to routinely calculate likelihood ratios (even if only roughly, in your head) and note them in the margins. The likelihood ratios are what you should try to remember because they provide the most useful summary of a test's accuracy.[50]

Using likelihood ratios to calculate the probability that a person has a particular diagnosis

From the moment a person presents for a physiotherapy consultation most physiotherapists will begin to make guesses about the probable diagnosis. For example, a young adult male may attend physiotherapy and begin to describe an ankle injury incurred the previous weekend. Even before he describes the injury, his physiotherapist may have arrived at a provisional diagnosis. It may be obvious from the way in which the patient walks into the room that he has an injury of the ankle. Most commonly, injuries to the ankle are ankle sprains or ankle fractures. But it is rare that someone can walk soon after an ankle fracture, so the physiotherapist's suspicion is naturally directed towards an ankle sprain. This simple scenario provides an important insight into the process of diagnosis: physiotherapists usually develop hypotheses about the likely diagnosis very early in the examination. Thereafter, most of the examination is directed towards confirming or refuting those diagnoses. Additional pieces of information are accrued with the aim of proving or disproving the diagnosis. Thus we can think of the examination as a process of progressive refinement of the probability of a diagnosis.

> The real value of likelihood ratios is that they tell us *how much* to change our estimates of the probability of a diagnosis on the basis of a particular test's finding.[51]

---

[48] Alternatively, if sensitivity and specificity are calculated as proportions, you can insert 1 instead of 100 in the equations.

[49] The use of likelihood ratios extends easily to tests that have more than two categories of outcomes. (A common example is tests whose outcomes are given as positive, uncertain or negative.) In that case there is a likelihood ratio for each possible test outcome.

[50] If you find it too hard to remember the numerical value of likelihood ratios, try and commit to memory a qualitative impression of the accuracy of the test: are the likelihood ratios such that the test is weakly discriminative, or moderately discriminative, or highly discriminative?

[51] More generally, likelihood ratios tell us about *strength of evidence*, or the degree to which the evidence favours one hypothesis over another. This is the basis of the likelihood approach to statistical inference (Royall 1997).

If we want to use likelihood ratios to refine our estimates of the probability of a diagnosis, we need first to be able to quantify probabilities. Probabilities can lie on a scale from 0 (no possibility) to 1 (definite) or, more conveniently, on a scale of 0% to 100%. Consider the following case scenarios:

Case 1: A 23-year-old male reports that 3 weeks ago he twisted his knee during an awkward tackle while playing soccer. Although he experienced only moderate pain at the time, the knee swelled immediately. In the 3 weeks since the injury, the swelling has only partly subsided. The knee feels unstable and there have been several occasions of giving way.

What probability would you assign to the diagnosis of a torn anterior cruciate ligament? Most physiotherapists would assign a high probability, perhaps between 70% and 90%, implying that most patients presenting like this are subsequently found to have a tear of the anterior cruciate ligament. For now, let us assign a probability of 80%. Because we have not yet formally tested the hypothesis that this patient has a torn anterior cruciate ligament, we will call this the *pre-test* probability (Sox et al 1988). That is, we estimate that the pre-test probability this patient has a torn anterior cruciate ligament is 80%.

It appears likely that this patient has a torn anterior cruciate ligament, but the diagnosis is not yet sufficiently likely that we can act as if that diagnosis is certain. The usual course of action would be to test this diagnostic hypothesis, probably with an anterior draw test, or Lachman's test, or the pivot shift test (Magee 2002). Clearly, if these tests are positive we should be more inclined to believe the diagnosis of anterior cruciate ligament tear, and if the tests are negative we should be less inclined to believe that diagnosis. The question is, if the test is positive *how much* more inclined should we be to believe the diagnosis? And if the test is negative *how much* less inclined should we be to believe the diagnosis? Likelihood ratios provide a measure of how much more or how much less we should believe a particular diagnosis on the basis of particular test findings (Go 1998).

A recent systematic review of diagnostic tests for injuries of the knee (Solomon et al 2001) concluded that the positive likelihood ratio for the anterior draw test was 3.8 (this is higher than 1, which is necessary for the test to be of any use at all, and high enough to make it diagnostically useful). The negative likelihood ratio was 0.3 (this is less than 1, which is necessary for the test to be of any use, and low enough to be useful).

Now we need to combine three pieces of information: our estimate of the pre-test probability; our test finding (whether or not the test was positive); and information about the diagnostic accuracy of the test (the positive or negative likelihood ratio, depending upon whether the test was positive or negative). The easiest way to combine these three pieces of information is with a likelihood ratio nomogram, such as Figure 6.8, reproduced from Davidson (2002), after Fagan (1975). The nomogram contains three columns. Reading from left to right, the first is the pre-test probability, the second is the likelihood ratio for the test, and the third is what we want to know: the probability that the person has the diagnosis (the 'post-test probability').

Figure 6.8 Example of a likelihood ratio nomogram. Reproduced with permission from Davidson (2002), after Fagan (1975).

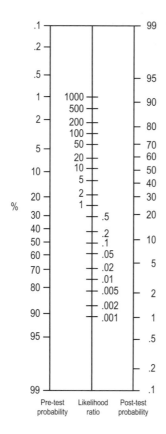

All we need do is draw a line from the point on the first column that is our estimate of the pre-test probability. The line should pass through the second column at the likelihood ratio for the test (we use the positive likelihood ratio if the test was positive and the negative likelihood ratio if the test was negative). When we extrapolate the line to the right-most column it intersects that column at the post-test probability. What we have done is to estimate the probability that the person has the condition on the basis of our estimate of the pre-test probability, the test result (positive or negative), and what we know about the properties of the test (expressed in terms of its likelihood ratios). We have used mathematical rules to combine these three pieces of information.[52]

Returning to our example, we find that the young man with the suspected anterior cruciate ligament tear tests positive with the anterior draw test. By using the nomogram, we can estimate a revised (post-test) probability of anterior cruciate ligament lesion given the positive test finding. The post-test probability is 94%. If the test had been negative, we would use the negative likelihood ratio in the nomogram and we would conclude that this man's post-test probability of having an anterior cruciate ligament tear is 55%.

---

[52] An important assumption underlying this approach is that likelihood ratios remain constant across pre-test probabilities.

This illustrates a central concept in diagnosis.

The proper interpretation of a diagnostic test can only be made after consideration of pre-test probabilities.

Theoretically, these pre-test probabilities could be 'evidence-based'.[53] However, good evidence of pre-test probabilities is rarely available. More often pre-test probabilities are based on clinical intuition and experience – the physiotherapist estimates the pre-test probability based on the proportion of people with such a presentation who, in his or her experience, have subsequently been found to have this diagnosis. Thus *rational* diagnosis is inherently *subjective* and *experience-based*.

Some physiotherapists feel suspicious about the inherent subjectivity of this approach to diagnosis. (The approach is sometimes called a 'Bayesian' approach.) Subjectivity, where it produces variation in practice, is probably undesirable. However, the alternatives (such as ignoring what intuition says about pre-test probabilities and making uniform assumptions about pre-test probabilities like 'all pre-test probabilities are 50%') are likely to produce much less accurate diagnoses. So, for the foreseeable future, it seems sensible to retain the subjective elements of rational diagnosis; the process of diagnosis will remain as much an art as a science.

Viewed in this way, the process of diagnosis is one in which intuition-based estimates of the probability of a diagnosis are replaced with progressively more objective estimates based on test findings. Indeed, if, after conducting a test, the diagnosis remains uncertain (that is, if the post-test probability is neither very high nor very low), the post-test probability can be used as a refined estimate of the next pre-test probability. Sequential testing can proceed in this way, the post-test probability of one test becoming the pre-test probability of the next test, until the post-test probability becomes very high or very low and the diagnosis is confirmed or rejected. The diagnosis is confirmed once the post-test probability has become very high, and the diagnosis is rejected once the post-test probability has become very low.

A consequence is that a given test finding should be interpreted quite differently when applied to different people, because different people will present with different pre-test probabilities. To illustrate this point, consider a second case.

Case 2: A 32-year-old netball player reports that she twisted her knee in a game three weeks ago. At the time her knee locked and she was unable to fully straighten it. She does not recall significant swelling, and reports no instability. However, in the 3 weeks since her injury there have been several occasions when the knee locked again. Between locking episodes the knee appears to function near normally.

This is not a classic presentation of an anterior cruciate ligament lesion. A more likely explanation of this woman's knee symptoms is that she has

---

[53] For example, pre-test probabilities could be based on epidemiological data about the prevalence of the condition being tested for in the population to whom the test is applied. The prevalence, or the proportion of people in this population who have the condition, provides us with an empirical estimate of the pre-test probability of having the condition.

a meniscal tear. We might estimate the pre-test probability of an anterior cruciate ligament lesion for this woman to be 15%. If she tests positive to the anterior draw test, we would obtain a post-test probability of 40%. (Try it and see if you get the same answer.) In other words, there is a 60% probability (100 − 40%) that she does *not* have an anterior cruciate ligament lesion, even though she tested positive with the anterior draw test. This illustrates that a positive anterior draw test should be considered to be much less indicative of an anterior cruciate ligament lesion when the pre-test probability is low. Perhaps that is not clever statistics, just common sense!

If we had used a more accurate test (of which Lachman's test may be an example – one study estimated that its positive likelihood ratio was 42; Solomon et al 2001), we should have expected further to modify our estimates of the probability of the diagnosis. With a positive likelihood ratio of 42 and pre-test probability of 15%, a positive Lachman test gives a post-test probability of 88%. This illustrates simply that discriminative tests (those with high positive likelihood ratios or low negative likelihood ratios) should influence the diagnosis more than tests with low discrimination.

References

Ada L, Foongchomcheay A 2002 Efficacy of electrical stimulation in preventing or reducing subluxation of the shoulder after stroke: a meta-analysis. Australian Journal of Physiotherapy 48:257–267

Albert H, Godskesen M, Westergaard J 2001 Prognosis in four syndromes of pregnancy-related pelvic pain. Acta Obstetrica et Gynecologica Scandinavica 80:505–510

Altman DG (1998) Confidence intervals for the number needed to treat. BMJ 317:1309–1312

Anonymous 1981 How to read clinical journals: II. To learn about a diagnostic test. Canadian Medical Association Journal 124:703–710

Armitage P, Berry G 1994 Statistical methods in medical research, 3rd edn. Blackwell, Oxford

Assendelft WJJ, Morton SC, Yu EI et al 2003 Spinal manipulative therapy for low back pain: a meta-analysis of effectiveness relative to other therapies. Annals of Internal Medicine 138:871–882

Barnett V 1982 Comparative statistical inference. Wiley, New York

Berghmans LC, Hendriks HJ, Bo K et al 1998 Conservative treatment of stress urinary incontinence in women: a systematic review of randomized clinical trials. British Journal of Urology 82:181–191

Brookes ST, Whitely E, Egger M et al 2001 Subgroup analyses in randomized trials: risks of subgroup-specific analyses; power and sample size for the interaction test. Journal of Clinical Epidemiology 57:229–236

Bunketorp L, Stener-Victorin E, Carlsson J 2004 Neck pain and disability following motor vehicle accidents. A cohort study. European Spine Journal, July 6 [published electronically ahead of print]

Cambach W, Chadwick-Straver RV, Wagenaar RC et al 1997 The effects of a community-based pulmonary rehabilitation programme on exercise tolerance and quality of life: a randomized controlled trial. European Respiratory Journal 10:104–113

Campbell DT, Stanley JC 1966 Experimental and quasi-experimental designs for research. Rand McNally, Chicago

Cates C 2003 Visual Rx, version 1.7 (software). Freely available at http://www.nntonline.net

Cohen J 1988 Statistical power analysis for the behavioral sciences. Erlbaum, Hillsdale NJ

Counsell CE, Clarke MJ, Slattery J et al 1994 The miracle of DICE therapy for acute stroke: fact or fictional product of subgroup analysis? BMJ 309:1677–1681

Davidson M 2002 The interpretation of diagnostic tests: A primer for physiotherapists. Australian Journal of Physiotherapy 48:227–233

Deehan DJ, Salmon LJ, Webb VJ et al 2000 Endoscopic reconstruction of the anterior cruciate ligament with an ipsilateral patellar tendon autograft. A prospective longitudinal five-year study. Journal of Bone and Joint Surgery [Br] 82:984–991

Deeks JJ, Altman DG 2001 Effect measures for meta-analysis of trials with binary outcomes. In: Egger M, Davey Smith G, Altman DG (eds) Systematic reviews in health care: meta-analysis in context. BMJ Books, London

de Gruttola VG, Clax P, DeMets DL et al 2001 Considerations in the evaluation of surrogate endpoints in clinical trials: summary of a National Institutes of Health workshop. Controlled Clinical Trials 22:485–502

Dini D, Del Mastro L, Gozza A et al 1998 The role of pneumatic compression in the treatment of postmastectomy lymphedema. A randomized phase III study. Annals of Oncology 9:187–190

Echt DS, Liebson PR, Mitchell LB et al 1991 Mortality and morbidity in patients receiving encainide, flecainide, or placebo. The Cardiac Arrhythmia Suppression Trial. New England Journal of Medicine 324:781–788

Efron B, Tibshirani RJ 1993 An introduction to the bootstrap. Chapman & Hall, New York

Fagan TJ 1975 Nomogram for Bayes theorem. New England Journal of Medicine 293:257

Ferreira ML, Ferreira PH, Latimer J et al 2003 Efficacy of spinal manipulative therapy for low back pain of less than three months' duration. Journal of Manipulative and Physiological Therapeutics 26:593–601

Furukawa TA, Guyatt GH, Griffith LE 2002 Can we individualize the 'number needed to treat'? An empirical study of summary effect measures in meta-analyses. International Journal of Epidemiology 31:72–76

Gardner MJ, Altman DG 1989 Statistics with confidence. Confidence intervals and statistical guidelines. BMJ Books, London

Giacomini M, Cook D, Guyatt G 2002 Qualitative research. In: Guyatt G, Rennie D and the Evidence-based Medicine Working Group (eds) Users' guide to the medical literature. A manual for evidence-based clinical practice. [Book with CD-ROM.] American Medical Association, Chicago

Gigerenzer G, Swijtink Z, Porter T et al 1989 The empire of chance: how probability changed science and everyday life. Cambridge University Press, New York

Glasziou PP, Irwig LM 1995 An evidence based approach to individualising treatment. BMJ 311:1356–1359

Go AS 1998 Refining probability: an introduction to the use of diagnostic tests. In: Friedland DJ, Go AS, Davoren JB et al (eds) Evidence-based medicine. A framework for clinical practice. Lange/McGraw-Hill, New York, pp 11–33

GRADE Working Group 2004 Grading the quality of evidence and the strength of recommendations. BMJ 328:1490

Greenhalgh T 2001 How to read a paper. BMJ Books, London

Guyatt GH, Berman LB, Townsend M et al 1987 A measure of quality of life for clinical trials in chronic lung disease. Thorax 42:773–778

Guyatt GH, Feeny DH, Patrick DL 1993 Measuring health-related quality of life. Annals of Internal Medicine 118:622–629

Guyatt GH, Sackett DL, Cook DJ 1994 Users' guides to the medical literature. II. How to use an article about therapy or prevention. B. What were the results and will they help me in caring for my patients? JAMA 271:59–63

Hajiro T, Nishimura K 2002 Minimal clinically significant difference in health status: the thorny path of health status measures? European Respiratory Journal 19: 390–391

Hedges LV, Olkin I 1980 Vote-counting methods in research synthesis. Psychological Bulletin 88: 359–369

Hedges LV, Olkin I 1985 Statistical methods for meta-analysis. Academic Press, Orlando

Herbert RD 2000a Critical appraisal of clinical trials. I: estimating the magnitude of treatment effects when outcomes are measured on a continuous scale. Australian Journal of Physiotherapy 46:229–235

Herbert RD 2000b Critical appraisal of clinical trials. II: estimating the magnitude of treatment effects when outcomes are measured on a dichotomous scale. Australian Journal of Physiotherapy 46:309–313

Herbert RD 2005 Diagnostic accuracy. In: Gass E, Refshauge K (eds) Musculoskeletal physiotherapy: clinical science and evidence-based practice. Butterworth-Heinemann, London (in press)

Herbert RD, Gabriel M 2002 Effects of pre- and post-exercise stretching on muscle soreness, risk of injury and athletic performance: a systematic review. BMJ 325: 468–472

Hjort I, Lundberg E, Ekegård H et al 1999 Motivation for home exercise in patients with rheumatoid arthritis. Nordisk Fysioterapi 3:31–37

Hovelius L, Augustini BG, Fredin H et al 1996 Primary anterior dislocation of the shoulder in young patients. A ten-year prospective study. Journal of Bone and Joint Surgery [Am] 78:1677–1684

Jaeschke R, Singer J, Guyatt GH 1989 A comparison of seven-point and visual analogue scales. Data from a randomized trial. Controlled Clinical Trials 11:43–51

Jones A, Pill R, Adams S 2000 Qualitative study of views of health professionals and patients on guided self management plans for asthma. BMJ 321:1507–1510

Jull G 2002 Use of high and low velocity cervical manipulative therapy procedures by Australian manipulative physiotherapists. Australian Journal of Physiotherapy 48:189–193

Katrak P, Bowring G, Conroy P et al 1998 Predicting upper limb recovery after stroke: the place of early shoulder and hand movement. Archives of Physical Medicine and Rehabilitation 79:758–761

Laakso EL, Robertson VJ, Chipchase LS 2002 The place of electrophysical agents in Australian and New Zealand entry-level curricula: is there evidence for their inclusion? Australian Journal of Physiotherapy 48:251–254

Lauritzen JB, Petersen MM, Lund B 1993 Effect of external hip protectors on hip fractures. Lancet 341(8836): 11–13

Lilford R, Royston G 1998 Decision analysis in the selection, design and application of clinical and health services research. Journal of Health Services and Research Policy 3:159–166

Linton SJ, van Tulder MW 2001 Preventive interventions for back and neck pain problems: what is the evidence? Spine 26: 778–787

Lotters F, van Tol B, Kwakkel G et al 2002 Effects of controlled inspiratory muscle training in patients with COPD: a meta-analysis. European Respiratory Journal 20:570–576

McAlister FA, Straus SE, Guyatt GH et al 2000 Users' guides to the medical literature: XX. Integrating research evidence with the care of the individual patient. JAMA 283:2829–2836

McDonagh MJN, Davies CTM 1984 Adaptive response to mammalian skeletal muscle to exercise with high loads. European Journal of Applied Physiology 52:139–155

McIlwaine PM, Wong LT, Peacock D, Davidson AGF 2001 Long-term comparative trial of positive expiratory pressure versus oscillating positive expiratory pressure (flutter) physiotherapy in the treatment of cystic fibrosis. Journal of Pediatrics 138:845–850

Magee D 2002 Orthopedic Physical Assessment. Saunders, Philadelphia

Malterud K 2001 Qualitative research: standards, challenges, and guidelines. Lancet 358:483–489

Meyer K, Steiner R, Lastayo P et al 2003 Eccentric exercise in coronary patients: central hemodynamic and metabolic responses. Medicine and Science in Sports and Exercise 35:1076–1082

Moseley AM, Stark A, Cameron ID et al 2004 Treadmill training and body weight support for walking after stroke. In: The Cochrane Library, issue 3. Wiley, Chichester

Moyé LA (2000) Statistical reasoning in medicine: the intuitive p-value primer. Springer, New York

Olsen MF, Hahn I, Nordgren S et al 1997 Randomized controlled trial of prophylactic chest physiotherapy in major abdominal surgery. British Journal of Surgery 84:1535–1538

O'Sullivan PB, Twomey LT, Allison GT 1997 Evaluation of specific stabilizing exercise in the treatment of chronic low back pain with radiologic diagnosis of spondylolysis or spondylolisthesis. Spine 22:2959–2967

Outpatient Service Trialists 2004 Therapy-based rehabilitation services for stroke patients at home. In: The Cochrane Library, Issue 3. Wiley, Chichester

Pope C, Mays N (eds) 2000 Qualitative research in health care, 2nd edn. BMJ Books, London

Pope R, Herbert RD, Kirwan J 2000 Effects of pre-exercise stretching on risk of injury in army recruits: a randomized trial. Medicine and Science in Sports and Exercise 32:271–277

Rothman KJ, Greenland S 1998 Modern epidemiology. Williams and Wilkins, Philadelphia

Royall RM 1997 Statistical evidence: a likelihood paradigm. Chapman and Hall, New York

Sackett DL, Haynes RB, Tugwell P 1985 Clinical epidemiology: a basic science for clinical medicine. Little, Brown, Boston

Sackett DL, Straus SE, Richardson WS et al 2000 Evidence-based medicine. How to practice and teach EBM, 2nd edn. Churchill Livingstone, Edinburgh

Sand PK, Richardson DA, Staskin DR et al 1995 Pelvic floor electrical stimulation in the treatment of genuine stress incontinence: a multicenter, placebo-controlled trial. American Journal of Obstetrics and Gynecology 173:72–79

Schmid CH, Lau J, McIntosh MW 1998 An empirical study of the effect of control rate as a predictor of treatment efficacy in meta-analysis of clinical trials. Statistics in Medicine 17:1923–1942

Schofield JW 2002 Increasing the generalisability of qualitative research. In: Huberman AM, Miles MB (eds) The qualitative researcher's companion. Sage, Thousand Oaks CA

Schonstein E, Kenny DT, Keating J et al 2003 Physical conditioning programs for workers with back and neck pain: a Cochrane systematic review. Spine 28:E391–395

Second International Study of Infarct Survival Collaborative Group 1988 Randomised trial of intravenous streptokinase, oral aspirin, both, or neither among 17 187 cases of suspected acute myocardial infarction: ISIS-2. Lancet 2(8607):349–360

Sherrington C, Lord SR, Herbert RD 2004 A randomized controlled trial of weight-bearing versus non-weight-bearing exercise for improving physical ability after hip fracture and completion of usual care. Archives of Physical Medicine and Rehabilitation 85:710–716

Solomon DH, Simel DL, Bates DW et al 2001 Does this patient have a torn meniscus or ligament of the knee? Value of the physical examination. JAMA 286:1610–1620

Sox HC, Blatt MA, Higgins MC et al 1988 Medical decision making, 2nd edn. Butterworths: Stoneham MA

Steen E, Haugli L 2001 From pain to self-awareness: a qualitative analysis of the significance of group participation for persons with chronic musculoskeletal pain. Patient Education and Counseling 42:35–46

Straus SE, Sackett DL 1999 Applying evidence to the individual patient. Annals of Oncology 10:29–32

te Slaa RL, Wijffels MP, Brand R et al 2004 The prognosis following acute primary glenohumeral dislocation. Journal of Bone and Joint Surgery (Br) 86:58–64

Tijhuis GJ, de Jong Z, Zwinderman AH et al 2001 The validity of the Rheumatoid Arthritis Quality of Life (RAQoL) questionnaire. Rheumatology 40:1112–1119

van der Windt DAWM, van der Heijden GJMG, van den Berg SGM et al 2004 Ultrasound therapy for acute ankle sprains. In: The Cochrane Library, Issue 3. Wiley, Chichester

van Poppel MN, Koes BW, Smid T et al 1997 A systematic review of controlled clinical trials on the prevention of back pain in industry. Occupational and Environmental Medicine 54:841–847

Widhe T, Aaro S, Elmstedt E 1988 Foot deformities in the newborn: incidence and prognosis. Acta Orthopedica Scandinavica 59:176–179

Yusuf S, Wittes J, Probstfield J et al 1991 Analysis and interpretation of treatment effects in subgroups of patients in randomised clinical trials. JAMA 266:93–98

Chapter **7**

Clinical guidelines as a resource for evidence-based physiotherapy

OVERVIEW

This chapter describes what clinical guidelines
are, why they are important in current health
care provision and how methods for guideline
development have evolved over the last 20 years.
The chapter discusses how to assess the quality and
trustworthiness of a clinical guideline to determine
whether it should be used in practice. It highlights
the importance of patient involvement in the
development of a 'good' guideline and describes
how recommendations can be developed in a
systematic and rigorous way even when there is
limited high quality clinical research. The legal
implications of developing and using clinical
guidelines are set out. Finally, there are some
reflections on current and possible future guideline
development activity in physiotherapy.

WHAT ARE CLINICAL GUIDELINES?

Many clinical problems are complex and require the synthesis of findings from several kinds of research. Management of a particular patient's condition may require information about diagnosis, prognosis, effects of therapy and attitudes. It is time-consuming to explore the evidence relating to each aspect of the management of each clinical problem separately. Clinical guidelines provide an efficient alternative. They provide a single source of information about the management of clinical conditions. Evidence-based clinical guidelines integrate high quality clinical research with contributions from clinical experts and patients, in order to formulate reliable recommendations for practice. Where there are practice issues relevant to the guideline topic for which there is little or no evidence, a rigorous and systematic process is used to reach consensus about best practice.

> The purpose of a clinical guideline is to provide a ready-made resource of high quality information for both practitioner and patient, so they can discuss together the different options for treatment and the different degrees of benefit or risk that interventions may have for that patient. A shared and informed decision can then be made about how to proceed with treatment.

Field and Lohr's description of clinical guidelines (Institute of Medicine 1992) has stood the test of time. It is now an internationally accepted definition:

> Clinical guidelines are systematically developed statements to assist practitioner and patient decisions about appropriate health care for specific circumstances.

In Chapter 3 we saw that systematic reviews provide a way of synthesizing evidence. There are some similarities between systematic reviews and clinical guidelines. At the heart of both is a comprehensive, rigorous review of high quality clinical research. However, there are also a number of differences. A summary of these is presented in Table 7.1.

Some people are concerned that clinical guidelines, because they include recommendations for practice, become recipes for health care that take away the individual practitioner's autonomy to make his or her own decisions about treatment. But clinical guidelines are not there to be slavishly implemented without thought being given to the implications of the recommendations for individual patients. It may be that the patient has a co-morbidity or a social situation that means that the recommendations are not applicable *in those circumstances*, or that even though the patient is aware of the evidence described in the guideline, his or her preference is for a different approach or specific treatment. It is a patient's right to make such decisions, and it is the physiotherapist's responsibility to facilitate those decisions by providing relevant, accurate and accessible information. However, if a recommendation in a guideline is based on

Table 7.1 Differences between systematic reviews and clinical guidelines

Systematic review	Clinical guideline
Focus is likely to be on a single clinical question, or a limited aspect of patient care	Usually covers the whole process of disease management, with many clinical questions, so may require a number of systematic reviews
Likely to be developed by a small group of researchers	Developed by a wide range of stakeholders: patients, clinical experts, researchers, professional groups
Conclusions of the review are based on results from high quality clinical research alone	Conclusions (recommendations) are based on a complex synthesis of high quality clinical research, but also expert opinion, patient experience and consensus views
Patients have a limited role or no role in production of the review. Rarely, patients may be involved in framing review question(s) and helping with the assessment and interpretation of evidence	Patients have a key role in production of the guidelines. They may participate in framing of questions, interpretation of evidence and, with the rest of the guideline development group, making judgements about information from patients and health care practitioners
Validity of conclusions depends on methodological rigour	Validity of conclusions (recommendations) depends on methodological rigour and judgements made by guideline development group
Can be developed relatively quickly (evidence can be very current)	Take a longer time to develop (risk of evidence being out of date at time of publication)
Typically published as a technical report for health professionals	Patient versions often produced, in addition to a publication for health professionals

strong and relevant evidence, it may reasonably be expected that the recommendations should be implemented unless there is a patient-related reason not to do so. So, while the implementation of clinical guidelines is not mandatory, a decision not to implement guideline recommendations ought to be justified, and it would be wise to document such decisions. The legal implications of clinical guidelines for users are discussed in more detail later in the chapter.

HISTORY OF CLINICAL GUIDELINES AND WHY THEY ARE IMPORTANT

Since the early 1990s, more and more has been written about what clinical guidelines are, and how they should be developed. There are a number of reasons why they have become popular. The introduction of the notion of 'evidence-based' clinical guidelines links closely to the development of evidence-based medicine and evidence-based practice, described in Chapter 1. This led to a greater awareness of the importance of utilizing the results of high quality clinical research in practice. Also, the exponential increase in the volume of published literature means that it is increasingly difficult to keep up to date with new research. Clinical guidelines, which provide summaries of high quality clinical research, patient views and clinical expertise, provide a more manageable resource for busy practitioners.

In some countries, such as the United Kingdom, there have been calls from the government and from the general public for more consistency in the provision of health care for any particular condition or clinical problem. The goal is to ensure that people can expect the same (excellent) health care, regardless of where they live. This can only be achieved if what constitutes excellent health care is known. Recommendations for practice need to be developed in a systematic, reliable and credible way if they are to be applied across a whole population. In countries such as the United States, insurance companies want to define the content of the specific health care package they will pay for. So they, too, need to know what is the most effective course of action in relation to a particular group of patients.

Lastly, but of equal importance, patients increasingly request information about what treatments will work best for them, what options they may have, and the basis for the information health care professionals give them.

Physiotherapists have always wanted to know that they are doing the best for their patients, and many look to their peers for guidance on what is expected 'best practice'. This could be a personal network of one or more colleagues of perceived similar or greater expertise, or local colleagues working in the same service, or an organized regional, national or international group of specialists.

But how reliable is such guidance? On what is it based? Is it based on opinion and experience, or is it based on high quality clinical research? Many 'guidelines' are based on informal consensus, which in turn is based on a combination of opinion and shared experience. Is this reliable enough? How do we know if the recommendations really reflect effective practice that will lead to health benefits for patients? How can we discern what is effective practice without looking *systematically* at the available evidence and considering its implications for practice?

Before the early 1990s, most clinical guidelines in health care were developed informally, often by groups from a single health care profession, who produced, by informal consensus, statements of 'best practice'. But over the following few years a literature developed which described a more systematic and evidence-based approach to developing guidelines.

There was a common view about the key processes required in the development of a good guideline (Grimshaw & Russell 1993, Grimshaw et al 1995):

- The scientific evidence is assembled in a systematic fashion.
- The panel that develops the guideline includes representatives of most, if not all, relevant disciplines.
- The recommendations are explicitly linked to the evidence from which they are derived.

There was an acknowledgement (Grimshaw & Russell 1993) that those guidelines that were not supported by a literature review may be biased towards reinforcing *current* practice, rather than promoting *evidence-based* practice. And there were concerns that guidelines developed using non-systematic literature reviews may suffer from bias and provide 'false reassurance'.

The literature on clinical guideline development suggests that, from 2000 onwards, a more systematic approach to guideline development methodology has become accepted in many countries (Burgers et al 2003). Developments in methods have, more recently, tended to focus on the difficult problem of formulating recommendations where there is limited research evidence – a situation that most guideline developers find themselves in. Methodological initiatives have focused on the impact of people on guideline development, as opposed to the research literature focus of the 1990s. For example, important recent initiatives have concerned guideline development group dynamics, the beliefs and values of participants in the development process, and how these can impact on making appropriate judgements as free from bias as possible.

WHERE CAN I FIND CLINICAL GUIDELINES?

Only a minority of clinical guidelines are published in journals, so the major databases such as MEDLINE, EMBASE and CINAHL provide a poor way of locating practice guidelines. The most complete database of evidence-based practice guidelines relevant to physiotherapy is PEDro. PEDro was described in some detail in Chapter 4.

PEDro only archives *evidence-based* practice guidelines. Evidence-based practice guidelines are defined by the makers of PEDro as guidelines in which:

1. a systematic review was performed during the guideline development *or* the guidelines were based on a systematic review published in the 4 years preceding publication of the guideline, and
2. at least one randomized controlled trial related to physiotherapy management is included in the review of existing scientific evidence, and
3. the clinical practice guideline must contain systematically developed statements that include recommendations, strategies, or information that assists physiotherapists or patients to make decisions about appropriate health care for specific clinical circumstances.

At the time of writing there are 444 clinical guidelines on the database.

To find clinical practice guidelines on PEDro, use the *Advanced Search* option, and choose *Clinical Guidelines* in the drop-down menu of the 'Methods' field. You can add additional search terms and combine them with AND or OR to refine your search.

Another database, of clinical guidelines relevant to rehabilitation, can be found at www.health.uottawa.ca/EBCpg/english/. Here, guidelines have been quality assessed using the AGREE instrument, discussed in subsequent sections of this chapter. A National Guidelines Clearing House can be found at www.guideline.gov/. This contains mostly guidelines developed in North America. Criteria for inclusion in the database include the presence of a systematic literature review based on published, peer-reviewed evidence and systematically developed statements that include recommendations to assist health care decision-making.

Some countries have national clinical guideline programmes, which produce multiprofessional clinical guidelines. Many of these will include reference to physiotherapy management. Sites of national clinical guideline programmes and information include:

- (in Scotland) www.show.scot.nhs.uk/sign/
- (in England) www.nice.org.uk
- (in Australia) www.nhmrc.gov.au/publications
- (in New Zealand) www.nzgg.org.nz
- (in the USA) www.guideline.gov

The Guidelines International Network (G-I-N) is an international association of organizations involved in clinical guidelines. Its aims include facilitating the sharing of information and knowledge and working between guideline programmes, and improving and harmonizing methodologies for guideline development. You can find more information about G-I-N at http://www.g-i-n.net/index.cfm?fuseaction=homepage

HOW DO I KNOW IF I CAN TRUST THE RECOMMENDATIONS IN A CLINICAL GUIDELINE?

With the growing number of clinical guidelines being developed by many different international, national and local organizations, it is important for physiotherapists to be able to distinguish between high and low quality clinical guidelines.

Two studies (Shaneyfelt et al 1999, Grilli et al 2000) examined published medical guidelines to determine their quality. Both concluded there were widespread quality problems. Grilli's study looked specifically at clinical guidelines published by specialist societies, while Shaneyfelt looked at guidelines published by specialist societies and by other organizations. Grilli argues for agreed, common standards of reporting clinical guidelines, similar to the CONSORT statement for randomized controlled trials (Begg et al 1996). The authors acknowledge their assessment was based on the *report* of the guideline development and that further information might have been elicited if they had known more about what was actually done in the development process. However, as readers of guidelines do not usually have the luxury of obtaining further insights into the guideline development process, this seems a reasonable position to have taken.

In 1999, Cluzeau et al argued for the development of criteria for the critical appraisal of guidelines, following the same principles as work that was already becoming established to assess the quality of a randomized controlled trial or systematic review (Cluzeau et al 1999). Such criteria would allow an assessment to be made to determine whether the guideline developers had taken a rigorous approach to minimizing potential biases in the guideline development process, providing reassurance concerning the validity of the guideline's recommendations.

> **Box 7.1   Domains of the AGREE instrument**
>
> Scope and purpose
> Stakeholder involvement
> Rigour of development
> Clarity and presentation
> Applicability
> Editorial independence

A checklist was developed containing 37 items (Cluzeau & Littlejohns 1999, Cluzeau et al 1999) addressing different aspects of guideline development. The results of this development project suggested good reliability for the instrument and acceptable face validity.

Later, this instrument was further developed and validated by an international group of researchers from 13 countries, known as the **A**ppraisal of **G**uidelines, **RE**search and **E**valuation (AGREE) Collaboration (The AGREE Collaboration 2003). The instrument is divided into six theoretical quality domains (Box 7.1) where

> the 'quality' of guidelines is defined as 'the confidence that the biases linked to the rigour of development, presentation, and applicability of a clinical practice guideline have been minimized and that each step of the development process is clearly reported' (p 18).

In the next sections we consider how to use the AGREE appraisal tool to assess the quality of a clinical guideline. The tool can be found at www.agreecollaboration.org. One of the key features of a good clinical guideline is that the way it has been developed should be transparent. In other words, the guideline development process has been thoroughly documented and is available for the reader of the guideline to assess for themselves its credibility, reliability and relevance to their practice. In appraising a clinical guideline, evidence is sought, primarily from the guideline document itself, about whether or not the criteria in the instrument have been met (as for a research study). The AGREE instrument and its accompanying User Guide provides a framework for the assessment of the quality of a clinical guideline and an explanation for each of the criteria respectively. The headings in the following sections broadly follow those used in the instrument.

SCOPE AND PURPOSE

The overall objectives of the guideline are specifically described

Before beginning the guideline development process, developers should be clear about the overall objective(s), including the guideline's potential impact on society and populations of patients.

A scoping document is sometimes written, detailing the background epidemiology (describing the health problem to be addressed), the population the guideline will be relevant to (and any exceptions), the health care settings and the interventions that will and will not be considered in the guideline. This information should be presented in the guideline document. The scoping document should have been available for consultation with a range of interested parties (stakeholders, see below) to ensure key areas have not been missed or misinterpreted, and that important issues for different groups, particularly patients, have been considered.

Clinical questions covered by the guideline are specifically described

There should be a clear and detailed description of the clinical questions covered by the guideline, and how these were formulated (normally a role of the guideline development group).

The significance of clearly articulated clinical questions is twofold:

1. Clear clinical questions break the scope of the guideline down into more specific and detailed components.
2. Clear clinical questions help the information scientist develop focused search strategies, including the identification of key words and which databases to search.

The patients to whom the guideline is meant to apply are specifically described

There should be a clear description of the population to whom the guideline recommendations will apply.

STAKEHOLDER INVOLVEMENT

The guideline should describe all those who have been involved at some stage of the development process. Some will have been part of the guideline development group, which carries out the guideline development process. Others will have been involved at particular consultation stages of the development process, or as an expert adviser at a particular point in the development process.

The guideline development group includes individuals from all relevant professional groups

The membership of the guideline development group is important on two counts:

1. The content and rigour of the guidelines depend, in part, on the expertise and range of experiences brought to the guideline development process.
2. To have a good chance of being successfully implemented, a guideline must have credibility with its readers. The names of those who were involved in the guideline development process may provide, or compromise, some of that credibility.

A number of authors describe the importance of having representatives from a range of different backgrounds in a guideline development group. This is thought to be critical to ensure potential biases are balanced (Shekelle et al 1999). A group with diverse values, perspectives and interests is less likely to skew judgements, particularly during the stage of formulating recommendations, than if group members consist solely of like-minded people (Murphy et al 1998).

Guideline developers should describe the process through which they considered who the key stakeholders are and on whom the guideline will impact. Stakeholders include any groups of health professionals involved with the care of patients for the topic being considered, patients themselves, people with technical skills that will support the rigour of the guideline development process, and those who have responsibility for the successful implementation of the guideline. The following groups should be considered:

- Acknowledged clinical experts in the clinical area in which the guidelines are being written. If there are different schools of thought, or protagonists for particular modalities or techniques, it will be important that as many of these are represented as possible, to ensure that all perspectives are considered, and that a balanced outcome can be achieved.

- More junior guideline users may be more 'hands on' than the 'acknowledged experts' (above), and may be able to contribute views about the practicalities of implementation and ensure the guideline sits in the context of the average health facility, not just specialist centres.

- Service managers, who may also need to contribute perspectives about the practicability of implementation, particularly if there are resource issues.

- Researchers in the clinical area. They can contribute knowledge of the current research base and *in-progress* research.

- A range of professionals involved with the care of the patient population that the guideline applies to. This may be one or more professional groups directly involved with the care of the patient as part of a team, or professions from whom patients are referred, or are referred to.

- Patients. It is essential that the views of patients are available at every point of the guideline development process. The rationale for this, and the process of involving patients, is described in more detail in the next section.

- Technical experts, including information scientists and systematic reviewers, who will carry out the all-important evidence review that inform the guideline's recommendations, and a project manager who will keep the guideline development project on track.

- A group leader with high level group process skills, to ensure full and equal participation of members of the guideline development group (Box 7.2).

It is not usually practical to include representatives from all of these groups in the guideline development group itself. In considering the quality of the guideline, you will need to consider whether there has been adequate involvement from different perspectives.

> **Box 7.2** Participants in a guideline development group
>
> *Clinical experts*
> Patients
> Acknowledged experts
> Researchers
> A range of professionals involved in the care of patients for whom the guideline is intended
>
> *Technical experts*
> Information scientists
> Systematic reviewers
> Project managers
> Group leaders

Patients' views and preferences have been sought

Just as with health care professionals, it is important that patients feel some ownership of clinical guidelines. The knowledge that patients were involved in the guideline development process will add credibility for those other patients who need to use the guidelines as a source of information.

Patients provide a valuable source of evidence about what constitutes clinically effective health care (Duff et al 1996). In clinical guideline development the involvement of patients is an increasingly established part of the process. A number of studies have been conducted to evaluate the ways in which patients and users can contribute most effectively to the guideline development process. Some are described below in order to provide those appraising a guideline with an idea of what to look for in descriptions of patient involvement in clinical guidelines.

In 1996, Duff and colleagues held a seminar for patient representatives, health professionals, researchers and patients. The aims were to identify the means by which patients and users of services could most effectively be involved in the development of clinical guidelines, and the key factors influencing effective involvement. Among the many recommendations were that patients should be involved throughout the whole process of guideline development, from identifying the topic (for example, having a view on the priorities for care) to educating groups who interpret and implement the guidelines. The significance of involving patients in guideline development was investigated in the Netherlands by Pijnenborg & van Veenendaal (2003). The authors concluded that the involvement of patients resulted in formulation of questions that were more relevant to patients, and there had been better considered judgement[1] of the evidence. It was

---

[1] Considered judgement (also discussed on p 193) describes the process that guideline development groups undertake in deciding what recommendations can be made on the basis of the available evidence. It is perhaps the most difficult part of the whole guideline development process and requires the exercise of judgement based on experience as well as knowledge of the evidence and the methods used to generate it (Scottish Intercollegiate Guidelines Network 2004). There should be clear documentation in the guideline which makes the link between the evidence and recommendation, explaining how and why the group has exercised its judgement in the interpretation of the evidence.

deemed important to provide supporting information for patients and patient representatives, for example on how to consult with fellow patients.

Target users of the guideline are clearly defined

The target users should be clearly defined in the guideline so that it is clear for which health professionals and patients the guideline is relevant.

The guideline has been piloted among target users

A pilot process should have taken place to test the feasibility and practicality of implementing the guideline. The pilot should also test the clarity, understandability and effectiveness of presentation of the guideline, as well as the acceptability of the rationale for the recommendations. This is likely to be a theoretical rather than a practical process so, for example, it might involve, at a local level, individuals or teams being asked to read the guideline. This would be followed by discussion in order to clarify understanding of the evidence base, the rationale for the recommendations, the acceptability of recommendations and perceptions of the practicalities for, and likelihood of, implementation.

The guideline developers should document the process of piloting, providing brief examples of comments received and how these have impacted on the final version of the guideline.

RIGOUR OF DEVELOPMENT

Systematic methods were used to search for and select the evidence, and these are clearly described

Readers of clinical practice guidelines need to be satisfied that the evidence is based on an up-to-date and rigorous review. Appraisal of systematic reviews has already been discussed in Chapters 5 and 6, and the same principles can be applied when considering the quality of the methods used for the evidence review in a clinical guideline.

Most clinical guidelines categorize 'levels of evidence', based on the strength and reliability of the evidence used. Typically, the hierarchies place high quality systematic reviews of randomized controlled trials at the top of the list, as these studies offer the most trustworthy information about the size of the effect of an intervention. This is usually followed by single randomized controlled trials, then cohort and other observational studies. Consensus and the views of expert groups are placed at the bottom of the hierarchy, as providing the least reliable evidence. This type of hierarchy, however, fails to recognize that different clinical questions lend themselves to different research designs. For example, evidence about diagnostic tests may draw on cross-sectional studies, yet such studies are not represented in the typical hierarchy. Similarly unrepresented is information about patients' experiences, discerned by qualitative research. However, readers should appreciate that the hierarchies used to categorize levels of evidence in clinical guidelines are usually only applicable to evidence about intervention, and they typically refer to the strength of evidence for the effects of interventions.

A typical hierarchy, or grading of evidence, likely to be found in many clinical guidelines, is set out in Table 7.2.

Table 7.2 An example of levels of evidence used in guideline development

Level	Type of evidence
Ia	Evidence obtained from a systematic review of randomized controlled trials
Ib	Evidence obtained from at least one randomized controlled trial
IIa	Evidence obtained from at least one well-designed controlled study without randomization
IIb	Evidence obtained from at least one other type of well-designed quasi-experimental study
III	Evidence obtained from well-designed non-experimental descriptive studies, such as comparative studies, correlation studies and case studies
IV	Evidence obtained from expert committee reports or opinions and/or clinical experience of respected authorities

Adapted from National Institute for Clinical Excellence (2001). (This hierarchy has subsequently been revised.)

There are, however, differences and shortcomings in the grading systems which can be confusing and even misleading. Ferreira et al (2002) highlighted the importance of using consistent criteria for defining levels of evidence in systematic reviews, finding that the use of different criteria could lead to markedly different conclusions being reached. New hierarchies are now evolving that aim to indicate more explicitly 'the extent to which one can be confident that an estimate of effect is correct' (GRADE Working Group 2004). The GRADE approach takes into account study design, study quality, consistency and directness in judging the quality of evidence for each important outcome. Further developments towards a common understanding and application of a transparent and explicit system for grading levels of evidence can be expected over the coming years.

The methods used for formulating the recommendations are clearly described

This criterion reflects one of the most difficult, but important, elements in guideline development. It concerns the judgements that are made about what the evidence really means for patients – its quality, reliability and relevance, including an assessment of relative benefits, harms and risks. The results of such judgements are then translated into meaningful recommendations for practice, which include an indication of the strength of the recommendation. The appraiser of a guideline must be satisfied that the process of formulating recommendations described in the guideline is transparent, free of bias and accurate.

Many clinical guidelines include a system for grading the strength of recommendations. For example, a 'Grade A' recommendation might be one that is based on at least one randomized controlled trial as part of a body of literature, and a 'Grade C' recommendation one that is based on expert opinion or clinical experience of respected authorities (National Institute for Clinical Excellence 2001). While this is logical, in the sense that a high quality randomized controlled trial is likely to provide more reliable evidence of effectiveness than expert opinion, there are several factors that should be considered before recommendations are made. The GRADE Working Group (2004) suggests that recommendations should consider four main factors:

- The balance between benefits and harms, taking into account the estimated size of the effect for the main outcomes, the confidence limits around those estimates, and the relative value placed on each outcome.
- The quality of evidence.
- Translation of the evidence into practice in a specific setting.
- Uncertainty about baseline risk for the population.

Based on these four criteria, the following categories for recommendations are suggested:

- 'Do it' or 'Don't do it', indicating 'a judgement that most well-informed people would make'.
- 'Probably do it' or 'Probably don't do it', indicating 'a judgement that a majority of well-informed people would make, but a substantial minority would not'.

Methods for grading the strength of recommendation in clinical practice guidelines are evolving rapidly. It is hoped this will produce grading methods with explicit criteria, empirically evaluated in an international collaboration.

For guideline developers, formulation of recommendations is difficult for two reasons. First, there is unlikely to be sufficient high quality clinical research on which to base clear recommendations for the whole range of interventions or care processes described in the guideline scope, so other methods have to be used to gather information that can be used as a reliable resource. Second, formulating recommendations for practice from the available information, whether high quality clinical research or consensus or expert views, requires a degree of judgement and interpretation by the guideline development group which is potentially open to the biases of the guideline development group participants and the group process.

These are difficult areas, about which relatively little has been written to date, yet they are crucial to the development of a clinical guideline. In order to help those appraising a guideline, we have gone into more detail in the following paragraphs to explain techniques used for consensus development and how to minimize the likelihood of bias in the formulation of recommendations. This will help readers and users of guidelines recognize the processes used by a guideline development group, as described in the guideline, and to make an assessment about the rigour of that process.

When developing clinical guidelines it is almost inevitable that it will not be possible to find high quality research evidence on which to base at least some recommendations. There may be only poor quality studies whose results are not reliable, or there may be no studies at all. What are guideline developers to do? The choice is to:

- limit the guideline recommendations to those areas where there *is* good evidence

- abort the development of the guideline
- supplement the evidence with expert views, consensus statements or judgements made by the guideline development group.

Limit the guideline recommendations to areas where there is good evidence

Guidelines based on pockets of good evidence will be both brief and disjointed. Such guidelines do not provide the basis for the decision-making that clinicians and policy makers need. For this reason they could be conceived as almost worthless. Eccles et al (1996) observed that such restrictions on guideline recommendations would 'limit their value to clinicians and policy makers who need to make their decisions in the presence of imperfect knowledge'. Trickey et al (1998) further observed that limiting the development of guidelines to areas where there is sufficient research would imply a reduction in the potential to improve health care in areas that, by their nature, do not lend themselves to randomized controlled trials.

Abort the development of the guideline

Aborting the guideline development process because there is a dearth of evidence might sound a logical step, yet there will never be as much high quality clinical research as would be ideal to formulate clear recommendations. The outcome would therefore be that there would be no guidelines with which to help patients and professionals make decisions.

Supplement the evidence with expert views, consensus and judgement

The pragmatic solution to the lack of evidence is to try to combine what evidence there is with a consensus process that will be as systematic, rigorous and free of bias as the assessment of the research evidence attempts to be. Consensus can be used to fill evidence gaps. Grimshaw et al (1995) observed that 'the effectiveness of clinical guidelines depends at least as much on the quality of the consensus development as on the quality of the evidence base'.

Over the last five years, there has been increasing interest in how to mix expert opinion with scientific literature. Some authors have identified factors that might introduce bias, such as the composition and dynamics of the guideline development group, and personal values and beliefs of guideline development group members. Murphy et al (1998) have reviewed the use of formal consensus methods in guideline development, including Delphi techniques, nominal group technique and consensus conferences. These techniques are not described here, but interested readers are referred to the review. The review suggests that the most commonly used consensus method for clinical guideline development is a modified nominal group technique. Its main characteristic is that the views of individuals involved in the guideline development process are initially sought privately, often via a mailed questionnaire, after which the group meets together, the results are fed back to the group and discussed, before individuals again complete a questionnaire privately. For example, Rycroft-Malone (2001) described how they brought together research evidence, patient evidence ('expert patient opinions') and clinical expertise using a modified nominal group technique, to develop clinical guidelines on the prevention and management of pressure ulcers. Participants, who were a heterogeneous, multiprofessional group, were sent a summary of evidence and asked to vote on 200 predetermined questions. The group members, who had been chosen for their expertise in the subject area and who were acknowledged experts with credibility and status among their peers, then met. They discussed the results of the voting, focusing primarily on areas where there was the greatest disagreement, and they then re-voted secretly. Scores were used to determine the 'consensus' position. Factors that were reported as significant in making the process successful included the expertise of the facilitator in maintaining an environment conducive to good decision-making and encouraging the group to view the task as research-based, rather than opinion-based. Although the influence of psychosocial factors (conformity, persuasion, etc.) on the group process was not evaluated, it was considered these were minimized, for example by having private rating rounds.

Whether recommendations are based on high quality research, or consensus in the absence of evidence, there is a broad acknowledgement that value judgements also play a key role in the decision-making process about the preferred course of action. Consequently, it is important that guidelines document how the guideline development group's final conclusions were made (for example, how disagreements were handled and how information was synthesized). Cook et al (1997) sum up the importance of documenting processes: 'If guideline developers do not indicate how they identified and summarized the evidence and integrated different values, clinicians cannot adequately evaluate the rigour of the guidelines and the extent to which research evidence supports the recommendations.'

In another model, the Scottish Intercollegiate Guidelines Network (SIGN) describes a process of 'considered judgement', during which the guideline development group decides what recommendations can be made from the evidence that has been presented to the group. The guidance can be found at http://www.show.scot.nhs.uk/sign/guidelines/fulltext/50/annexd.html

The key factors are described as:

● The *nature of the evidence* – its quantity, quality and consistency. This determines the degree of susceptibility to bias to which the evidence may be exposed.

● The *applicability of the evidence* to the scope of the guideline, including the population, settings and available resources and systems within which health care is provided. For example, if the evidence suggests a particular piece of equipment is effective, but it is impracticable to use in the primary care setting for which the guideline is being written, it would not make sense for it to be recommended.

- The *generalizability of the evidence* to the population and settings being considered in the guideline. For example, studies of lifestyle modification carried out in Japan might not be applicable to a European population. There could be cultural issues that make it difficult to assume that the same study carried out in the UK would have produced similar results.

- *Clinical and cost impact*. The incremental health gains for patients if the guideline recommendations are implemented need to be balanced against incremental costs of implementation to health care providers and patients. Cost-effectiveness of an intervention should be weighed against the cost-effectiveness of its alternatives. For example, if a community-based rehabilitation programme was to be recommended, what other services would need to be cut back as a result?

- *Impact of beliefs and values on decision-making*. From the discussion above, it is clear that for each of the issues described, a degree of judgement is required to be able to draw conclusions that are balanced and well thought through. Bias can be minimized by having a group that includes a wide range of interested parties, including patients, and a group that is well facilitated to avoid undue authority being given to some members than others. Other external sources of information can also be utilized to support decision-making, for example reported patient concerns or qualitative studies that shed light on the acceptability for patients of specific procedures, or data on the likelihood of patient or professional adherence to particular strategies. Consensus views, collected in a systematic way, such as that described earlier in the chapter, also need to be considered at this stage.

The guideline development group should document the process of evidence review and considered judgement in order that the recommendations can be clearly tracked back to the evidence and subsequent discussions about it. This should include a description of the key issues raised within the group and how these were resolved. This will assist the users of the guideline to be able to make their own judgement about the robustness of the process and therefore the reliability of the guideline recommendations.

It is inevitable that the interpretation of the evidence will be influenced by the values of individual panel members. Grimshaw and colleagues (1995) urged the establishment of programmes of research and development that give at least as much thought to the psychology of the group dynamics as to the science of systematic reviews. However, few, if any attempts have been made to investigate the role of group dynamics. Reports on such studies are eagerly awaited.

Health benefits, side-effects and risks have been considered in formulating the recommendations

The guideline should consider the health benefits, side-effects and risks of the recommendations. This allows patients and physiotherapists to understand the relative benefits and risks of different options for intervention, so that shared decisions can be made.

There is an explicit link between the recommendations and the supporting evidence

The guideline should be clear about the evidence, whether high quality clinical research, consensus or expert views, on which each recommendation has been based. Each recommendation should have a list of references on which it is based.

The guideline has been externally reviewed by experts prior to its publication

There should be evidence of an external review process in the guideline document. The guideline, at final draft stage, should be sent to experts in the clinical area of the guideline topic and to guideline methodologists for peer review. Clinical and academic experts in the topic area should be asked to assess the evidence presented. For example, has any evidence of significance been missed, are the judgements that have been made about the interpretation of the evidence sound? Methodologists should be asked to review the rigour of the whole guideline development process and assess any potential for bias in the conclusions reached.

The results of the external review process should be documented in the guideline and examples given of discussion and changes made as a result.

A procedure for updating the guideline is provided

There should be a clear statement in the guideline about the procedure for updating the guideline. A time scale may be given, but arrangements should also be in place to act sooner if it is known that new high quality clinical research will soon be published, particularly if it is possible that the new evidence could significantly change the guideline recommendations. A formal or informal monitoring process should be set up so that the developers are made aware of new research.

CLARITY AND PRESENTATION

The recommendations are specific and unambiguous

Recommendations should be as precise and clear as possible, identifying specific patient populations and specific circumstances when recommendations apply. Dosages should be included if these can be supported by the evidence.

The different options for management of the condition are clearly presented

Clear options for management will enhance patient choice and facilitate decision-making.

Key recommendations are easily identifiable

The AGREE instrument suggests that guideline developers highlight the most important recommendations for practice in some way, to allow guideline users to find them easily. This might be in the form of a flow chart, or box. These recommendations should relate back to the key clinical questions identified at the start of the guideline development process.

The guideline is supported with tools for application

The implementation of clinical guidelines is not as easy as might be thought, as we will see in the next chapter. Additional materials, for example a quick reference guide, educational tools or patient leaflet, are often disseminated with the guideline to facilitate implementation.

APPLICABILITY

The potential organizational barriers in applying the recommendations have been discussed

Guideline recommendations may, directly or indirectly, require organizational, as well as individual practitioner change. If this is the case, those able to influence and facilitate organizational change should have been involved in the guideline development process.

The potential cost implications of applying the recommendations have been considered

Clinical guidelines should discuss the cost implications of the guideline recommendations, for example requirements for more staff or new equipment. The guideline should include a discussion on the potential impact on resources.

The guideline presents key review criteria for monitoring and/or audit purposes

Audit criteria provide the means by which health professionals can measure their adherence to the guideline recommendations, thus enhancing the guideline's successful use in practice. If there are many recommendations, the review criteria may need to focus on the key recommendations.

EDITORIAL INDEPENDENCE

The guideline is editorially independent from the funding body

If the guideline is not editorially independent from a funding body there could be the potential for the funding body to influence the content of the guideline. This may arise, for example, if the producer of therapeutic equipment, or a service provider, or a physiotherapy association funds the guideline development. These groups may have a vested interest in guideline recommendations. In general, it is better if the process of guideline development is independent of influence from funding bodies. The guideline should include a statement about its editorial independence.

Conflicts of interest of guideline development group members have been recorded

Members of the guideline development group should be asked to declare any interests that might affect their judgements during the guideline development process. The results of this should be documented in the guideline.

WHAT DO THE RESULTS OF THE CRITICAL APPRAISAL MEAN FOR MY PRACTICE?

By the end of the assessment of a clinical guideline using the AGREE instrument, you will have formed a judgement about whether the guideline is 'good enough' to apply to your patients. The key factors will be:

- Is the purpose of the guideline clear?
- Is the patient population to which the guideline applies similar to your own patients?
- Are the settings to which the guideline applies similar to the settings of your patients?
- Has the development process been systematic and rigorous?
- Is the guideline generally, and the recommendations in particular, clear?

LEGAL IMPLICATIONS OF CLINICAL GUIDELINES

Many health professionals, including physiotherapists, have concerns that, with the increasing number of clinical guidelines being developed, their autonomy to use professional judgement and make their own decisions about a patient's care will be compromised. The concern centres on the legal basis of clinical guidelines, with fears that, should they be sued and found not to have been following an available, relevant high quality clinical guideline, this would leave the health professional vulnerable.

Much of the literature about the legal implications of clinical guidelines goes back to the mid-1990s, before the methodology for the development of rigorous, systematic evidence-based clinical guidelines had become more widely used. The literature is almost entirely restricted to that related to medical practitioners. However, there is nothing to suggest the principles that apply to doctors would not apply equally to physiotherapists, or that the legal position of clinical guidelines has changed in more recent years.

The literature is clear on two counts:

- There is little case law in relation to the use (or not) of clinical guidelines. In the United States, where the incidence of litigation is high, clinical guidelines play 'a relevant or pivotal role in the proof of negligence' in only 7% of cases (Hyams 1995, cited by Hurwitz 1995). Despite an explosion of clinical guideline development since the 1990s, it appears that the courts are more likely to focus on the facts of the case than refer to clinical guidelines (Samanta et al 2003).

- There has been no suggestion that the presence of a clinical guideline takes away the responsibility of the practitioner for using professional judgement in relation to a particular patient. Rather, there is an expectation that the user of clinical guidelines will not accept recommendations at face value, but will first consider their relevance and acceptability for any individual patient (Mann 1996). Indeed, the practitioner could be deemed to have been negligent to apply the recommendations in a clinical guideline if the patient's condition contraindicated its application.

CLINICAL GUIDELINES OR 'REASONABLE CARE': WHICH DO THE COURTS CONSIDER MORE IMPORTANT?

Perhaps surprisingly, the courts seem to take the view that the status of clinical guidelines is secondary to the reasonableness of a group of respected health professionals. In UK law and elsewhere, the 'Bolam test' still dominates. The Bolam test was derived from a legal ruling in 1957, in the case of *Bolam* v. *Friern Hospital Management Committee*. The judgement was that 'a doctor will not be guilty of negligence if he has acted in accordance with a practice accepted as proper by a responsible body of medical men skilled in that particular art'. Further, the test also recognizes that there can be more than one school of thought, so doctors can often rebut a charge of negligence by claiming to conform to the practice of another body of responsible doctors (Hurwitz 1999).

Concerns have been expressed (Chalmers 1994) that courts may consider 'usual practice' more 'reasonable' than an evidence-based practice that has not necessarily gained general professional acceptance. Justice Denning, acknowledging the rapidly increasing volume of literature, ruled in 1953 'it would be quite wrong to suggest that the medical man is negligent because he does not at once put into operation the suggestion that some contributor or other might make to a medical journal … The time may come in a particular case when a new recommendation may be so well proved and so well known, and so well accepted that it should be adopted, but that was not so in this case' (*Crawford* v. *Board of Governors of Charing Cross Hospital* (1953), cited in Hurwitz 1995). So, if clinical guidelines make recommendations that are evidence-based, but do not at the time of publication constitute 'customary practice', those recommendations may be challenged in a court by the existing 'customary professional care', or by expert witnesses.

However, clinical guidelines developed by a responsible body have also been used to support practice and protect the practitioner. In the case of Tony Bland, a young man in a persistent vegetative state (PVS), the court accepted the British Medical Association's guidelines on discontinuing life support to patients in PVS and agreed that hydration and nutrition should be withdrawn (Hurwitz 1995). In another case reported by Hurwitz (*Early* v. *Newham Health Authority* (1994)), where there was a failure to intubate successfully, it was agreed that the anaesthetist had followed locally developed guidelines produced by a 'competent medical authority who applied its mind to this problem and came up with a reasonable solution' and was not, therefore, deemed to have been negligent (Samanta et al 2003).

In France, clinical guidelines published by the Agence Nationale pour le Développement de l'Evaluation Médicale constitute an enforceable agreement between doctors and the social security administration. In Germany, guidelines have no direct legal status but courts may consider they represent the standard of medical care, so a physician may need to justify their deviation from the 'expected standard'. In Norway, clinical guidelines are considered to represent the standard of medical practice and are an important factor in medicolegal cases. Deviations from guidelines are expected to be explained and documented. Guidelines have no legal force in Australia, but patient care could be viewed as less than reasonable where clinical guidelines are available but not followed, unless it can be justified on appropriate clinical grounds. A law requiring physicians in the Netherlands to treat patients according to a professional standard was passed in 1995. Dutch guidelines do not have direct legal status, but in 2001 the Netherlands Supreme Court ruled that medical protocols are part of the medical professional standard. Not following them could be judged an 'accountable shortcoming' (Damen et al 2003).

DOCUMENTING THE USE OF A CLINICAL GUIDELINE IN PRACTICE: LEGAL IMPLICATIONS

There are two issues in relation to documentation:

1. If a clinical guideline is available, but the recommendations are not followed, an explanation of the rationale for the variance should be documented.

2. It may be prudent for each practice to keep an archive of versions of documents that have been used over time, and the dates during

which they were in use. This is so that reference can be made to the recommendations that were in current usage at any particular point in time, for example by a court, which would need to have access to the version of a clinical guideline in use at the time of the episode under scrutiny.

REFLECTIONS ON THE FUTURE OF GUIDELINE DEVELOPMENT

WHO SHOULD DEVELOP CLINICAL GUIDELINES?

Grimshaw et al (1995) observed that the development of valid guidelines requires considerable resources. They argued for greater co-ordination nationally on guideline development, to avoid duplication, and felt that national programmes would reduce the costs of local guideline development. They concluded that expertise was needed for conducting systematic reviews, synthesizing the evidence and developing valid guidelines. Sudlow & Thomson (1997) reached similar conclusions, stressing that the development of guidelines requires considerable skills and resources not likely to be available at a local level. At a local level, the expertise required was in appraising and adapting national guidelines and identifying local resource constraints and barriers to implementation.

COLLABORATION IN GUIDELINE DEVELOPMENT

Between guideline developers and systematic reviewers

The development of clinical guidelines relies on making use of existing systematic reviews and/or the formulation of new reviews as part of the guideline development process. This suggests close alliances and partnerships should be developed between systematic review generators and clinical guideline developers, to share common methodologies, problems and solutions, and also to share actual reviews, to avoid duplication. An increasing number of commentators are acknowledging this. Indeed it has been suggested that there should be a database of evidence tables available that both systematic reviewers and guideline developers can access. In the Netherlands, partnerships are already established between the Dutch Cochrane Centre and guideline centres. In physiotherapy in the Netherlands, this has led to collaboration in guideline development between the professional body (Royal Dutch Society for Physiotherapy, KNGF) and the Cochrane Rehabilitation and Related Therapies Field in Maastricht.

International collaboration

A growing number of commentators are also discussing international collaboration in guideline development as a way of avoiding duplication and unnecessary resource use. These calls acknowledge that different health care settings, systems and resources may mean that recommendations are not generalizable in different countries. However, there is a growing desire for evidence reviews to be shared across countries.

In physiotherapy, there is already discussion taking place between the Netherlands (KNGF) and the UK (Chartered Society of Physiotherapy, CSP) about future collaboration on guideline development, particularly the evidence review component. The World Confederation of

Physical Therapy (Europe) has agreed a common position on guideline development methodology in physiotherapy (J. Mead & P. van der Wees, unpublished work 2004) and it is hoped this will be adopted worldwide, providing a common basis for guideline development processes in physiotherapy. International networks of guideline developers urgently need to be established so that those less familiar with guideline development can explore methodological issues with more experienced colleagues. This in turn could lead to a wider sharing of the work of developing clinical guidelines, allowing the profession to extend the coverage of topics.

Between guideline developers and researchers

Clinical guidelines, if developed rigorously, provide a systematic review of the available evidence in a particular clinical area. Their development can provide a valuable opportunity to highlight the most clinically relevant gaps in the evidence, including those that are most important for patients. Researchers should consider clinical guidelines a source of clinically relevant research topics when identifying priorities for research programmes.

UNIPROFESSIONAL OR MULTIPROFESSIONAL GUIDELINE DEVELOPMENT?

Most published physiotherapy guidelines are developed by physiotherapists for physiotherapists. Yet it may be preferable for a multiprofessional group, including patients or their representatives, to develop clinical guidelines. This would enhance the credibility of the guidelines and ensure that a variety of views have been considered. So physiotherapy guidelines may benefit from being developed in a way that is more integrated with other health care providers and patients. When multiprofessional guidelines *are* developed, even with physiotherapists involved in the process, the recommendations relevant to physiotherapists have tended to be scant, even where there is strong evidence of effectiveness. The recommendations tend to be restricted to broad statements which do not help physiotherapists 'make decisions about appropriate health care' (Institute of Medicine 1992). For example, in a clinical guideline for multiple sclerosis, published by the National Institute for Clinical Excellence in 2003 (http://www.nice.org.uk/pdf/CG008guidance.pdf), one Grade A recommendation states: 'Physiotherapy treatments aimed at improving walking should be offered to a person with multiple sclerosis who is, or could be, walking.' While this is based on high level evidence, it provides no guidance on what types of treatments might be more effective than others in improving walking, or even whether the improvements that can be expected are in the quality of gait, distance walked or speed of walking. Why do multidisciplinary guidelines often lack specific recommendations? Perhaps this is in part related to time pressures of multiprofessional guideline developers. Developers may not have the time to look in detail at every aspect of a guideline's scope. Alternatively, there may be a lack of high quality evidence. Or it may be that the relevant systematic reviews contain heterogeneous studies which are not easily interpreted except by a reviewer with specific knowledge of each clinical issue. Indeed, the individual studies may have to be re-analysed in order to be able to draw relevant conclusions – a complex and time-consuming exercise. Physiotherapists, or professional bodies, may need to go back to the evidence of a national multiprofessional guideline to look in more detail at the evidence, and develop consensus where gaps are identified or uncertainties lie, in order to present more meaningful findings.

To conclude, high quality clinical guidelines provide a valuable resource for practice in the form of recommendations for practice based on a systematic evidence review integrated with information from a consensus process and expert judgement. However, clinical guidelines are expensive and time-consuming to develop. A real challenge for the years ahead will be to set up international collaborations of organizations that will trust each others' work sufficiently to avoid the current duplication of guidelines developed across countries. A second challenge will be to determine with more clarity whether clinical guidelines actually lead to health benefits for patients. Finally, optimal mechanisms for facilitation and implementation of guidelines need to be found and used.

Chapter 8 will describe what is currently known about strategies for the successful implementation of clinical guidelines.

References

Begg C, Cho M, Eastwood S et al 1996 Improving the quality of reporting of randomized controlled trials: the CONSORT statement. JAMA 276:637–639

Bolam v. Friern Hospital Management Committee [1957] 2 All ER 118–128, 122.

Burgers J, Grol R, Klazinger N et al 2003 Towards evidence-based clinical practice: an international survey of 18 clinical guidelines programs. International Journal for Quality in Health Care 15(1):31–45

Chalmers I 1994 Why are the opinions about the effects of health care so often wrong? Med Leg J 62(Pt 3):116–123; discussion 124–130

Cluzeau FA, Littlejohns P, Grimshaw JM et al 1999 Development and application of a generic methodology to assess the quality of clinical guidelines. International Journal for Quality in Health Care 11(1):21–28

Cluzeau FA, Littlejohns P 1999 Appraising clinical practice guidelines in England and Wales: the development of a methodological framework and its application to policy. Joint Commission Journal on Quality Improvement 25(10):514–521

Cook DJ, Greengold NL, Ellrodt AG et al 1997 The relation between systematic reviews and practice guidelines. Annals of Internal Medicine 127(3):210–216

Damen J, van Diejen D, Bakker J et al 2003 Legal implications of clinical practice guidelines. Intensive Care Medicine 29:3–7

Duff LA, Kelson M, Marriott S et al 1996 Clinical guidelines: involving patients and users of services. Journal of Clinical Effectiveness 1(3)

Eccles M, Clapp Z, Grimshaw et al 1996 Developing valid guidelines: methodological and procedural issues from the North of England Evidence Based Guideline Development Project. Quality in Health Care 5:44–50

Ferreira PH, Ferreira ML, Maher CG et al 2002 Effect of applying different 'levels of evidence' criteria on conclusions of Cochrane reviews of interventions for low back pain. Journal of Clinical Epidemiology 55:1126–1129

GRADE Working Group 2004 Grading quality of evidence and strength of recommendations. BMJ 328:1490–1497

Grilli R, Magrini N, Penna A et al 2000 Practice guidelines developed by speciality societies: the need for a critical appraisal. Lancet 355:103–106

Grimshaw J, Russell I 1993 Achieving health gain through clinical guidelines I: developing scientifically valid guidelines. Quality in Health Care 2:243–248

Grimshaw J, Eccles M, Russell I 1995 Developing clinically valid practice guidelines. Journal of Evaluation of Clinical Practice 1(1):37–48

Hurwitz B 1995 Clinical guidelines and the law: advice, guidance or regulation? Journal of Evaluation in Practice 1(1):49–60

Hurwitz B 1999 Legal and political considerations of clinical practice guidelines. BMJ 318:661–664

Institute of Medicine 1992 Guidelines for clinical practice: from development to use (Field MJ, Lohr KN, eds). National Academy Press, Washington DC

Mann T 1996 Clinical guidelines: using clinical guidelines to improve patient care within the NHS. Department of Health, London

Murphy MK, Black NA, Lamping DL et al 1998 Consensus development methods, and their use in clinical guideline development. Health Technology Assessment 2(3):1–88

National Institute for Clinical Excellence 2001 Information for national collaborating centres and guideline development groups. The Guideline Development Process Series No. 3. NICE, London

Pijnenborg L and van Veenendaal H 2003 Patient involvement. Guidelines International Network Conference, Edinburgh

Rycroft-Malone J 2001 Formal consensus: the development of a national clinical guideline. Quality in Health Care 10:238–244

Samanta A, Samanta J, Gunn M 2003 Legal considerations of clinical guidelines: will NICE make a difference? Journal of the Royal Society of Medicine 96:133–138

Scottish Intercollegiate Guidelines Network. SIGN 50: A guideline developers' handbook, Annex D: Synthesising evidence and making recommendations. http://www.show.scot.nhs.uk/sign/guidelines/fulltext/50/annexd.html

Shaneyfelt TM, Mayo-Smith MF, Rothwangl J 1999 Are guidelines following guidelines? The methodological quality of clinical practice guidelines in the peer-reviewed medical literature. JAMA 281:1900–1905

Shekelle PG, Woolf SH, Eccles M et al 1999 Developing guidelines. BMJ 318:593–596

Sudlow M, Thomson R 1997 Clinical guidelines: quantity without quality. Quality in Health Care 6:60–61

The AGREE Collaboration 2003 Development and validation of an international appraisals instrument for assessing the quality of clinical practice guidelines: the AGREE project. Quality and Safety in Health Care 12:18–23

Trickey H, Harvey J, Wilcock G et al 1998 Formal consensus and consultation: a qualitative method for development of a guideline for dementia. Quality in Health Care 7:192–199

Chapter **8**

Making it happen

CHAPTER CONTENTS

OVERVIEW

Producing high quality clinical research does not necessarily result in improved quality of care. The translation of research into practice is difficult for many reasons. This chapter focuses on implementing evidence-based physiotherapy. Barriers to change for physiotherapists are presented, and some theories of change are discussed. The chapter provides an overview of what is known about evidence-based implementation of evidence-based care, with a specific emphasis on guideline implementation. The use of evidence is one factor that can affect the quality and effectiveness of interventions. The practice of evidence-based physiotherapy should be viewed in the context of a range of other organizational and individual quality improvement activities.

WHAT DO WE MEAN BY 'MAKING IT HAPPEN'?

Making evidence-based physiotherapy happen implies implementing practices informed by high quality clinical research. Implementation can be achieved and promoted in many ways. The underlying assumption is that producing high quality clinical research is not enough on its own to ensure improvement in practice behaviour. Gaps between research and practice exist, so the translation of research into practice is an important issue. Traditionally, passive diffusion of research has been regarded as a way of closing the research–practice gap. A more active strategy, often called dissemination, involves targeting the message to defined groups. Implementation is even more active, planned and tailored. 'Implementation involves identifying and assisting in overcoming the barriers to the use of the knowledge obtained from a tailored message. It is a more active process still, which uses not only the message itself, but also organizational and behavioural tools that are sensitive to constraints and opportunities of health professionals in identified settings' (Lomas 1993). This implies that implementation is an active process that addresses and overcomes barriers to change.

As discussed in Chapter 1, there are a number of motivators for informing practice by high quality clinical research, but we also know there are barriers to changing practice behaviour. Making evidence-based physiotherapy happen is a challenge to both individuals and organizations, so action is needed from several perspectives. Up to now this book has focused on how individual physiotherapists can identify, appraise, interpret and use high quality clinical research. But bringing about change is a responsibility not just of practising physiotherapists. Often implementation programmes are initiated 'top-down'. For example, there may be a national or local strategy to improve physiotherapy for low back pain or for the management of osteoporosis. This means someone is responsible at a management level for the implementation of a specific practice change or a guideline. Such management activities are important because individuals need support, access to resources and a culture ready for change, to make evidence-based practice happen. That is why we have focused on a broader perspective of implementation in this book. The target group for this chapter is, therefore, primarily physiotherapy and health service leaders, managers of health services and policy-makers.

TWO APPROACHES

Evidence-based physiotherapy can be made to happen in two main ways. The first is by implementing the five steps of evidence-based practice (described in Chapter 1) as an integral part of everyday practice. This involves physiotherapists formulating questions of relevance for practice, searching, critically appraising research and informing current practice with high quality clinical research. In the clinical decision-making process this information is combined with practice knowledge and patient preferences. These 'steps' provide the infrastructure for, or foundations of, evidence-based physiotherapy. Application of the steps requires the skills to ask questions, search, appraise and interpret the evidence. It also requires access to equipment or technology, for example a computer, access to the internet and journals. Chapter 9 will consider how you can evaluate whether or not you are implementing the steps in your own pratcice.

A second approach to making evidence-based physiotherapy happen is through the implementation of a personal and/or organizational practice or behaviour change related to a specific condition. This may be necessary because there is current variation in practice, or because that practice needs to be improved or changed in a particular area. A typical example is the implementation of new strategies for management of low back pain. Organizations have to decide which strategies to use to improve professional performance and quality of care, and on what to base these decisions.

CHANGING IS HARD

Change is always difficult, in every area of human life. We guess you will have experienced how hard it can be. Most physiotherapists provide a good service for their patients. Where there are large variations in practice among physiotherapists, or gaps between current practice and high quality clinical research, there is generally a good reason. It may be that the patient or the physiotherapist has strong preferences for, or positive experiences of, a certain treatment, or it may simply be due to a lack of knowledge by the physiotherapist. Sometimes, however, there are other reasons. Clinical behaviour, like other behaviours (for example physical activity, sexual behaviour or smoking habits) is determined by a number of factors, and the link between knowledge and behaviour is often weak. Anyone who has tried to change patient behaviour, or one's own behaviour, will recognize how difficult it is. Knowledge alone is often not sufficient for behaviour change. When it comes to physiotherapists' behaviour there might be a number of factors that determine practice patterns. For example, factors related to resources, social support, practice environment, prevailing opinions and personal attitudes might all act as barriers to desired change.

Before moving on to a discussion of barriers that have been identified in physiotherapy, it will be useful to consider some theories of change.

THEORIES OF CHANGE

Implementation research has been defined as the scientific study of methods to promote the uptake of research findings for the purpose of improving the quality of care. It includes the study of factors that influence the behaviour of health care professionals and organizations, and the interventions that enable them to use research findings more effectively. Research in this area has followed two related tracks: the transfer or diffusion of knowledge and behaviour change (Agency for Healthcare Research and Quality 2004).

Theories of change can be used both to understand the behaviour of health professionals and to guide the development and implementation of interventions intended to change behaviour. Numerous theories of behaviour change have developed from a variety of perspectives: psychology, sociology, economics, marketing, education, organizational behaviour and others. The theories relate to changing the behaviours of patients, professionals and organizations. One type of theory is often called the classical, or descriptive, model (Agency for Healthcare Research and Quality 2004) and the most referred to is Rogers' Diffusion of Innovation Theory (Rogers 1995). This is a passive model that describes the naturalistic process of change. The innovation–decision process is derived from Rogers' theory and consists of five stages that potential adopters pass through as they decide to adopt an innovation. Rogers developed the model of adopter types in which he classified people as innovators (the fastest adopter group), early adopters, the early majority, the late majority and laggards (the slowest to change). However, these classical models provide little information about how to actually accelerate and promote change.

Other types of theory are often called planned change models (Agency for Healthcare Research and Quality 2004). They aim to explain how planned change occurs and how to alter ways of doing things in social systems. Most of these are based on social cognitive theories. Three examples of planned change theories are Green's precede–proceed model, the social marketing model and the Ottawa Model of Research Use.

The precede–proceed model outlines steps that should precede an intervention and gives guidance on how to proceed with implementation and subsequent evaluation (Green et al 1980). The 'precede' stage involves identifying the problem and the factors that contribute to it. The factors are categorized as predisposing, enabling or reinforcing. The key 'proceed' stages are implementation and evaluation of the effect the intervention had on behaviour change, and on predisposing, enabling and reinforcing factors.

Social marketing provides a framework for identifying factors that drive change. According to this model, change should be carried out in several stages (Kotler 1983). The first stage is a planning and strategy development stage. The next stage involves selecting the relevant channels and materials for the intervention. At this stage the target group is 'segmented' to create homogeneous subgroups based, for example, on individuals' motivations for change. Subsequently, materials are developed and piloted with the target audience. Finally, there is implementation, evaluation and feedback, after which the intervention may be refined. Social marketing has largely focused on bringing about health behaviour change at a community level, but it has also been used as the basis for other quality improvement strategies, for example academic detailing or outreach visits, discussed later in this chapter.

The *Ottawa Model of Health Care Research* requires quality improvement facilitators to conduct an assessment of the barriers to implementing evidence-based recommendations. They then identify the potential adopters, and look at the practice environment to determine factors that might hinder or support the uptake of recommendations (Agency for Healthcare Research and Quality 2004). The information is then used to tailor interventions to overcome identified barriers or enhance the supporters. Finally, the impact of the implementation is evaluated and the interactive process begins again.

Motivational theories, including the social cognition model, propose that motivation determines behaviour, and therefore the best predictors of behaviour are factors that predict motivation. This assumption is the basis for *social psychological* theories. *Bandura's social cognitive theory* is one example (Bandura 1997). This theory proposes that behaviour is determined by incentives and expectations. Self-efficacy expectations are beliefs about one's ability to perform the behaviour (for example, 'I can start being physically active') and have been found to be a very important construct and predictor of behaviour change. A refinement of social cognitive theory is *stage models* of behaviour, which describe the factors thought to influence change in different settings. Individuals are thought to go through different stages to achieve a change, and different interventions are needed at different stages. Such theory might be applied to the types of change required for evidence-based practice. One model (Prochaska & Velicer 1997) involves five stages: pre-contemplation, contemplation, preparation, action and maintenance. One can easily understand that a person who is in a pre-contemplation stage (someone for whom no reason for change has been given) would need strategies to raise awareness and acknowledge information needs. In contrast, a person at an action or maintenance stage needs easy access to high quality clinical research, and reminders to keep up the achieved behaviour. This theory is widely used, as in a study to improve physical activity (Marcus et al 1998). Nonetheless a recent systematic review found that there was little evidence to support the use of stage model theories for smoking cessation (Riemsma et al 2003).

Most of the theories described above focus on individuals, but organizational factors play an important role in change processes as well. One type of *organizational theory* is *rational system models*, which focus on the internal structure and processes of an organization (Agency for Healthcare Research and Quality 2004). These models describe four stages in the process of organizational change and different perspectives that need to be addressed in each stage. The stages relate to awareness of a problem, identification of actions, implementation and institutionalization of the change. *Institutional models* assume that management has the freedom to implement change and the legitimacy to ask for behaviours to drive the implementation. Institutional models can explain important factors of quality improvement involving *total quality management*, an organizational intervention that is carried out by a range of philosophies and activities. All organizational models emphasize the complexity of organizations and the need to take account of multiple factors that influence the process of change.

Learning theory from educational research emphasizes the role of intrinsic personal motivation. From these theories have developed activities based on consensus development and problem-based learning. In contrast, *marketing approaches* are widely used to target physician behaviour (for example prescribing) and also to promote health to the general public, as in health promotion campaigns.

As demonstrated here, there are many theories of change. All have shortcomings because implementation is a complex process. Only by testing these out in clinical and practice settings can evidence on whether they work be generated. There is much debate about how they should be evaluated. There is also a growing call on future implementation research developing a better theoretical basis for implementation strategies than seen up until now (Grimshaw et al 2004).

BARRIERS TO CHANGE

In the introduction to this chapter we presented two different approaches to 'making it happen'. The first was through implementation of the 'steps' of evidence-based physiotherapy in everyday practice. The second approach was by implementing a desired change in current practice for a particular patient group. The outcome measures for the first approach would be measures of the extent to which physiotherapists formulate questions, search and read papers critically and use high quality clinical research to inform their everyday practice. The outcome measure for the second approach would be the extent to which current practice is matched to high quality clinical research. Both approaches require a change in behaviour, but the barriers to using the steps for evidence-based physiotherapy as part of everyday practice might differ from the barriers to achieving a desired practice for a patient group. The barriers might also differ between patient groups and cultures. There are no one-size-fits-all or universal barriers to good practice (Oxman & Flottorp 1998). Specific barriers have to be identified for every implementation project, which might then not be relevant to other settings or circumstances.

The identification of barriers to implementation of evidence-based physiotherapy is often carried out with qualitative research methods, as the aim is to explore attitudes, experiences and meanings. Many of us will have a limited insight into barriers to using evidence in our own practices. Critical reflection is the starting point for identifying determinants for practice.

Barriers to implementing the steps of evidence–based practice

Several studies have tried to identify barriers to evidence-based practice among health professionals (Freeman & Sweeny 2001, Young & Ward 2001). In a survey of Australian general practitioners, 45% stated that the most common barrier was 'patients' demand for treatment despite lack of evidence for effectiveness' (Young & Ward 2001). The next three highest-rated barriers were all related to lack of time. This was rated as a 'very important barrier' by significantly more participants than lack of skills.

Humphris et al (2000) used qualitative methods to identify barriers in occupational therapy and followed this qualitative study with a survey to evaluate the importance of the identified factors. The three most discouraging factors were workload pressure, time limitations and insufficient staff resources. Another survey, carried out with dieticians, occupational therapists, physiotherapists and speech and language therapists, identified barriers related to skills, understanding research methodology, and having access to research and time. The relevance of research and institutional barriers seemed to be less of a problem (Metcalfe 2001). More specifically, the top three barriers were 'statistical analysis in papers is not understandable', 'literature not compiled in one place' and 'literature reports conflicting results'. More than one-third (38%) of the physiotherapists felt that doctors would not co-operate with implementation, and 30% felt that they did not have enough authority to change practice.

A well-conducted study was carried out in the Wessex area of the UK with the aim of identifying physiotherapists' attitudes and experiences related to evidence-based physiotherapy (Barnard & Wiles 2001). Junior physiotherapists and physiotherapists working in hospital settings felt that they had the skills needed to appraise research findings prior to implementation. Others, particularly senior physiotherapists working in community settings, felt that they did not. Community physiotherapists also felt that they were not able to engage in evidence-based practice, due to poor access to library facilities and difficulties in meeting with peers. Some physiotherapists also described problems with the culture working against evidence-based physiotherapy where senior staff were resistant to change.

Barriers to implementing a change in specific practice behaviour

One study from the Netherlands was carried out to identify barriers to implementation of a guideline for low back pain (Bekkering et al 2003). One hundred randomly selected physiotherapists were invited to participate and asked, in a survey, to identify any difference between the guideline recommendations and their current practice. The survey revealed a number of issues, highlighted by discrepancies between guideline recommendations and practice, that might be regarded as barriers to implementation. The most important of these was lack of knowledge or skills of physiotherapists in both the diagnosis and treatment processes. In the treatment process this was due to differences between traditional and evidence-based treatment (for example, passive interventions were traditionally used, but were discouraged by the guidelines). The second most important difference was an organizational one involving problems with getting the co-operation of the referring physicians (mostly general practitioners). There was also an issue about the expectations of patients. The authors conclude that, since skills and knowledge were the most important barriers, there is a need for continuing postgraduate education to keep knowledge and skills up to date.

In Scotland, a stroke therapy evaluation programme was carried out as a multidisciplinary project. One part of this project was the implementation of evidence-based rehabilitation. Pollock et al (2000) conducted a study to identify barriers to evidence-based stroke rehabilitation among health professionals, of whom 31% were physiotherapists. The study started with focus groups identifying perceived barriers, followed by a postal questionnaire to rate participants' agreement with the identified barriers. The barriers were divided into three areas: ability, opportunity and implementation. The key barriers identified across professionals were lack of time, lack of ability/need for training, and difficulties relating to the implementation of research findings. Physiotherapists felt less put off by statistics than occupational therapists and nurses. Sixty-seven percent of all respondents agreed that they needed more training in appraisal and interpretation of studies, and only 8% agreed that they had sufficient time to read. Barriers to implementation appeared to be a lack of confidence in the validity of research findings and in the transferability of research findings to an individual's working environment.

What do these studies tell us? There are big variations in the barriers reported, but the main barriers to implementing evidence-based practice relate to time, skills and culture. One barrier that was not identified in the studies reported, but which we believe is relevant, is the lack of high quality clinical research in many areas. If you go through the steps of formulating a question and searching for evidence without identifying high quality studies, this must be a barrier to evidence-based practice.

Barriers to implementation of specific behaviour changes are more complex in nature, and specific to the topic under study. Overall, the conclusion seems to be that barriers need to be identified for each project and setting, because different approaches seem to be needed to address them.

EVIDENCE-BASED IMPLEMENTATION

WHAT HELPS PEOPLE TO CHANGE PRACTICE?

A range of strategies exists to change the behaviour of health care professionals, with the aim of improving the quality of patient care. Box 8.1 provides examples of interventions that have been evaluated in systematic reviews with a focus on improving practice. The interventions are classified by the Cochrane Collaboration's Effective Practice and Organization of Care group (EPOC; http://www.epoc.uottawa.ca/). The focus of the EPOC group's work is on reviews of interventions designed to improve professional practice and the delivery of effective health services.

Box 8.1   Examples of interventions to promote professional behaviour change (based on EPOC taxonomy; www.epoc.uottawa.ca)

- **Educational materials**   Distribution of published or printed recommendations for clinical care (such as clinical practice guidelines, audio-visual materials, electronic publications)
- **Didactic educational meetings**   Lectures with minimal participant interaction
- **Interactive educational meetings**   Participation of health care providers in workshops that include discussion or practice
- **Educational outreach visits**   A personal visit by a trained person to a health care provider in his or her own setting to give information with the intent of changing practice
- **Reminders (manual or computerized)**   Patient or encounter-specific information, provided verbally, on paper or on a computer screen, which is designed or intended to prompt a health professional to recall information
- **Audit and feedback**   Any summary of clinical performance of health care over a specified period of time. The summary may also have included recommendations for clinical action
- **Local opinion leaders**   Health professionals nominated by their colleagues as being educationally influential are recruited to promote implementation
- **Local consensus process**   Inclusion of health professionals in discussions to agree to an approach to managing a clinical problem that they have selected as important
- **Patient mediated interventions**   Specific information sought from or given to patients
- **Multifaceted interventions**   A combination of two or more interventions

EPOC reviews produce information about the effectiveness of interventions. The focus includes various forms of continuing education, quality assurance, informatics, and financial, organizational and regulatory interventions that can affect the ability of health care professionals to deliver services more effectively and efficiently.

As discussed in the introduction to this chapter, implementation of evidence-based practice can be promoted in different ways or stages. Implementing the steps of evidence-based practice is one option that might lead to changes in specific behaviours.

Implementing the steps of evidence–based practice

One systematic review focused on teaching critical appraisal in health care settings (Parkes et al 2004). This review included only one randomized study, carried out among nurses. The study indicated that the participants improved their knowledge, but professional behaviour was not assessed. There is a need for more research to find ways of implementing the steps effectively. Currently, much of the teaching of the steps involves interactive educational meetings with small group discussions and practice-related questions. There is a close link from here to issues related to self-evaluation, discussed in the next chapter.

Implementing a change in specific practice behaviour

The effects of implementation strategies could be assessed by measuring either of two types of outcome. Outcomes can be measured at the level of professional performance, for example by measuring the frequency with which ultrasound is used to treat carpal tunnel syndrome or physiotherapists' compliance with a guideline for the treatment of ankle sprains. Outcome can also be measured at the level of the patient, for example by measuring changes in pain, disability or time away from work. Studies have evaluated effects of implementation interventions on both types of outcome.

Several interventions have been evaluated, although most studies (approximately 90%) are carried out among physicians. The studies have been carried out in both primary care and hospitals, and the focus has often been on improvement in one or more aspects of practice behaviour or compliance with a guideline. However, as we will discuss later in this chapter, it remains unclear how best to implement and sustain evidence-based practice, especially among physiotherapists.

The following section provides an overview of systematic reviews of the effects of interventions aimed at changing professional practice. The overview is based on two high quality evidence-based reports (Grimshaw et al 2001, Effective Health Care Bulletin 1999). We have added information from systematic reviews that were published subsequently and not included in these reports. The systematic reviews were identified by the EPOC group. We have also identified a doctoral thesis from the Netherlands that includes an evaluation of an implementation strategy for low back pain guidelines (Bekkering 2004).

To provide an overview of the findings, we have summarized the reviews and graded the evidence into four categories. The summary and categories are shown in Table 8.1. The grades are based on the quality and

Table 8.1   The effects of various implementation strategies

1. Systematic reviews show that:[a]	■ No intervention works in all settings ■ Passive strategies alone, such as the distribution of educational materials, conferences and didactic talks do not improve professional practice or patient outcomes (Oxman et al 1995*, Bero et al 1998, Thomson O'Brien et al 2004a) ■ Teaching critical appraisal improves knowledge in health professionals (Parkes et al 2004)
2. Systematic reviews point towards:[b]	■ Educational meetings that include interactive teaching and small group discussions might have a moderate effect on professional practice or patient outcomes (Davis et al 1995, Thomson O'Brien et al 2004a) ■ Educational outreach visits might have a small to moderate effect on professional practice or patient outcomes, at least on short term follow-up (Thomson O'Brien et al 2004b) ■ Audit and feedback on performance might have a small to moderate effect on professional practice or patient outcomes (Jamtvedt et al 2004).
3. Systematic reviews are not consistent with regard to whether:[c]	■ Strategies to implement guidelines improve professional practice or patient outcomes (Grimshaw et al 2004, Thomas et al 2004) ■ The use of opinion leaders improves professional practice or patient outcomes (Thomson O'Brien et al 2004c) ■ Reminders, electronic or other, improve professional practice or patient outcomes (Bero et al 1998, Effective Health Care Bulletin 1999) ■ Multifaceted interventions work better than single interventions (Grimshaw et al 2004, Jamtvedt et al 2004)
4. There is a lack of systematic reviews on the following topic:[d]	■ The effect of mass media, quality improvement interventions and organizational interventions on professional practice or patient outcomes (Foxcroft & Cole 2004, Grilli et al 2004) ■ Effect of incentives (Gosden et al 2004, Guiffrida et al 2004) ■ Effect of teaching critical appraisal in health care settings on professional practice or patient outcomes (Parkes et al 2004)

[a] At least one updated systematic review of high quality which includes at least two high quality studies with consistent results.
[b] One updated systematic review of high or moderate quality that includes at least one high quality study or two studies of moderate quality with consistent results.
[c] Systematic reviews of variable quality with heterogeneous results.
[d] No systematic review identified that covers this topic, or systematic review identified with no relevant studies included.
* This review needs to be updated; there might be newer relevant studies that could change the conclusion.

number of the systematic reviews, the quality and number of primary studies included, and the consistency of the results across primary studies. You need to bear in mind that these results are mainly based on studies carried out among physicians in different settings, but this is the only high quality evaluation of implementation strategies available.

The title of a systematic review of implementation strategies published in 1995 declared there are 'no magic bullets' when it comes to translating research into practice (Oxman et al 1995). This still seems to be the case. Although no intervention seems to work in all settings, small to moderate improvements can be achieved by many interventions. Overall, it seems that passive strategies, such as the distribution of educational materials and lectures alone, do not change practice much. Active interventions, such as workshops and outreach visits that involve discussion, reflection and practice seem to be able to make modest to moderate improvements. There is a need for more implementation research within physiotherapy and other allied health professions.

IMPLEMENTING CLINICAL GUIDELINES

As outlined in Chapter 7, clinical guidelines are an increasingly common resource used to improve physiotherapy practice and health care outcomes. Guidelines have the potential to improve quality and achieve better practice by promoting interventions of proven benefit and discouraging ineffective interventions. But do we know whether they are worth the costs and resources spent on their development and on implementation strategies?

Although many countries have developed clinical guidelines in physiotherapy over the last years, very few have evaluated their impact on practice or health care outcome. Our impression is that physiotherapy bodies and groups have put a lot of effort and resources into the development process, but very few have followed this up with systematic implementation and evaluation processes. In most cases clinical guidelines have been implemented by passive interventions, such as dissemination by post and by articles in national physiotherapy publications. Sometimes the guidelines have only been available by actively purchasing them from organizations. There are also some examples of more active implementation strategies. In Australia, the implementation of guidelines for low back pain was carried out as a 'road show' and a lot of marketing and advertising was put into the process. In the UK, physiotherapists identified as opinion leaders have been involved in the guideline development process. This has been seen as both a strategy for improving the quality and relevance of the guidelines and a way of giving the guidelines credibility.

There are many reasons why we do not see robust evaluations of the effects on practice after guideline development and dissemination in physiotherapy, but lack of resources is certainly a common factor. Another reason might be a belief that passive dissemination of guidelines and presentation at conferences alone will have an impact on practice and change behaviour if needed. But we do not know if this approach works, and we have to admit we have limited knowledge of the effects of guidelines in physiotherapy. Just as all interventions carried out in physiotherapy should be evaluated for their effect, there is a need to look in the same way at implementation strategies. A randomized controlled trial is needed to see if the implementation strategies have an impact on practice or patients' health. (That is also the case when it comes to other quality improvement strategies.)

Implementation of physiotherapy guidelines for low back pain

As far as we know, only one implementation study including a robust evaluation design has been carried out in physiotherapy. This study evaluated the implementation of a guideline on low back pain (Bekkering 2004). The guideline was developed as part of a continuous quality programme by the Royal Dutch Society of Physiotherapy. The whole project was carried out as a collaboration between physiotherapists and researchers. An active implementation strategy was developed based on a study that had identified the perceived barriers to using the guidelines among clinicians, and the difference between the guideline recommendations and current practice (Bekkering et al 2003). The strategy was built on a theoretical model for changing behaviour, together with the findings from systematic reviews of the effect of implementation strategies. The intervention consisted of two training sessions comprising education, role play and discussion, addressing the perceived barriers. This strategy was evaluated in a cluster-randomized controlled trial where the control group only received the guidelines by mail. Outcome measures were the process of care or adherence to the guidelines, and patient outcomes. The study showed that physiotherapists who received the active strategy adhered more to guideline recommendations than control physiotherapists, but the strategy did not result in demonstrable effects on patient outcome. The physiotherapists in the control group already adhered to the guideline considerably which may have decreased the contrast between groups on patient outcome.

Effectiveness of guideline implementation in professions allied to medicine

In a Cochrane review, Thomas et al (2004) focused on guideline implementation in professions allied to medicine. The searches were conducted only up to 1996, so there might be several newer studies published since this review was conducted. Eighteen studies involving more than 450 professionals were included. In all but one study the professionals were nurses. The remaining study was aimed at dieticians. Three of five studies observed improvement in the process of care and six of eight studies observed improvement in some outcome of care. The authors conclude that there is some evidence that guideline-driven care is effective in changing the process and outcome of care provided by professionals allied to medicine, primarily among nurses. These results should be viewed with caution because of the generally poor methodological quality in the studies included in this review. And we should bear in mind that the findings might not be relevant to other professions, such as physiotherapy and related therapies.

Overviews of effectiveness of guideline implementation

Grimshaw et al (2004) conducted a systematic review of the effectiveness and costs of different guideline development, dissemination and implementation strategies from studies published up to 1998. They identified 235 studies that evaluated guideline dissemination and implementation among medically qualified health care professionals. No study was carried out in physiotherapy; 39% of the studies were carried out in primary care. Seventy-three percent of the comparisons evaluated multifaceted interventions, defined as more than one implementation strategy. Commonly evaluated single interventions were reminders, dissemination of educational materials and audit and feedback. The evidence base for the guideline recommendations was not clear in 94% of the studies.

An overview of the findings of the review is presented in Tables 8.2 and 8.3 (Grimshaw et al 2004, Ekeland & Jamtvedt 2004). Overall the majority of the studies observed improvements in care, but there were big variations both within and across interventions. The improvements were small to moderate, with a median improvement in care of 10% across all studies. One important result, that many will find surprising, is that multifaceted interventions did not appear more effective than single interventions. Only 29% of the comparisons reported any economic

Table 8.2 Effect of single interventions on implementation of guidelines

Effect size*	Intervention	Based on
Moderate positive	Patient-mediated interventions	17 studies
Modest-to-moderate positive	Reminders	38 studies
Modest positive	Distribution of educational materials	18 studies
Modest positive	Audit and feedback	10 studies
Small-to-modest positive	Educational meetings	3 studies

*Size of effect (absolute difference across post-intervention measures) for process outcomes: small = effect sizes <5%; modest = ≥5% and <10%; moderate = ≥10% and <20%; large = ≥20%.

Table 8.3 Effect of multifaceted interventions on implementation of guidelines

Effect size*	Intervention	Based on
Moderate positive	Reminders and patient-mediated interventions	6 studies
Modest-to-moderate positive	Distribution of educational materials, educational meetings and educational outreach visits	4 studies
Modest positive	Distribution of educational materials and educational meetings	10 studies
Modest positive	Distribution of educational materials and audit and feedback	4 studies
Small positive	Distribution of educational materials, educational meetings and audit and feedback	8 studies
Small positive	Distribution of educational materials, educational meetings and organizational interventions	6 studies
No effect	Distribution of educational materials and educational outreach visits	8 studies

*Size of effect (absolute difference across post-intervention measures) for process outcomes: small = effect sizes <5%; modest = ≥5% and <10%; moderate = ≥10% and <20%; large = ≥20%.

data, and the majority of these reported only the cost of treatment. Very few studies reported costs of guideline development, dissemination or implementation.

The generalizability of the findings from this review to other behaviours, settings or professions is uncertain. Most studies provided no rationale for their choice of intervention and gave only limited descriptions of the interventions and contextual data (Grimshaw et al 2004). The authors of the review wrote that there is a need for a robust theoretical basis for understanding health care provider and organizational behaviour, and that future research is needed to develop a better theoretical base for the evaluation of guideline dissemination and implementation (Grimshaw et al 2004).

EVIDENCE–BASED PHYSIOTHERAPY IN THE CONTEXT OF CONTINUOUS QUALITY IMPROVEMENT

Making evidence-based physiotherapy happen should have benefits for patients, as they receive more effective care, which should in turn lead to better health outcomes. However, in the real world, evidence-based physiotherapy is only one dimension of quality improvement and should not be implemented in a way that is isolated from an overall organizational quality improvement system. Whether the 'organizational system' is a sole practitioner practice, a 1000-bed hospital, or a community service in a remote setting, there will always be a range of processes or pathways of care for patients. For example, a pathway could extend from the point of entry of a patient into the health care system, to the identification of needs, referral, tests (single or multiple), treatment by a single or team of practitioners, social support, identification of a longer-term plan or strategy for ongoing care or prevention of recurrence … and so on. The pathway crosses departments and organizations horizontally – it is not hierarchical in nature. The physiotherapist's application of evidence-based physiotherapy needs to be seen in the context of, and must be sensitive to, the whole care pathway.

Good organizations strive to continually improve their processes of care (continuous quality improvement) and physiotherapists should engage in this process. As people actually working in a particular setting, they often know which services function best and what the problems with services are. They are therefore well placed to make improvements. A progressive organization will empower staff to identify the potential for improvement and instigate change. The culture of an organization is all-important. A good organization will have a culture of striving for improvement and places high importance on staff learning.

Continual improvement requires leaders who can support and nurture individuals and who believe that individuals want to do better, to learn and to develop. Donald Berwick, a pioneer of continuous quality improvement, once famously said 'Every process is perfectly designed to achieve exactly the results it delivers,' which suggests that if a process is not working it ought to be changed.

The theme of continuous improvement can also be applied at an individual practitioner level. As discussed at the beginning of this book, part of the responsibility attached to being an autonomous practitioner is a responsibility for keeping up to date and striving for improvement through learning. Physiotherapists can set up their own continuous improvement cycles through the measurement of their practice (audit, outcomes evaluation) and by reflective practice and peer review. We will discuss these more in Chapter 9.

References

Agency for Healthcare Research and Quality 2004 Closing the quality gap: a critical analysis of quality improvement strategies. AHRQ, Rockville

Bandura A 1997 Self-efficacy: towards a unifying theory of behaviour change. Psychological Review 84:191–215

Barnard S, Wiles R 2001 Evidence-based physiotherapy. Physiotherapy 87:115–124

Bekkering GE 2004 Physiotherapy guidelines for low back pain. Development, implementation, and evaluation. PhD thesis, Vrije Universiteit, Amsterdam

Bekkering T, Engers AJ, Wensing M et al 2003 Development of an implementation strategy for physiotherapy guidelines on low back pain. Australian Journal of Physiotherapy 49:208–214

Bero LA, Grilli R, Grimshaw JM et al 1998 Closing the gap between research and practice: an overview of systematic reviews of interventions to promote the implementation of research findings. BMJ 317:465–468

Davis DA, Thomson MA, Oxman AD et al 1995 Changing physician performance. A systematic review of the effects of continuing medical education strategies. JAMA 274:700–705

Effective Health Care Bulletin 1999 Getting evidence into practice. Effective Health Care Bulletin 5:1 NHS Centre for Reviews and Dissemination, York. (www.york.ac.uk/inst/crd/ech51.pdf)

Ekeland E, Jamtvedt G 2004 Tiltak for faglig ajourføring i fysioterapi. Norwegian Research Centre for Health Services, Oslo

Foxcroft DR, Cole N 2004 Organisational infrastructures to promote evidence based nursing practice (Cochrane review). In: The Cochrane library, issue 2. Wiley, Chichester

Freeman AC, Sweeney C 2001 Why general practitioners do not implement evidence: qualitative study. BMJ 323:1100

Giuffrida A, Gosden T, Forland F et al 2004 Target payments in primary care: effects on professional practice and health care outcomes (Cochrane review). In: The Cochrane library, issue 2. Wiley, Chichester

Gosden T, Forland F, Kristiansen IS et al 2004 Capitation, salary, fee-for-service and mixed systems of payment: effects on the behaviour of primary care physicians (Cochrane review). In: The Cochrane library, issue 2. Wiley, Chichester

Green L, Kreuter M, Deeds S 1980 Health education planning: a diagnostic approach. California: Mayfield, Mountain View CA

Grilli R, Ramsay C, Minozzi S 2004 Mass media interventions: effects on health services utilisation (Cochrane review). In: The Cochrane library, issue 2. Wiley, Chichester

Grimshaw JM, Shirran L, Thomas R et al 2001 Changing provider behaviour. An overview of systematic reviews of interventions. Medical Care 39(suppl 2): II2–II45

Grimshaw JM, Thomas R, Maclennan G et al 2004 Effectiveness and efficiency of guideline dissemination and implementation strategies. Health Technology Assessment 8(6):1–72

Humphris D, Littlejohns P, Victor CJ et al 2000 Implementing evidence-based practice: factors that influence the use of research evidence by occupational therapists. British Journal of Occupational Therapy 11:516–522

Jamtvedt G, Young JM, Kristoffersen DT et al 2004 Audit and feedback: effects on professional practice and health care outcomes (Cochrane review). In: The Cochrane library, issue 2. Wiley, Chichester

Kotler P 1983 Social marketing of health behaviour. In: Fredriksen L, Solomon L, Brehony K (eds) Marketing health behaviour: principles, techniques and applications. Plenum Press, New York

Lomas J 1993 Diffusion, dissemination, and implementation: who should do what? Annals of the New York Academy of Sciences 703:226–235

Marcus BH, Emmons KM, Simkin-Silverman et al 1998 Motivationally tailored vs standard self-help physical activity interventions at the workplace: a prospective randomized, controlled trial. American Journal of Health Promotion 12(4):246–253

Metcalfe C, Lewin R, Wisher S et al 2001 Barriers to implementing the evidence base in four NHS therapies. Physiotherapy 87:443–441

Oxman A, Flottorp S 1998 An overview of strategies to promote implementation of evidence based health care. In: Silagy C, Haines A (eds) Evidence based practice in primary care. BMJ Books, London

Oxman AD, Thomson MA, Davis DA et al 1995 No magic bullets: a systematic review of 102 trials of interventions to improve professional practice. Canadian Medical Association Journal 153(10):1423–1431

Parkes J, Hyde C, Deeks J et al 2004 Teaching critical appraisal skills in health care settings (Cochrane review). In: The Cochrane library, issue 2. Wiley, Chichester

Pollock A, Legg L, Langhorne P et al 2000 Barriers to achieving evidence-based stroke rehabilitation. Clinical Rehabilitation 14:611–617

Prochaska JO, Velicer WF 1997 The transtheoretical model of health behavior change. American Journal of Health Promotion 12(1):38–48

Riemsma PR, Pattenden J, Bridle C et al 2003 Systematic review of effectiveness of stage based interventions to promote smoking cessation. BMJ 326:1175–1177

Rogers E 1995 Diffusion of innovation, 4th edn. Free Press, New York

Thomas L, Cullum N, McColl E et al 2004 Guidelines in professions allied to medicine (Cochrane review). In: The Cochrane library, issue 2. Wiley, Chichester

Thomson O'Brien MA, Freemantle N, Oxman AD et al 2004a Continuing education meetings and workshops: effects on professional practice and health care outcomes (Cochrane review). In: The Cochrane library, issue 2. Wiley, Chichester

Thomson O'Brien MA, Oxman AD, Davis DA et al 2004b Educational outreach visits: effects on professional practice and health care outcomes (Cochrane review). In: The Cochrane library, issue 3. Wiley, Chichester

Thomson O'Brien MA, Oxman AD, Haynes RB et al 2004c Local opinion leaders: effects on professional practice and health care outcomes (Cochrane review). In: The Cochrane library, issue 2. Wiley, Chichester

Young J, Ward JE 2001 Evidence-based medicine in general practice: beliefs and barriers among Australian GPs. Journal of Evaluation in Clinical Practice 7:201–210

Chapter 9

Am I on the right track?

OVERVIEW

In this chapter we consider how physiotherapists can evaluate their practice. Evaluation could involve evaluation of either outcomes or process of practice. Measurement of outcomes potentially provides some insights into the effectiveness of practice. However, clinical measures of outcome need to be interpreted cautiously because they are potentially misleading. We argue that clinical measures of outcome are most useful when there is little strong evidence of the effects of intervention and when outcomes are extreme (either very good or very poor). When the evidence is strong, or when outcomes are less extreme, it is more useful to evaluate processes. Evaluation of the process of clinical practice could involve a formal process audit, peer review of clinical performance, or reflective practice. Finally, we consider the audit of the steps of practising evidence-based physiotherapy, discussed in Chapter 1.

The process of evidence-based physiotherapy begins and ends by questioning one's own practice. Having asked a clinical question, sought out and critically appraised evidence, and implemented evidence-based practice, it is constructive to reflect on whether the process was carried out well and produced the best outcome for the patient. We refer to this as evaluation.

In this chapter we separately consider how to evaluate the *outcomes* of evidence-based practice and to audit the *process*.

ASSESSING PATIENT OUTCOMES: CLINICAL MEASUREMENT

Historically, outcome measurement was not a feature of routine clinical practice. Physiotherapists (and, for that matter, most other health professionals) did not systematically collect data on patients' outcomes. Typically, physiotherapists obtained information about the effectiveness of their practice incidentally, from their impressions of clinical outcomes or from patients' comments about their satisfaction (or dissatisfaction) with physiotherapy services.

In more recent times there has been pressure on physiotherapists to become more accountable for their practices. The pressure has come from makers of health care policies, those who allocate and fund health care (government, insurers, managers), and from within the physiotherapy profession. One of the driving forces has been the perception that physiotherapists must justify what they do. It is thought that by providing evidence of good clinical outcomes physiotherapists can demonstrate that what they do is worthwhile.

In the last two decades the physiotherapy profession has taken up the call for more and better clinical measurement. An early landmark was the publication, in 1985, of *Measurement in Physical Therapy* (Rothstein 1985). More recently, there has been a proliferation of textbooks, journal features and web sites documenting clinical outcome measures and their measurement properties (Wade 1992, Koke et al 1999, Maher et al 2000, Finch et al 2002; see also the excellent web site and on-line database produced by the Chartered Society of Physiotherapy at http://www.csp.org.uk/effectivepractice/outcomemeasures.cfm and the regular feature entitled Meten in de Practijk in the *Nederlands Tijdschrift voor Fysiotherapie*). In some countries at least, a large proportion of physiotherapists routinely document clinical outcomes using validated tools. In New South Wales, Australia, the public provider of rehabilitation services for work-related injuries pays an additional fee to practitioners who adequately document measures of clinical outcomes.

The evolution of a culture in which physiotherapists routinely measure clinical outcomes with validated tools may well have produced an increase in the effectiveness of physiotherapy practice, because systematic collection of outcome data focuses both patients and therapists on outcomes. To our knowledge, however, there have been no randomized trials of the effects of routine measures of outcomes on outcomes of care.

Perhaps it is unfortunate that the physiotherapy profession has responded to the perception that physiotherapists must justify what they do by routinely measuring clinical outcomes. The implication is that measures of outcome can provide justification for intervention. Arguably that is not the case.

HOW CAN WE INTERPRET MEASUREMENTS OF OUTCOME?

Outcome measures measure outcomes. They do not measure the effects of intervention. Outcomes of interventions and effects of interventions are very different things.

In Chapter 3 we saw that clinical outcomes are influenced by many factors other than intervention, including the natural course of the condition, statistical regression, placebo effects, polite patient effects, and so on. The implication is that a good outcome does not necessarily indicate that intervention was effective (because a good outcome may have occurred even without intervention). And a poor outcome does not necessarily indicate that intervention was ineffective (because the outcome may have been worse still without intervention). Consequently, we look to randomized trials to find out about the effects of intervention. This implies a belief that clinical outcome measures should not be relied upon to provide dependable information about the effectiveness of interventions. It is illogical, on the one hand, to look to randomized controlled trials for evidence of effects of interventions, while on the other hand to seek justification for the effectiveness of clinical practice with uncontrolled measurement of clinical outcomes.

Taken further, this line of reasoning suggests that, at least in some circumstances, measures of a patient's clinical outcome should have no role in influencing decisions about treatment for that patient. According to this view, randomized trials provide better information about the effects of intervention than measures of clinical outcomes. So decisions about intervention for a particular patient should be based entirely on the findings of randomized trials, without regard to the apparent effects of treatment suggested by measures of clinical outcome on that patient. For example, if a randomized trial suggests that, on average, an intervention produces effects that a patient considers would be worthwhile, the implication is that intervention should continue to be offered even if the patient's outcomes are poor. The reasoning goes that the best we can know of the effects of a treatment (from randomized trials) tells us that this intervention typically produces clinically worthwhile effects. The patient may be one of the unlucky patients who does not benefit from (or is harmed by) this intervention, or it may be that the patient's poor outcomes might have been worse still without the intervention. We cannot discriminate between these scenarios so we act on the basis of what we think is most likely to be true: on average the intervention is helpful. Consequently we continue to provide the intervention, even though the outcome of intervention is poor.

This view is completely antithetical to the empirical approach to clinical practice exemplified by some authors (notably Maitland et al 2001). In the fully empirical approach, intervention is always followed by assessment. If outcomes improve, the intervention may be continued until the problem is completely resolved. If outcomes do not improve or worsen, the intervention is modified or discontinued. This approach appears to be reasonable, but it involves making clinical decisions on the basis of information that is very difficult to interpret. The empirical approach, in which clinical decisions are based on careful measurement of outcomes, is not evidence-based physiotherapy. If we base clinical decisions about intervention exclusively on high quality clinical research, measures of clinical outcome can have little role in clinical decision-making or in justifying clinical practice. Interventions can be recommended without consideration of their outcomes.

Is there any role for clinical outcome measures in clinical decision-making? We think that, when there is evidence of effects of intervention from high quality clinical trials, a sensible approach to clinical decision-making lies somewhere between the two extremes of the fully empirical approach and a hard-line approach in which clinical decision-making is based only on high quality clinical research without regard to outcome.[1] As a consequence, extreme clinical observations (very good or very poor outcomes) are likely to be 'real' (bias is unlikely to have qualitatively altered the clinical picture). On the other hand, the qualitative interpretation of typical observations (small improvements in outcome) could plausibly be altered by bias.

> In other words, this approach suggests that clinical decision-making should be influenced by observations of very good and very poor outcomes, but should not be influenced by less extreme observations.

What does this mean in practice? It means, first of all, that there is value in careful measurement of clinical outcomes, because extreme clinical outcomes influence clinical decision-making. It also means that the degree of regard we pay to measures of clinical outcomes depends on how extreme the outcomes are. When outcomes are *very* poor we *should* discontinue the intervention, even if the best clinical trials tell us that the intervention is, on average, effective: a *very* poor outcome is unlikely to be explicable only by confounding effects such as the natural course of the condition, statistical regression, polite patients and so on – it probably also reflects that this person truly responded poorly to the intervention. On the other hand, less extreme poor outcomes might reasonably be ignored, and an intervention might be persisted with, regardless of moderately poor outcome, if the best clinical trials provide strong evidence that the intervention produces, on average, a clinically worthwhile effect.[2] In all circumstances, clinical decision-making should be informed by patients' preferences and values.

Clinical outcome measures become more important when there is little or no evidence from high quality randomized trials. In that case, the alternatives are either not to intervene at all, or to intervene in the absence of high quality evidence and use (potentially misleading) clinical outcome measures to guide decisions about intervention. In contrast, when randomized trials provide clear evidence of the effects of an intervention from high quality clinical trials, clinical outcome measures

---

[1] The essence of this approach is that it recognizes that person-to-person variability in response to an intervention is likely to be far greater than the bias in inferences about effects of interventions based on measures of clinical outcomes. The degree of person-to-person variability can be estimated in cross-over trials which use outcomes measured with little or no error. In that case the width of the 95% prediction interval describing the person-to-person variability in response to intervention is $\sqrt{n} \times$ the 95% confidence interval for the mean effect of treatment. Try this out! You will find that person-to-person variability in response to an intervention is almost always enormous.
[2] This theoretical position may be very difficult to maintain in practice. It could be hard to continue a treatment that you expect is effective if clinical observations suggest it is not. And, conversely, it could be hard to resist provision of a treatment when outcomes associated with the treatment are good.

become relatively unimportant and measures of the process of care become more useful.

> When evidence of effects of interventions is strong, we should use process audit to evaluate practice. When there is little or no evidence (i.e. when practice cannot be evidence-based) we should use measures of clinical outcomes to evaluate practice.

The preceding discussion assumes that it is not possible rigorously to establish the effects of therapy on a single patient. But, as we saw in Chapter 4, there is one exception: single case experimental designs (n-of-1 studies) can establish, with a high degree of rigour, the effects of intervention on a single patient. Unfortunately, n-of-1 trials are difficult to conduct as part of routine clinical practice and are, at any rate, suited only to certain conditions (Chapter 4). A more practical approach is to use less rigorous designs, such as the so-called ABA' design. In ABA' designs, the patient's condition is monitored prior to intervention (period A), during intervention (period B) and following intervention (period A'). The magnitude of the improvement seen in the transition from period A to period B and the magnitude of the decline seen in the transition from period B to period A' provide an indication of the effect of intervention on that patient, although this approach should be considered less rigorous than properly designed n-of-1 trials. Smith et al (2004) provide a nice example of how the ABA' approach can be used in practice, in this case to test the effects of low-Dye taping on plantar fasciitis pain.

Before completing the discussion of the role of clinical measurement, we note that there is another role for measurement of outcomes, other than its limited role in telling us about the effects of intervention. Routine standardized outcome measurements potentially provide us with other useful data. They can be used to generate practice-specific estimates of prognosis. For example, a physiotherapist who routinely assesses the presence or absence of shoulder pain in stroke patients at discharge following an upper limb rehabilitation programme can use those data to generate practice-specific prognoses about the risk of developing shoulder pain by the time of discharge. It is important to recognize that these data have useful prognostic value, but they do not provide good evidence of the effectiveness or otherwise of intervention.

We have argued that clinical outcome measures have two roles. First, they provide limited information about the effects of an intervention on a particular patient; such measures are most useful when there is little or no evidence of the effects of intervention and when extreme outcomes are observed. Second, if standardized outcome data are routinely collected, they potentially provide practice-specific prognostic data. Where physiotherapists measure clinical outcomes for these purposes they ought to use appropriate measurement tools. That is, they should choose tools that are reliable (precise) and valid. We will not consider how to ascertain whether a clinical measurement tool has these properties, as that is the topic of other more authoritative texts (Rothstein 1985, Feinstein 1987, Streiner & Norman 2003).

ASSESSING THE PROCESS OF CARE: AUDIT

AUDIT OF CLINICAL PRACTICE

Clinical audit

Clinical audit has been defined as a 'quality improvement process that seeks to improve patient care and outcomes through systematic review of care against explicit criteria and the implementation of change' (National Institute for Clinical Excellence 2002). Put simply, audit is a method of comparing what is actually happening in clinical practice against agreed standards or guidelines. Audit criteria should be based on high quality clinical research. As we saw earlier in this chapter, when evidence of the effects of an intervention is strong, audit of process is a more appropriate way to evaluate practice than the use of measures of clinical outcome.

Clinical audit is a cyclical process. The key components of the process are:

- The setting of explicit standards or criteria for practice
- Measurement of actual performance against the pre-determined criteria
- Review of performance, based on the measurements
- Agreement about what practice improvements are needed (if any)
- Action taken to implement agreed improvements
- Measurement of actual performance repeated to confirm improvement (or not)
- Continuation of the cycle.

We present an 'evidence based' audit cycle in Figure 9.1, which includes all the components discussed above. Additionally, it includes a requirement that the standards or criteria (the foundation of the audit process) have been developed from evidence derived from high quality clinical research, following the steps described in this book. This means that, if there is adherence with the standards and criteria, practice will be based on an evidence-based process of care.

Audit can also be used to assess whether the recommendations of a high quality clinical guideline are being adhered to. Here, the guideline recommendations provide the basis for criteria against which to measure clinical practice. One example, described in Chapter 8, is a project that assessed compliance with guidelines for low back pain in The Netherlands (Bekkering et al 2003).

Audit of practice can be carried out by the individual practitioner (self-audit), but is better undertaken by someone else so the data is collected systematically, objectively and without bias. Usually, the source of the data is the patient or physiotherapy record. The auditor (or data collector) examines a sample of records to see if practice, as recorded, met the evidence-based standards or criteria. The data is then used to review practice, and there is consideration of the extent to which practice adhered to the criteria. If there was a discrepancy between the criteria and practice, there is consideration of why this occurred. An action plan, or recommendations, can then be drawn up and implemented, after which another data collection exercise can be carried out to see if adherence is greater.

More commonly, audit of a service is carried out as part of an organization's quality assurance systems. This can provide valuable feedback to individual physiotherapists about their use of evidence in practice. The

Figure 9.1   An evidence-based audit cycle.

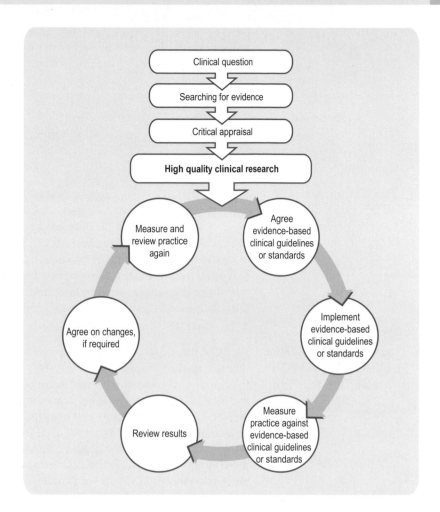

greatest impact for patients will occur in organizations where there is a culture of continuous improvement and willingness to change. Still, there is a need to evaluate the impact of quality improvement activities on process and patient outcomes, and there is an ongoing debate on how to run these projects (Øvretveit & Gustafson 2003).

Peer review

Another form of audit is peer review, which is assessment of clinical performance undertaken by another physiotherapist (a peer). It provides an opportunity for an individual's practice to be evaluated by someone with similar experience, ideally by a trusted colleague whom the individual has selected. The review process should be approached by both parties with commitment and integrity, as well as trust (Chartered Society of Physiotherapy 2000). The process can be a learning opportunity for both parties and can be used in particular to enhance skills in clinical reasoning, professional judgement and reflective skills, all of which are difficult to evaluate in more objective ways. It is normally carried out by the peer selecting a random set of patient notes or physiotherapy records. The peer reviews the notes, and the physiotherapist being reviewed may re-familiarize himself or herself with the records. This is followed by a discussion that focuses on the physiotherapist's clinical reasoning skills. The discussion may consider assessment and diagnosis, decisions about intervention, and evaluation of each stage of the episode of care (Chartered Society of Physiotherapy 2000). The use of evidence to support decision-making can also be reviewed. Following discussion, the peer has the responsibility for highlighting areas for further training, learning or development for the individual. A timed action plan should be agreed upon.

Reflective practice

Reflective practice is a professional activity in which practitioners think critically about practice. As a result, they may modify their actions, behaviours or learning needs. Reflective practice involves reviewing episodes of practice to describe, analyse and evaluate activity. It enables learning at a subconscious level to be brought to a level where it can be articulated and shared with others. The opportunity to re-think practices becomes a tool for professional learning and contributes to an individual's practice knowledge and clinical expertise (Gamble et al 2001).

AUDIT OF THE PROCESS BY WHICH QUESTIONS ARE ANSWERED

We hope this book will encourage you to practise evidence-based physiotherapy so that you become not only a reader of research but also a user of high quality clinical research. As we have seen, evidence-based physiotherapy involves formulating questions, searching for evidence, critical appraisal, implementation and evaluation.

One way of evaluating your performance is to reflect on questions related to each step of the process of evidence-based practice. This part of the chapter will describe the domains in which you might want to evaluate your performance. A summary is found in Box 9.1. Sackett and colleagues (2000) provide further reading on this issue.

To become a user of research you first have to acknowledge your information needs and reflect on your practice. This implies a process that might start with raising awareness and discussing different sources of information, and ends up by framing questions and finding and applying evidence. Do you think there is a need for high quality clinical research to inform physiotherapy practice? Do you challenge your colleagues by asking what they base their practice on?

You can also evaluate your performance by asking questions. One way of doing this is by recording the questions you ask and checking whether the questions were answerable and translated into a search for literature. Do you classify your question as a question of therapy, prognosis, diagnosis or experiences (Chapter 2)? In our experience, when physiotherapists have learned that there are different types of questions, asking and searching become much easier. When you become more skilled in formulating questions, you might also start asking your colleagues questions and promoting an 'asking environment' in your workplace.

To be able to carry out searches for evidence you need to have access to an information infrastructure. A first step might be to get access to the internet so you can search PEDro, PubMed and, in some countries, the

Box 9.1   Evaluating performance of the process of evidence-based physiotherapy

Reflection on practice/raising awareness
- Do I ask myself why I do the things I do at work?
- Do I discuss with colleagues the basis for our clinical decisions?

Asking questions
- Do I ask clinical questions?
- Do I ask well-formulated questions?
- Do I classify questions into different types (effect of interventions, prognosis, aetiology, etc.)?
- Do I encourage my colleagues to ask questions?

Searching for evidence
- Do I search for evidence?
- Do I know the best sources for different types of questions?
- Do I have access to the internet?
- Am I becoming more efficient in my searching?
- Do I start by searching for systematic reviews?

Critical appraisal
- Do I read papers at all?
- Do I use critical appraisal guides or checklists for different designs?
- Have I improved my interpretation of effect estimates (e.g. numbered needed to treat)
- Do I promote the reading of research articles at my workplace?

Implementing high quality clinical research
- Do I use high quality research to inform or change my practice?
- Do I use this approach to help resolve disagreement with colleagues about the management of a problem?

Self-evaluation
- Have I audited my evidence-based practice-performance?

Cochrane Library (Chapter 4). Refine your search strategies, for example by routinely looking first for systematic reviews. You might need to improve your searching performance by asking a librarian. Librarians are useful people and very important collaborators for evidence-based practice. Perhaps you need to undertake a course to update your literature searching skills, or ask a librarian to repeat a search that you have already done, and compare that with yours.

Next, consider how you read papers. Do you start by assessing the validity of the study (Chapter 5), or do you only read the conclusion? Reading and discussing a paper together with peers is useful, and can be fun, and you can learn a lot. Do you have a journal club at your workplace? Different checklists are available as useful tools for appraisal. Do you know where to find checklists for different kinds of studies? By reading more studies (and this book) you will become more skilled in interpreting measures of effect (Chapter 6). Do you feel more confident in reading and applying the results that are presented in research papers?

The most important question of all is perhaps this one: 'Do I use the findings from high quality research to improve my practice?' If you go through the steps without applying relevant high quality research to practice then you may have wasted time and resources. If this has happened, consider what barriers prevented you from using research in practice (Chapter 8). As outlined in Chapter 1, research alone does not make decisions so there can be many legitimate reasons for not practising as the evidence suggests you should. Informed health care decisions are made by integrating research, patient preferences and practice knowledge, so that practice is informed by high quality clinical research but adapted to a specific setting or individual patient. This can regarded as the optimal outcome of evidence-based practice.

CONCLUDING COMMENT

Evaluation satisfies more than a technical requirement for quantifying the quality and effects of care. It also provides an opportunity for reflecting on practice. With routine self-reflection, physiotherapists should be better able to combine evidence from high quality research with patient preferences and practice knowledge, so they should be better practitioners of evidence-based physiotherapy.

References

Bekkering T, Engers AJ, Wensing M et al 2003 Development of an implementation strategy for physiotherapy guidelines on low back pain. American Journal of Physiotherapy 49:208–214

Chartered Society of Physiotherapy 2000 Clinical audit tools. In: Standards of physiotherapy practice pack. CSP, London

Feinstein AR 1987 Clinimetrics. Yale University Press, New Haven

Finch E, Brooks D, Stratford P et al 2002 Physical rehabilitation outcome measures: a guide to enhanced clinical decision making (2nd edn). Lippincott, Williams and Wilkins, Philadelphia

Gamble J, Chan P, Davey H 2001 Reflection as a tool for developing professional practice knowledge and expertise. In: Higgs J, Titchen A (eds) Practice knowledge and expertise in the health professions. Butterworth-Heinemann, Oxford

Koke AJA, Heuts PHTG, Vlaeyen JWS et al 1999 Meetinstrumenten chronische pijn. Deel 1 functionele status. Pijn Kennis Centrum S, Maastricht

Maher C, Latimer J, Refshauge K 2000 Atlas of clinical tests and measures for low back pain. Australian Physiotherapy Association, Melbourne

Maitland GD, Hengeveld E, Banks K et al 2001 Maitland's vertebral manipulation. Butterworth-Heinemann, Oxford

National Institute for Clinical Excellence 2002 Principles for best practice in clinical audit. Radcliffe Medical Press, Abingdon

Øvretveit J, Gustafson D 2003 Using research to inform quality programmes. BMJ 326:759–761

Rothstein JM (ed) 1985 Measurement in physical therapy. Churchill Livingstone, New York

Sackett DL, Straus SE, Richardson W et al 2000 Evidence-based medicine: how to practice and teach EBM. Churchill Livingstone, Edinburgh

Smith M, Brooker S, Vicenzino B et al 2004 Use of anti-pronation taping to assess suitability of orthotic prescription: case report. Australian Journal of Physiotherapy 50:111–113

Streiner DL, Norman GR 2003 Health measurement scales: a practical guide to their development and use. Oxford University Press, Oxford

Wade DT 1992 Measurement in neurological rehabilitation. Oxford University Press, Oxford

Index